# New Paradigms in Reconstructive Surgery

# New Paradigms in Reconstructive Surgery

Edited by Marvin Trey

hayle medical
New York

Hayle Medical,
750 Third Avenue, 9th Floor,
New York, NY 10017, USA

Visit us on the World Wide Web at:
www.haylemedical.com



ISBN: 978-1-63241-771-8

The publisher's policy is to use permanent paper from mills that operate a sustainable forestry policy. Furthermore, the publisher ensures that the text paper and cover boards used have met acceptable environmental accreditation standards.



Printed in China.

**Cataloging-in-Publication Data**

New paradigms in reconstructive surgery / edited by Marvin Trey.
p. cm.
Includes bibliographical references and index.
ISBN 978-1-63241-771-8
1. Surgery, Plastic. 2. Surgery, Plastic--Technique. 3. Transplantation of organs, tissues, etc.
4. Operations, Surgical. I. Trey, Marvin.
RD118 .N48 2019
617.95--dc23

# Table of Contents

# Preface

Reconstructive surgery is a type of plastic surgery. It is concerned with the restoration of the form and function of some specific part of the body. Reconstructive surgery is often performed by plastic surgeons, maxillo-facial surgeons and otolaryngologists to reconstruct or restore the body parts after trauma or cancer. In reconstructive surgery, surgeons often use the concept of a reconstructive ladder in order to manage increasingly complex wounds. A reconstructive ladder includes techniques, like primary closure, skin graft, tissue expansion, random flap, axial flap, free flap, etc. The various advancements in reconstructive surgery are glanced at in this book and their applications as well as ramifications are looked at in detail. Most of the topics introduced herein cover new techniques and applications of reconstructive surgery. As this field is emerging at a rapid pace, the contents of this book will help the readers understand the modern concepts and applications of the subject.

Significant researches are present in this book. Intensive efforts have been employed by authors to make this book an outstanding discourse. This book contains the enlightening chapters which have been written on the basis of significant researches done by the experts.

Finally, I would also like to thank all the members involved in this book for being a team and meeting all the deadlines for the submission of their respective works. I would also like to thank my friends and family for being supportive in my efforts.

**Editor**

1

# Emerging applications of bedside 3D printing in plastic surgery

*Michael P. Chae[1,2], Warren M. Rozen[1,2], Paul G. McMenamin[3], Michael W. Findlay[1,4]*, Robert T. Spychal[1] and David J. Hunter-Smith[1,2]*

*[1] 3D PRINT Laboratory, Department of Surgery, Peninsula Health, Frankston, VIC, Australia, [2] Monash University Plastic and Reconstructive Surgery Group (Peninsula Clinical School), Peninsula Health, Frankston, VIC, Australia, [3] Department of Anatomy and Developmental Biology, Centre for Human Anatomy Education, School of Biomedical Sciences, Faculty of Medicine, Nursing and Health Sciences, Monash University, Clayton, VIC, Australia, [4] Department of Surgery, Stanford University, Stanford, CA, USA*

**Edited by:**
*Swee T. Tan,*
*Gillies McIndoe Research Institute,*
*New Zealand*

**Reviewed by:**
*Jan A. Plock,*
*University of Zurich, Switzerland*
*June Wu,*
*Columbia University, USA*

***Correspondence:**
*Michael W. Findlay,*
*3D PRINT Laboratory, Department of Surgery, Peninsula Health, 2 Hastings Road, Frankston, VIC 3199, Australia*
*mfindlay@stanford.edu*

**Specialty section:**
*This article was submitted to Reconstructive and Plastic Surgery, a section of the journal Frontiers in Surgery*

Modern imaging techniques are an essential component of preoperative planning in plastic and reconstructive surgery. However, conventional modalities, including three-dimensional (3D) reconstructions, are limited by their representation on 2D workstations. 3D printing, also known as rapid prototyping or additive manufacturing, was once the province of industry to fabricate models from a computer-aided design (CAD) in a layer-by-layer manner. The early adopters in clinical practice have embraced the medical imaging-guided 3D-printed biomodels for their ability to provide tactile feedback and a superior appreciation of visuospatial relationship between anatomical structures. With increasing accessibility, investigators are able to convert standard imaging data into a CAD file using various 3D reconstruction softwares and ultimately fabricate 3D models using 3D printing techniques, such as stereolithography, multijet modeling, selective laser sintering, binder jet technique, and fused deposition modeling. However, many clinicians have questioned whether the cost-to-benefit ratio justifies its ongoing use. The cost and size of 3D printers have rapidly decreased over the past decade in parallel with the expiration of key 3D printing patents. Significant improvements in clinical imaging and user-friendly 3D software have permitted computer-aided 3D modeling of anatomical structures and implants without outsourcing in many cases. These developments offer immense potential for the application of 3D printing at the bedside for a variety of clinical applications. In this review, existing uses of 3D printing in plastic surgery practice spanning the spectrum from templates for facial transplantation surgery through to the formation of bespoke craniofacial implants to optimize post-operative esthetics are described. Furthermore, we discuss the potential of 3D printing to become an essential office-based tool in plastic surgery to assist in preoperative planning, developing intraoperative guidance tools, teaching patients and surgical trainees, and producing patient-specific prosthetics in everyday surgical practice.

**Keywords: 3D printing, bedside, desktop application, plastic and reconstructive surgery, cost, preoperative planning, intraoperative guidance, education**

## Introduction

Advanced medical imaging has become an essential component of preoperative planning in plastic surgery. In breast reconstructive surgery, the introduction of computed tomographic angiography (CTA) has enabled surgeons to improve clinical outcomes (1) through accurate and reliable prospective selection of the donor site, flap, perforators, and the optimal mode of dissection (2, 3). Recent development of three-dimensional (3D) and 4D CTA techniques have enhanced spatial appreciation of the perforator vessels, their vascular territory, and dynamic flow characteristics preoperatively (4, 5). However, current imaging modalities are limited by being displayed on a 2D surface, such as a computer screen. In contrast, a 3D-printed haptic biomodel allows both the surgeon and the patient to develop a superior understanding of the anatomy and the procedure with the goal of improved operative planning through the ability to interact directly with a model of the patient-specific anatomy. Historically, the technically challenging nature of 3D software and the high prices of early 3D printers usually meant that clinicians keen to exploit these advantages had to outsource 3D printing and the cost of outsourcing often precluded it from being implemented widely. In this review, we analyze how recent advancements have enabled 3D printing to transition from the research and development laboratory to the clinical 'bedside' potentially making it a ubiquitous application in plastic surgery.

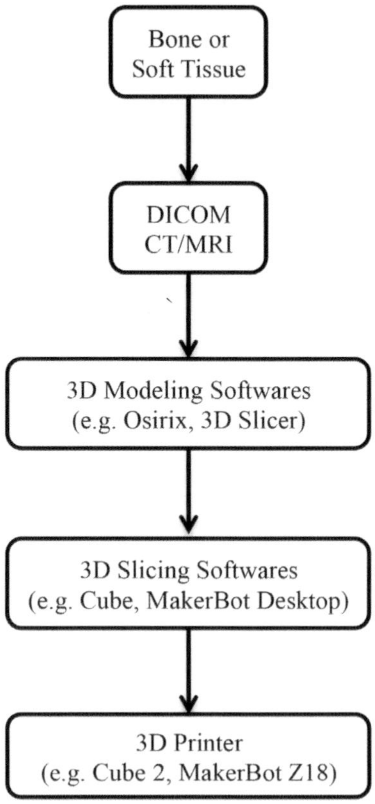


**FIGURE 1 | Steps involved from imaging to 3D-printed models.** Abbreviations: DICOM, digital imaging and communications in medicine; CT, computed tomography; MRI, magnetic resonance imaging.

## 3D Printing

3D printing, also known as rapid prototyping or additive manufacturing, describes a process by which a product derived from a computer-aided design (CAD) is built in a layer-by-layer fashion (**Figure 1**) (Video S1 in Supplementary Material) (6–8). In contrast to the conventional manufacturing processes like injection molding, 3D printing has introduced an era of design freedom and enabled rapid production of customized objects with complex geometries (9–11). One of the major advantages of 3D printing is the capacity to directly translate a concept into an end product in a convenient, cost-efficient manner. It eliminates the typical intermediary stages involved in a product development, such as development, production, assembly lines, delivery, and warehousing of parts (12), and the subsequent savings made from using fewer materials and labor lead to an overall reduction in the cost of production (13).

3D printing has been utilized in industrial design since the 1980s; however, it has only become adapted for medical application in the last decade (14). Imaging data from routine computed tomography (CT) or magnetic resonance imaging (MRI) can be converted into a CAD file using a variety of 3D software programs, such as Osirix (Pixmeo, Geneva, Switzerland) or 3D Slicer (Surgical Planning Laboratory, Boston, MA, USA) (**Figure 1**). These files are processed into data slices suitable for printing by proprietary softwares from the 3D printer manufacturers. While a range of 3D printing techniques have been developed for industrial use; stereolithography (SLA), multijet modeling (MJM), selective laser sintering (SLS), binder jetting, and fused deposition modeling (FDM) are the main approaches that have been explored in the clinical setting (**Table 1**). We will explore each of these to evaluate their current and potential applications in clinical practice for both bony reconstruction and soft tissue reconstruction.

## Types of 3D Printing

### Stereolithography

Stereolithography is the earliest 3D printing technology described for fabricating biomodels, where a layer of liquid photopolymer or epoxy resin in a vat is cured by a low-power ultraviolet (UV) laser (15). Excess raw materials and the supporting structures must be manually removed from the final product and cured in a UV chamber (16–18). Currently, SLA is considered the gold standard in 3D biomodel production and can yield resolutions of up to 0.025 mm. Moreover, its efficiency increases when constructing larger objects and is able to faithfully reproduce internal structural details (19). However, the need for manual post-build handling makes it labor-intensive and it still takes more than a day to produce a large model. Furthermore, in comparison to other 3D printing techniques, it is considered more expensive due to the high cost of the raw materials and for the printer upkeep (20, 21). Recently, a novel modification to SLA has been developed called continuous liquid interface production (CLIP). This simplifies traditional SLA and increases the production speed by harnessing oxygen

**TABLE 1 | A summary of the most commonly used 3D printing techniques in medical application.**

| 3D printing techniques | Pros | Cons |
|---|---|---|
| SLA | Current gold standard<br>High resolution<br>Increased efficiency with increase in print size<br>Detailed fabrication of internal structures | >1 day of printing time required<br>Require extensive post-production manual handling<br>High cost related to the materials, the printer, and the maintenance |
| MJM | High resolution<br>Minimal post-production manual handling<br>Multiple materials | High cost related to the material and printer<br>Poorer surface finishing than SLA |
| SLS | Not require support structures<br>Smooth surface finishing<br>Print delicate structures<br>Print in metal | Require post-production manual handling<br>High cost related to the materials, the printer, and the maintenance<br>Require expert handling of the printer |
| BJT | Not require support structures<br>Multiple colors<br>Multiple materials | Brittle<br>Require extensive post-production manual handling<br>Poor surface finish |
| FDM | Low cost<br>Minimal maintenance<br>High availability of printers | Require post-production manual removal of support structures<br>Poor surface finish<br>Mono-color and mono-material with the current technology |

*SLA, stereolithography; MJM, multijet modeling; SLS, selective laser sintering; BJT, binder jet technique; FDM, fused deposition modeling.*

inhibition of UV-curable resin photopolymerization (22). This emerging modality has yet to be evaluated in plastic and reconstructive surgery but holds promise due to its combination of speed, structural integrity, and ability to fabricate complex structures.

### MultiJet Modeling

Multijet modeling printing, also known as MultiJet Printing (3D Systems, Rock Hill, SC, USA) or Poly Jet Technology (Stratasys, Edina, MN, USA), is akin to SLA, but the liquid photopolymer is immediately cured by the UV light preventing the time-consuming post-processing in the UV chamber and the prototypes are built with gel-like support materials that are readily dissolvable in water (23). MJM can manufacture models with high resolution (16 μ) that is comparable to or better than SLA, with an added benefit of the capacity to print in multiple materials for the desired degree of tensile strength and durability. Furthermore, a MJM printer is easier to maintain than a SLA set-up. However, the high price of these printers makes MJM more suitable for large-scale productions than for office-based/bedside desktop application.

### Selective Laser Sintering

Selective laser sintering describes a process where powdered forms of thermoplastic, metal, glass, or ceramic material are sintered by high-power laser beams in a layer-by-layer fashion (24, 25). Similar to SLA, the unsintered powders must be brushed away from the final product; however, they provide support and eliminate the need for support structures. As a result, SLS yields models with smoother surface finish and facilitates the production of delicate structures with high accuracy. Furthermore, the unsintered powders can be reused leading to a reduction in cost compared to SLA (20, 26). However, SLS remains significantly more expensive than binder jet technique (BJT) (below) and FDM, due mainly to the cost of the printer. In addition, SLS printers can be potentially hazardous due to the presence of lasers, pistons, and gas chambers that can reach extremely high temperatures and hence, requires expert handling. These features have discouraged it from being widely implemented in non-industrial settings.

### Binder Jet Technique

Binder jet technique, or powder bed technique, is the first 3D printing approach that reduced the cost of 3D printers, thereby enabling a widespread consumerization of 3D printing (27). Similar to the SLS process, printer heads eject a binder material along with colored dye onto a layer of powder, fusing them layer-by-layer into a plaster model (28). Unfused powders provide adequate support for the "overhanging" designs and hence, simultaneous deposition of support structures is rarely required. Moreover, binder jet 3D printers can print in multiple colors and materials, and have multiple printer heads for faster printing. One of the major drawbacks of binder jetting is that the final product usually lacks strength and has a poorer surface finish than SLA or SLS. Hence, all models require post-production strengthening with materials such as melted wax, cyanoacrylate glue, or epoxy.

### Fused Deposition Modeling

Fused deposition modeling is the most commonly used consumer 3D printing technology available currently and is also the most affordable (21, 29, 30). A melted filament of thermoplastic material is extruded from a nozzle moving in the x-y plane and solidifies upon deposition on a build plate (31). After each layer, the build plate is lowered by 0.1 mm and the process is repeated until the final product is produced. Acrylonitrile-butadiene-styrene (ABS) and polylactic acid (PLA) are the most frequently used raw materials in FDM printers. A notable shortcoming for the use of FDM in medical applications is that most anatomical structures have complex shapes and hence, would require support structures. Although they are easy to remove manually, the aftermath generally leaves superficial damage to the model compromising its surface finish and esthetics. Hollow internal structures or blind-ended openings are particularly difficult to clean build material from. Furthermore, most household FDM printers are currently limited to fabricating in mono-color and mono-material. However, this can be overcome by recently developed dual-extruder technology, where two filaments of different color or material can be extruded from a common printer head. It is currently found in printers, such as MakerBot Replicator 2X Experimental (MakerBot Industries, New York, NY, USA), Cube 3 (3D Systems, Rock Hill, SC, USA), and Creatr x1 (Leapfrog, Emeryville, CA, USA). Moreover, the second extruder can be configured to build support structures using MakerBot Dissolvable Filament (MakerBot Industries), made up of high impact polystyrene (HIPS) (32). When the final product is immersed in water with limonene, a widely available citrus-scented solvent, the support structures selectively dissolve away within 8 to 24 h but these dual extruder printers have not yet become established in the mainstream.

## 3D Printing in Medicine

In the last decade or so, researchers have demonstrated a wide range of uses for 3D printing across numerous surgical disciplines. Clinically, 3D-printed haptic biomodels provide a tactile feedback and enable users to simulate complex anatomical movements, such as articulation at the temporomandibular joint, that are difficult to reproduce in a computer software (33). As a result, they facilitate an enhanced appreciation of the visuospatial relationship between anatomical structures for the surgeons (34). This can translate into shorter operative time, reduced exposure to general anesthesia, shorter wound exposure time and reduced intraoperative blood loss (18, 35, 36).

### Preoperative Planning

In preoperative planning, 3D-printed biomodels have been beneficial in orbital and mandibular reconstruction in maxillofacial surgery (21, 37–41); craniofacial, skull base, and cervical spine reconstruction in neurosurgery (35); prefabrication of bony fixation plates and planning excision of bony lesions in orthopedic surgery (42, 43); mapping complex congenital heart defects and tracheobronchial variation in cardiothoracic surgery and cardiac transplantation (26, 44–52) (**Figure 2**); endovascular repair of abdominal aortic aneurysm and aortic dissection in vascular surgery (53–55); partial nephrectomy for renal tumors in urology (56); osteoplastic flap reconstruction of frontal sinus defects in ear, nose, and throat surgery (57, 58); and hepatectomy and liver transplantation in general surgery (59–61).

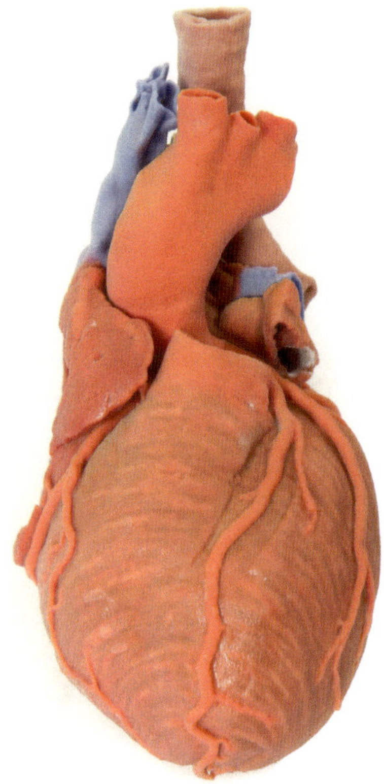

**FIGURE 2 | 3D-printed haptic model of a heart and the great vessels fabricated using Projet x60 series 3D printers**. Reproduced with permission from Centre for Human Anatomy and Education.

### Intraoperative Guidance

Furthermore, 3D softwares have been used to fabricate patient-specific surgical templates and intraoperative guidance devices to aid surgeons in maxillofacial surgery (62–67), neurosurgery (68), orthopedic surgery (69), hand surgery (70), and general surgery (71).

### Education

3D-printed haptic biomodels can be useful for educating patients during medical consultations and training surgical trainees (29, 45, 72–81).

### Customized Prosthesis

Moreover, 3D printing has enabled rapid and convenient production of customized implants. Investigators have manufactured patient-specific mandibular implants in maxillofacial surgery (82–84), cranial vault implants for cranioplasty in neurosurgery (85, 86), hip implants in orthopedic surgery (87, 88), and a bioresorbable airway splint for complex tracheobronchomalacia in pediatric cardiothoracic surgery (89).

### Allied Health

In other areas of medicine, 3D printing has revolutionized the manufacturing of hearing aids and currently 99% of all hearing aids in the world are 3D printed (90). Additionally, 3D printing has helped in making complex diagnoses in forensic medicine (91); reformed anatomy education (92); helped in planning repairs of Charcot's foot in podiatry (93); permitted the fabrication of custom-made dental implants in dentistry (94–96); produced patient-specific 3D-printed medication in pharmaceutical industry (97, 98); and assembled custom-design tissue scaffolds in regenerative medicine (99, 100).

## 3D Printing at the Bedside

Despite a vast potential scope of 3D printing in clinical practice and significant media interest with frequent reports of the latest innovative advancements made using this technology (101). The incorporation of 3D printing as a clinical bedside application has not been widespread (102). One potential barrier is the perception amongst clinicians that 3D printing is technically sophisticated and is reserved for planning intricate operations and devising highly specialized implants (102). As a result, 3D printing is often outsourced to an external company, which compounds the cost and time. This demonstrates a lack of awareness of the increasing accessibility of the 3D softwares and the declining cost of the 3D printers (102).

### 3D Reconstruction Software

In order to fabricate a 3D biomodel, two types of software are required; firstly, a "3D modeling" software that translates the

DICOM (digital imaging and communications in medicine) files from CT/MRI scans into a CAD file, and secondly, a "3D slicing" software that divides the CAD file into thin data slices suitable for 3D printing (103).

### 3D Modeling Software

A range of 3D modeling softwares is available (**Table 2**); however, early ones, such as Mimics (Materialise NV, Leuven, Belgium), would incur a high cost for the initial purchase and for the ongoing software updates. Driven by the consumerization of 3D printing and an increasing number of both professional and community software developers, free open-source softwares, such as Osirix (104) and 3D Slicer (105–107), have become widely utilized. Our group prefers using them due to the latter's expansive developer community base, called the Slicer Community, a plethora of plug-in functions, and a user interface that is intuitive to an individual with no engineering background (108, 109). An ideal 3D modeling software should be free; capable of highlighting the region of interest and eliminate undesired areas using the threshold and the segmentation function, respectively; export the 3D model as a CAD file in a universally accepted 3D file format, such as STL (standard tessellation language); and possess an easy-to-use interface. Encouragingly, there are numerous 3D modeling softwares available in the market currently that fit all of the criteria (**Table 2**).

### 3D Slicing Software

3D slicing softwares digitally "slice" a CAD file into layers suitable for 3D printing. However, they are also useful for altering the orientation of the CAD file relative to the printer build plate to give an optimal direction, which minimizes the requirement for the support structures and, in turn, reduces the amount of material used and therefore also reduces the printing time. This process can be readily performed using proprietary softwares that accompany the 3D printers at no extra cost and usually possess a simple graphic user interface, such as Cube software (3D Systems) and MakerBot Desktop (MakerBot Industries).

### 3D Printers

The cost of early 3D printers, consisting of mostly the SLA type described above, precluded widespread adoption of 3D printing in the initial years; however, the expiration of key patents surrounding SLA and FDM in the last decade has fueled a surge in the number of commercial developers leading to an increase in the availability and a significant reduction of the cost (**Table 3**). Several affordable SLA 3D printers have entered the market since then, such as Form 1+ (Formlabs, Somerville, MA, USA) and ProJet 1200 (3D Systems). However, they are capable of building only small designs (i.e., 12.5 cm × 12.5 cm × 16.5 cm) and hence, remain unsuitable for many applications. Similarly, current MJM and SLS 3D printers are generally bulky and expensive, and require specialized skills for safe handling of the hardware and its maintenance. Binder jet 3D printers are gradually being avoided due to the brittle quality of the end-products and the large size of the printer. Currently, FDM 3D printers are the preferred option as a desktop application in medicine for their affordability and practicality. The accuracy and the quality of FDM products are comparable to SLA, SLS, and binder jet (110–112). Furthermore, FDM incurs the least cost in maintenance from ongoing print materials (**Table 4**).

## 3D Printing in Plastic and Reconstructive Surgery

In plastic and reconstructive surgery, 3D-printed haptic biomodels can potentially play a significant role in preoperative planning, intraoperative guidance, training and teaching, and fashioning patient-specific prosthesis (**Table 5**).

### Preoperative Planning: Soft Tissue Mapping

Perforator flap surgery is routinely performed in the reconstruction of large soft tissue defects after trauma or an oncologic resection. Preoperative planning with CTA has revolutionized the field by enabling the reconstructive surgeon to identify an ideal donor site, flap, and perforator for a free flap transfer (3, 123), facilitating a greater flap success rate and an overall improvement in the

**TABLE 2 | A summary of 3D modeling softwares that can convert a DICOM data from a standard CT/MRI scans into a CAD file.**

| Name | Company | Free | Threshold/ segmentation | Export STL | Easy user interface | OS platform |
|---|---|---|---|---|---|---|
| 3D Slicer | Surgical Planning Laboratory | Y | Y | Y | Y | W, M |
| MITK | German Cancer Research Centre | Y | Y | Y | Y | W, M |
| Osirix | Pixmeo | Y | Y | Y | Y | M |
| MIPAV | NIH CIT | Y | Y | Y | N | W, M |
| MeVisLab | MeVis Medical Solutions AG | Y | Y | Y | N | W, M |
| InVesalius | CTI | Y | Y | Y | N | W, M |
| Mimics | Materialise NV | N | Y | Y | Y | W, M |
| Avizo/Amira | FEI Visualization Science Group | N | Y | Y | Y | W, M |
| 3D Doctor | Able Software | N | Y | Y | Y | W |
| Dolphin Imaging 3D | Dolphin Imaging and Management | N | Y | Y | Y | W |
| Analyze | AnalyzeDirect | N | Y | Y | N | W, M |
| GuideMia | GuideMia | N | Y | Y | N | W, M |
| OnDemand3D | CyberMed | N | N | Y | N | W, M |
| VoXim | IVS Technology | N | Y | Y | N | W |
| ScanIP | Simpleware | N | Y | Y | N | W |

*STL, standard tessellation language; OS, operating system; Y, yes; N, no; W, Windows OS; M, Mac OS.*

**TABLE 3 | A summary of commercially available 3D printers from ten leading 3D printing companies in the world.**

| Type | Name | Company | Cost (USD) | Print area (cm) | Print resolution (nm) | Printer size (cm) | Printer weight (kg) |
|---|---|---|---|---|---|---|---|
| SLA | Form 1+ | Formlabs | 3,999 | 12.5 × 12.5 × 16.5 | 25 | 30.0 × 28.0 × 45.0 | 8 |
| SLA | ProJet 1200 | 3D Systems | 4,900 | 4.3 × 2.7 × 15.0 | 30.5 | 22.9 × 22.9 × 35.6 | 9 |
| SLA | ProJet 6000 | 3D Systems | 200,000 | 25.0 × 25.0 × 25.0 | 50 | 78.7 × 73.7 × 183.0 | 181 |
| SLA | ProJet 7000 | 3D Systems | 300,000 | 38.0 × 38.0 × 25.0 | 50 | 98.4 × 85.4 × 183.0 | 272 |
| SLA | ProX 950 | 3D Systems | 950,000 | 150.0 × 75.0 × 55.0 | 50 | 220.0 × 160.0 × 226.0 | 1,951 |
| MJM | Objet 24 series | Stratasys | 19,900 | 23.4 × 19.2 × 14.9 | 28 | 82.5 × 62.0 × 59.0 | 93 |
| MJM | Objet 30 series | Stratasys | 40,900 | 29.4 × 19.2 × 14.9 | 28 | 82.5 × 62.0 × 59.0 | 93 |
| MJM | ProJet 3510 series | 3D Systems | 69,500 | 29.8 × 18.5 × 20.3 | 16 | 29.5 × 47.0 × 59.5 | 43.4 |
| MJM | Objet Eden | Stratasys | 123,000 | 49.0 × 39.0 × 20.0 | 16 | 132.0 × 99.0 × 120.0 | 410 |
| MJM | ProJet 5000 | 3D Systems | 155,000 | 53.3 × 38.1 × 30.0 | 32 | 60.3 × 35.7 × 57.1 | 53.8 |
| MJM | ProJet 5500X | 3D Systems | 155,000 | 53.3 × 38.1 × 30.0 | 29 | 80.0 × 48.0 × 78.0 | 115.7 |
| MJM | Connex series | Stratasys | 164,000 | 49.0 × 39.0 × 20.0 | 16 | 140.0 × 126.0 × 110.0 | 430 |
| MJM | Objet Connex series | Stratasys | 164,000 | 49.0 × 39.0 × 20.0 | 16 | 142.0 × 112.0 × 113.0 | 500 |
| MJM | Objet 1000 | Stratasys | 614,000 | 100.0 × 80.0 × 50.0 | 16 | 280.0 × 180.0 × 180.0 | 1,950 |
| SLS | sPro series | 3D Systems | 300,000 | 55.0 × 55.0 × 46.0 | 80 | 203.0 × 160.0 × 216.0 | 2,700 |
| SLS | ProX series | 3D Systems | 500,000 | 38.1 × 33.0 × 45.7 | 100 | 174.4 × 122.6 × 229.5 | 1,360 |
| BJT | ProJet 160 | 3D Systems | 40,000 | 23.6 × 18.5 × 12.7 | 100 | 74.0 × 79.0 × 140.0 | 165 |
| BJT | ProJet 260C | 3D Systems | 40,000 | 23.6 × 18.5 × 12.7 | 100 | 74.0 × 79.0 × 140.0 | 165 |
| BJT | ProJet 360 | 3D Systems | 40,000 | 20.3 × 25.4 × 20.3 | 100 | 122.0 × 79.0 × 140.0 | 179 |
| BJT | ProJet 460 Plus | 3D Systems | 40,000 | 20.3 × 25.4 × 20.3 | 100 | 122.0 × 79.0 × 140.0 | 193 |
| BJT | ProJet 4500 | 3D Systems | 40,000 | 20.3 × 25.4 × 20.3 | 100 | 162.0 × 80.0 × 152.0 | 272 |
| BJT | ProJet 660 Pro | 3D Systems | 40,000 | 25.4 × 38.1 × 20.3 | 100 | 188.0 × 74.0 × 145.0 | 340 |
| BJT | ProJet 860 Plus | 3D Systems | 40,000 | 50.8 × 38.1 × 22.9 | 100 | 119.0 × 116.0 × 162.0 | 363 |
| FDM | Huxley Duo | RepRapPro | 453 | 13.8 × 14.0 × 9.5 | 12.5 | 26.0 × 28.0 × 28.0 | 4.5 |
| FDM | Mendel | RepRapPro | 586 | 21.0 × 19.0 × 14.0 | 12.5 | 50.0 × 46.0 × 41.0 | 8 |
| FDM | Ormerod 2 | RepRapPro | 702 | 20.0 × 20.0 × 20.0 | 12.5 | 50.0 × 46.0 × 41.0 | 6 |
| FDM | Tricolor Mendel | RepRapPro | 863 | 21.0 × 19.0 × 14.0 | 12.5 | 50.0 × 46.0 × 41.0 | 8 |
| FDM | Cube 3 | 3D Systems | 999 | 15.3 × 15.3 × 15.3 | 70 | 33.5 × 34.3 × 24.1 | 7.7 |
| FDM | Buccaneer | Pirate 3D | 999 | 14.5 × 12.5 × 15.5 | 85 | 25.8 × 25.8 × 44.0 | 8 |
| FDM | Original + | Ultimaker | 1,238 | 21.0 × 21.0 × 20.5 | 20 | 35.7 × 34.2 × 38.8 | N/A |
| FDM | Replicator mini | MakerBot | 1,375 | 10.0 × 10.0 × 12.5 | 200 | 29.5 × 31.0 × 38.1 | 8 |
| FDM | Creatr | Leapfrog | 1,706 | 20.0 × 27.0 × 20.0 | 50 | 60.0 × 50.0 × 50.0 | 32 |
| FDM | Replicator 2 | MakerBot | 1,999 | 28.5 × 15.3 × 15.5 | 100 | 49.0 × 42.0 × 38.0 | 11.5 |
| FDM | LulzBot TAZ 4 | Aleph Objects | 2,195 | 29.8 × 27.5 × 25.0 | 75 | 668.0 × 52.0 × 51.5 | 11 |
| FDM | AW3D HDL | Airwolf 3D | 2,295 | 30.0 × 20.0 × 28.0 | 100 | 61.0 × 44.5 × 46.0 | 17 |
| FDM | Creatr HS | Leapfrog | 2,373 | 29.0 × 24.0 × 18.0 | 50 | 60.0 × 60.0 × 50.0 | 40 |
| FDM | Replicator 2x | MakerBot | 2,499 | 24.6 × 15.2 × 15.5 | 100 | 49.0 × 42.0 × 53.1 | 12.6 |
| FDM | Ultimaker 2 | Ultimaker | 2,500 | 23.0 × 22.5 × 20.5 | 20 | 35.7 × 34.2 × 38.8 | N/A |
| FDM | Replicator 5th gen | MakerBot | 2,899 | 25.2.19.9 × 15.0 | 100 | 52.8 × 44.1 × 41.0 | 16 |
| FDM | AW3D HD | Airwolf 3D | 2,995 | 30.0 × 20.0 × 30.0 | 60 | 61.0 × 44.5 × 46.0 | 17 |
| FDM | Cube Pro | 3D Systems | 3,129 | 20.0 × 23 × 27.0 | 100 | 57.8 × 59.1 × 57.8 | 44 |
| FDM | AW3D HDX | Airwolf 3D | 3,495 | 30.0 × 20.0 × 30.0 | 60 | 61.0 × 44.5 × 46.0 | 17 |
| FDM | AW3D HD2X | Airwolf 3D | 3,995 | 27.9 × 20.3 × 30.5 | 60 | 61.0 × 45.7 × 45.7 | 18 |
| FDM | Creatr xl | Leapfrog | 4,988 | 20.0 × 27.0 × 60.0 | 50 | 75.0 × 65.0 × 126.0 | 37 |
| FDM | Replicator Z18 | MakerBot | 6,499 | 30.5 × 30.5 × 45.7 | 100 | 49.3 × 56.5 × 85.4 | 41 |
| FDM | Xeed | Leapfrog | 8,705 | 35.0 × 27.0 × 60.0 | 50 | 101.0 × 66.0 × 100.0 | 115 |
| FDM | Mojo | Stratasys | 9,900 | 12.7 × 12.7 × 12.7 | 178 | 63.0 × 45.0 × 53.0 | 27 |
| FDM | uPrint | Stratasys | 13,900 | 20.3 × 15.2 × 15.2 | 254 | 63.5 × 66.0 × 94.0 | 94 |
| FDM | Objet Dimension series | Stratasys | 40,900 | 25.4 × 25.4 × 30.5 | 178 | 83.8 × 73.7 × 114.3 | 148 |
| FDM | Fortus series | Stratasys | 184,000 | 91.4 × 61.0 × 91.4 | 127 | 277.2 × 168.3 × 202.7 | 2,869 |

*Where a 3D printer series is characterized, the lowest cost, largest print area, lowest print resolution, largest printer size, and greater printer weight are selected for comparison.SLA, stereolithography; MJM, multijet modeling; SLS, selective laser sintering; BJT, binder jet technique; FDM, fused deposition modeling; cm, centimeter; kg, kilograms; nm, nanometers; N/A, not available.*

clinical outcomes (1, 2, 124). In addition to CTA, 3D biomodels can provide an additional layer of clinical information through visual and tactile examination.

In a recent report, our research group described a technique of fashioning a "reverse" model representing a soft tissue ankle defect that was utilized for planning a perforator flap-based reconstruction (**Figure 3**) (109). Routine CTA of the lower limbs (i.e., recipient site) and the forearms (i.e., donor site) were conducted and the DICOM data were converted into a CAD file using Osirix. The 3D image of the normal contralateral ankle was mirrored, superimposed over the image of the pathological side, and after digital subtraction using Magics software (Materialise

**TABLE 4 | A summary of average raw material cost of each 3D printing technique.**

| Type of 3D printing | Average cost of print material (USD) |
|---|---|
| SLA | 200 per L |
| MJM | 300 per kg |
| SLS | 500 per kg |
| BJT | 100 per kg |
| FDM | 50 per kg |

*SLA, stereolithography; MJM, multijet modeling; SLS, selective laser sintering; BJT, binder jet technique; FDM, fused deposition modeling; L, liter.*

**TABLE 5 | A summary of published application of 3D printing in Plastic and Reconstructive Surgery.**

| Application | | Example | Reference |
|---|---|---|---|
| Preoperative planning | Soft tissue mapping | Breast reconstruction | (108) |
| | | Ear reconstruction | (113, 114) |
| | | Nasal reconstruction | (115) |
| | | Mandibular soft tissue tumor resection | (116) |
| | | "Reverse" model of ankle defect | (109) |
| | | Sacral defect | (117) |
| | Vascular mapping | Internal mammary artery perforators | (118) |
| | | DIEA perforators | (7) |
| | Bony mapping | Basal thumb osteoarthritis | (7) |
| | 4D printing | Thumb movement | (119) |
| Intraoperative guidance | | Bone reduction clamp | (70) |
| Surgical training | | N/A | |
| Patient education | | N/A | |
| Patient-specific prosthesis | | Craniofacial implant | (120) |
| | | "Ear and nose library" | (121, 122) |

*DIEA, deep inferior epigastric artery; 4D, four dimensional; N/A, not available.*

NV), a "reverse" model representing the wound defect is created (**Figure 4**). This mirroring function can also be performed in free open-source softwares, such as Osirix and 3D Slicer. This helped the surgeon preoperatively appreciate the length, width, and depth of the free flap that needed to be harvested in order to adequately cover the defect. Both the pathological ankle and the "reverse" model were fabricated in PLA filaments using a Cube 2 printer (3D Systems) (**Figures 5** and **6**) (Table S1 in Supplementary Material).

We also recently demonstrated the utility of a 3D-printed biomodel for planning perforator flap reconstruction of a sacral wound defect post-oncologic resection (117). Likewise, we used Osirix to translate the preoperative sacral CTA data into a CAD file. Due to the maximal build dimensions of the Cube 2 printer (i.e., 16 cm × 16 cm × 16 cm), the 3D image of the sacral defect was scaled down using the Cube software. The haptic model still accurately represented the shape and depth of the defect and its relationship with the surrounding anatomical structures.

3D printing can potentially be a valuable tool in the assessment of soft tissue volume. Volumetric analysis is an essential component of breast reconstructive surgery and currently surgeons rely on 2D photography or 3D scanning technology, such as VECTRA (Canfield Imaging Systems, Fairfield, NJ, USA) (125), and subjective visual assessment. One of the main limitations of 3D photography like VECTRA is the inability to account for an underlying chest wall asymmetry that may

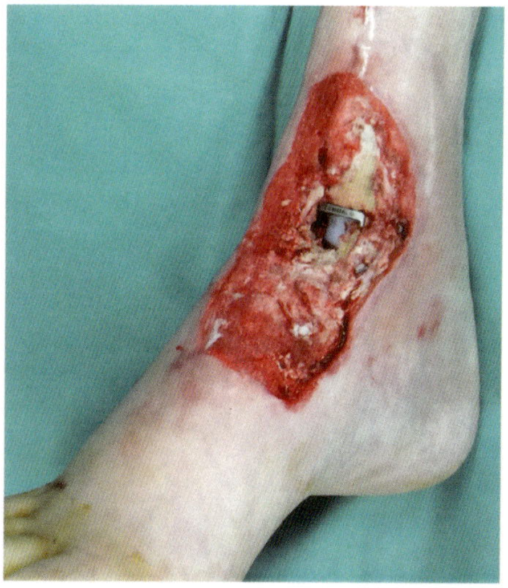

**FIGURE 3 | Photograph of the soft tissue ankle defect showing the exposed metal hardware from a previous ankle reconstruction.** Reproduced with permission from *Microsurgery* (109).

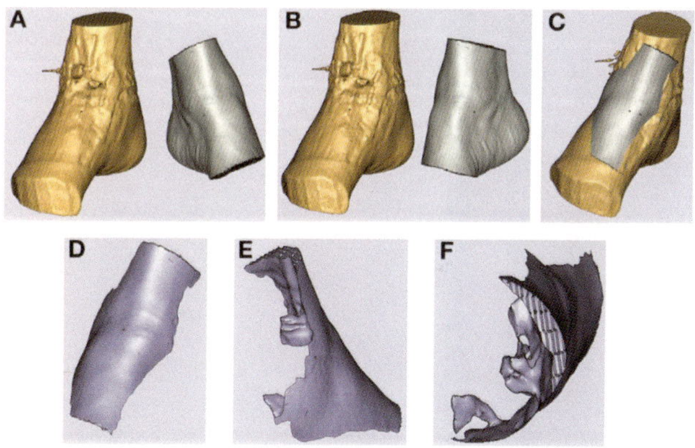


**FIGURE 4 | 3D images of the right (pathological) ankle is juxtaposed to the left (normal) ankle (A).** The left ankle is reflected **(B)** and superimposed on to the right ankle **(C).** These images are subtracted from each other to produce a "reverse" model of the soft tissue defect **(D-F).** Reproduced with permission from *Microsurgery* (109).

incorrectly lead to an asymmetrical appearance despite equal breast parenchymal volumes. Moreover, the accuracy of each scan is reliant on the patients standing with their back flat against a wall, which may not be feasible in certain conditions, such as kyphosis or scoliosis. Recently, we reported the use of a 3D-printed model of a patient with post-mastectomy breast asymmetry for preoperative planning (**Figure 7**) (108). Despite being scaled down to fit the build size of the printer, having an accurate physical replica helped surgeons appreciate the difference in the breast shape and volume. Furthermore, using the segmentation function in Osirix we were able to quantify the breast parenchymal volume difference.

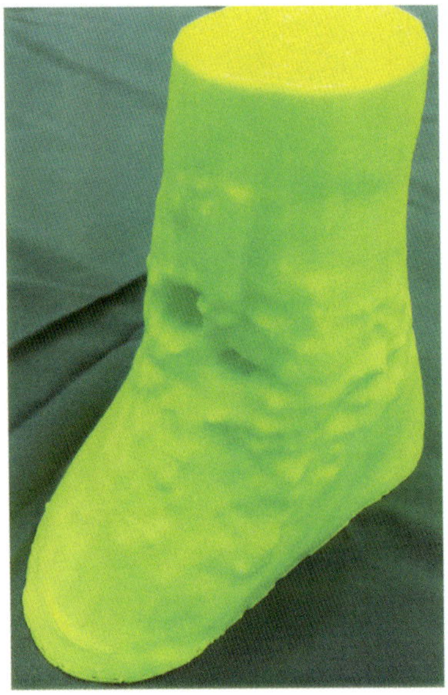

**FIGURE 5 | 3D-printed haptic model of the soft tissue ankle defect**. Reproduced with permission from *Microsurgery* (109).

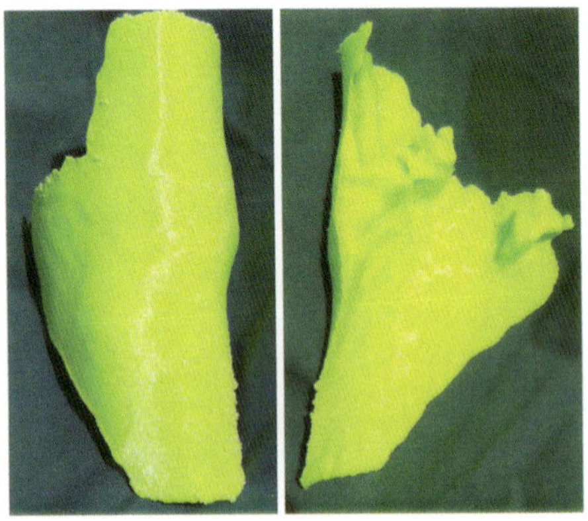

**FIGURE 6 | 3D-printed haptic model of the "reverse" image representing the wound defect**. Reproduced with permission from *Microsurgery* (109).

## Preoperative Planning: Vascular Mapping

Understanding the vascular anatomy of perforators and their relationship with the regional anatomical structures is critical in perforator flap surgery and to this effect, CTA is currently the gold standard preoperative investigation (1, 2, 123, 126). Recently, Gillis and Morris reported a cadaveric study where a model of internal mammary artery perforators and the neighboring ribs was fabricated using a binder jet 3D printer (ProJet x60 series, 3D Systems) (118). The authors demonstrated the benefits of physically interacting with the model and the ability to visualize it in multiple planes to aid dissection and identification of the dominant perforator. However, they also noted a significant cost associated with outsourcing the 3D printing (USD 400–1,200) and the print material was too delicate for small-size blood vessels that required post-production strengthening with wax coating.

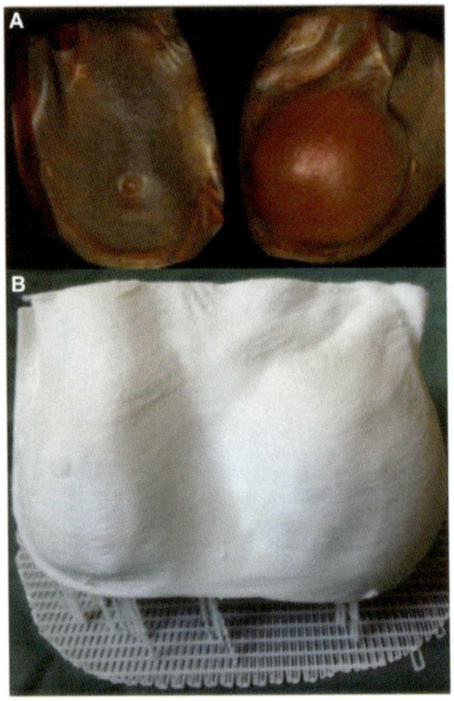



**FIGURE 7 | 3D reconstructed CT images of a patient with breast asymmetry post-mastectomy (A) and the 3D printed breast model of the same patient (B)**. Reproduced with permission from *Breast Cancer Research and Treatment* (108).

Likewise, our group 3D printed the perforator anatomy for planning a deep inferior epigastric artery perforator (DIEP) flap breast reconstruction. From the preoperative CTA, we created a CAD file of the deep inferior epigastric artery (DIEA) with the surrounding bony landmarks using 3D Slicer and the Cube 2 printer. Despite having to scale down the model to fit the printer dimensions, surgeons could intuitively discern the arterial anatomy from the replica. Interestingly, the current technique impeded the perforators of DIEA to be 3D printed. Considering that the DICOM data of the CTA and the Cube 2 printer have a resolution of 0.625 and 0.200 mm, respectively, and the mean diameter of a DIEA perforator ranges between 1 and 1.4 mm (127), this may be most likely explained as a limitation of the 3D modeling software, 3D Slicer. This may be prevented in the future by installing free add-on software functions, such as Vascular Modeling Toolkit (VMTK, Orobix, Bergamo, Italy) in 3D Slicer, that are designed to specifically segment vascular structures. Currently, these are still early in the development phase and are difficult to manipulate without significant computer engineering proficiencies. As the field advances, we would naturally expect the user interface of these softwares to become easier to use.

## Preoperative Planning: Bony Mapping

3D printing bony pathology in the forearm, wrist, and hand is another suitable utility of this technology in plastic and reconstructive surgery. CT scans have been the most commonly used imaging modality for medical 3D printing. Since they readily differentiate bones, 3D printing bony structures has become well established in various surgical disciplines, such as maxillofacial surgery (20, 21,

33, 128–130), neurosurgery (35, 68, 86), and orthopedic surgery (131–135). Using Osirix and Cube 2 printer, our research group 3D printed a model of a subluxed first carpometacarpal joint. Being able to visualize the model from various angles and the tactile feedback facilitated an intuitive understanding of the anatomical relationship between the first metacarpal and the trapezium. The information was useful for planning the optimal method of reduction.

## A New Evolution: 4D Printing

Recently, we described for the first time the concept of applying 3D printing to 4D CT scans, or 4D printing, where time is added as the fourth dimension to the standard 3D printing (119). 4D CT is a novel imaging modality developed to remove motion artifacts from organs, such as lungs, in order to enhance the image quality and facilitate precise delivery of radiotherapy (136, 137). In plastic surgery, investigators have utilized 4D CTA to assess the vascular territories and the dynamic flow characteristics of an individual perforator (4, 5). Using Osirix and Cube 2 printer, our group 3D printed the carpal and metacarpal bones of a patient in life-size at various stages of the thumb movement, such as thumb abduction (**Figure 8**). In contrast to the 3D reconstructions on a 2D computer screen and 3D models, 4D-printed haptic models accurately depicted the position of the carpal bones during each movement and enabled an instinctive appreciation of the spatiotemporal relationship between them. One of the major disadvantages was the reliance on the clinician reviewing the 4D CT data to select the scans most representative of the carpal bone transition during each movement for 3D printing. This can be overcome as 3D printers become faster thus allowing more models to be fabricated.

## Intraoperative Guidance

The convenience of 3D printing has propelled an innovation in custom designs of surgical templates and equipments that help guide the surgeon intraoperatively. In the literature, investigators have demonstrated the utility of 3D printing a modified army/navy surgical retractor (71); patient-specific orthognathic templates to guide osteotomy (66) and mandibular fracture reduction device (138) in maxillofacial surgery; screw fixation guide system in spinal neurosurgery (139); and drill templates to aid surgical correction of multilevel cervical spine instability in orthopedic surgery (69). In plastic and reconstructive surgery, Fuller et al. illustrated how 3D printing can expedite the development of a custom-made bone reduction clamp design for hand fractures, in comparison to the conventional processes that can become protracted and actually be discouraging to innovation (70). The authors collaborated with an engineer to produce 3D prototype designs and converted them into CAD files using free 3D softwares, such as SketchUp (Trimble Navigation, Sunnyvale, CA, USA) and MeshLab (ISTI-CNR, Pisa, Italy), respectively. 3D printing of the FDM prototypes was outsourced, costing USD 75 and 1–3 days for the delivery to arrive. The final design was manufactured in metal using an additive manufacturing technique, called direct metal laser sintering, and was again outsourced, costing USD 1,200 and 2 days for the delivery. The authors acknowledged that the 3D softwares for designing prototypes are currently not intuitive for clinicians with only basic computer proficiency. Furthermore, the final cost exceeded the cost of purchasing a standard equipment. However, as 3D printing technology advances and the 3D printing is performed "in-house", the difference may become minimal in the future.

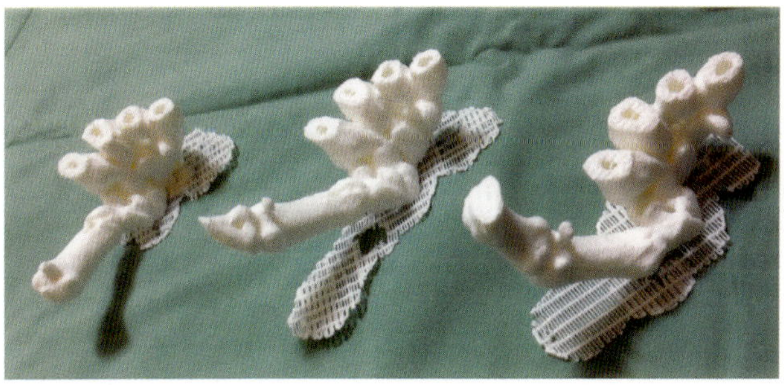

**FIGURE 8 | 4D-printed haptic models of carpal and metacarpal bones demonstrating thumb abduction (from left to right).** Reproduced with permission from *Journal of Reconstructive Microsurgery* (119).

## Surgical Training

Detailed knowledge of anatomical structures and their spatial relationships are essential assets of a plastic surgeon and objectives of a surgical training program. Through the standard medical training, a surgical aspirant can gain procedural experiences from performing dissections on human cadavers as a medical student and assisting senior surgeons in the operating theater as a resident, leading toward a gradual acquisition of competence. However, human cadavers are becoming relatively scarce from the anatomical education curricula due to high maintenance costs, cultural and social controversies, and safety issues associated with the formalin-containing embalming fluids (92, 140). Furthermore, the operative experience gained as an assistant to a senior surgeon is secondary to a primary operator experience. To this end, 3D-printed anatomical models can serve as an accurate, tactile visualization tool and a surgical simulation device. Moreover, 3D-printed haptic biomodels can be utilized to reproduce complex, patient-unique pathologies that facilitate the surgical trainees to preoperatively predict potential intraoperative challenges and postoperative outcomes and aid in their learning. Subsequent improvement in the surgeon's competence may lead to enhanced clinical outcomes and a reduced risk of complications. Investigators from various surgical disciplines have demonstrated the utility of 3D printing in training, such as neurosurgery (72–77, 141, 142), cardiothoracic surgery (54, 78–80, 143–145), urology (81, 146), and general surgery (29) However, one of the major limitations currently is the ability to print in materials that closely mimic the biomechanical properties and modulus of real human tissue as well as possessing realistic colors. As more materials enter the scope of 3D printing, future 3D-printed biomodels will be able to more closely reproduce true anatomy (50, 72, 74, 79).

## Patient Education

3D-printed replicas can be useful to facilitate the physician–patient interaction during a consultation with the aim of improved understanding of the intended procedure, its potential outcomes and complications and thus can form an important aspect of informed consent. Traditional CT/MRI scans are often difficult to comprehend for patients from a non-medical background. In recent times, plastic surgeons have utilized 3D scanning technology, such as

VECTRA (Canfield Imaging Systems), to accurately simulate potential outcomes from a cosmetic procedure on a computer screen (125). However, studies have consistently demonstrated that visual and tactile feedback from a 3D haptic model provides a superior understanding of anatomical details compared to 2D or 3D imaging techniques (34, 58, 147).

### Patient-Specific Prosthesis

As modern medicine ultimately progresses toward individualized treatment approaches, customizability of 3D printing can transform the manufacturing of patient-specific prostheses to being widely accessible and affordable. In comparison to a standard implant, a custom-made one is more likely to yield superior functional and esthetic outcomes (148, 149). Typical 3D printing materials can be sterilized using chemicals, such as Food and Drug Administration approved glutaraldehyde protocols (71), steam (20), and gas (150) for intraoperative handling. In the last decade, investigators have reported 3D-printed prostheses of nose (121, 151), ears (122, 152–155), eyes (156, 157), face (158, 159), and hand (6, 160). Furthermore, an Italian research group led by De Crescenzio and Ciocca has established an "Ear and Nose Library" where CAD files of 3D scanned ears and noses of normal university students are stocked (121, 122). When patients have pathology affecting both ears or the entire nose that impedes mirroring of the normal contralateral side to reconstruct the defect, the clinicians can select the most suitable CAD file from this database to fashion a prosthesis. In plastic surgery, standard breast implants are available in different volumes, but in a limited number of shapes. To this effect, 3D-printed breast implants customized to conform to the individual variations in the chest wall anatomy and the patient's desired breast shape and size may lead to a more esthetic and satisfactory outcome.

Most reports have indicated that 3D-printed custom prostheses provide superior esthetics in comparison to the traditional wax-based handcrafted prosthetics (152, 154, 155). Furthermore, customized implants eschew the need to intraoperatively modify and adjust associated with the standard implants, which can directly lead to improved clinical outcomes, such as a reduction in the length of surgery, reduced exposure to anesthetics, and a decreased risk of complications like infection (161, 162). Currently, one of the major drawbacks is that most custom implants are manufactured using expensive 3D printing techniques, such as MJM (157) and SLS (151, 160). In contrast, the affordable FDM 3D printers are used to fabricate negative molds for silicone or wax-based casts, which ironically increases the overall production time and cost (121, 122, 152–154, 156, 158). This is mainly because at present, only ABS and PLA filaments are available for FDM and their hard material characteristic makes them unsuitable for producing soft tissue prosthetics. However, as research and development in 3D printing continues to grow exponentially and more materials become available for FDM, we expect to be able to directly create a custom-made prosthesis affordably in the near future.

## Future and Conclusion

In the last decade, image-guided 3D-printed haptic biomodels have proven to represent a valuable adjunct to the conventional 2D imaging modalities in plastic surgery for preoperative planning, producing intraoperative guidance tools, educating surgical trainees and patients, and fashioning patient-specific implants. In the early years, the technical complexity of 3D softwares and the prohibitive cost of 3D printers restricted accessibility of 3D printing in medicine. The expiration of key 3D printing patents has fueled an exponential development in the field and a significant reduction in the cost. Ultimately, we envision that 3D printing has the potential to become ubiquitous and function as an essential clinical bedside tool for a plastic surgeon.

## Author Contributions

All authors contributed to the preparation of this manuscript. The manuscript has been seen and approved by all authors. The content of this article has not been submitted or published elsewhere.

## Acknowledgments

The authors would like to acknowledge Dr. Alexandra Rizzitelli at Peninsula Health for her support.

## References

1. Rozen WM, Anavekar NS, Ashton MW, Stella DL, Grinsell D, Bloom RJ, et al. Does the preoperative imaging of perforators with CT angiography improve operative outcomes in breast reconstruction? *Microsurgery* (2008) **28**:516–23. doi:10.1002/micr.20526
2. Rozen WM, Ashton MW, Grinsell D, Stella DL, Phillips TJ, Taylor GI. Establishing the case for CT angiography in the preoperative imaging of abdominal wall perforators. *Microsurgery* (2008) **28**:306–13. doi:10.1002/micr.20496
3. Rozen WM, Ashton MW, Stella DL, Phillips TJ, Grinsell D, Taylor GI. The accuracy of computed tomographic angiography for mapping the perforators of the deep inferior epigastric artery: a blinded, prospective cohort study. *Plast Reconstr Surg* (2008) **122**:1003–9. doi:10.1097/PRS.0b013e3181845994
4. Colohan S, Wong C, Lakhiani C, Cheng A, Maia M, Arbique G, et al. The free descending branch muscle-sparing latissimus dorsi flap: vascular anatomy and clinical applications. *Plast Reconstr Surg* (2012) **130**:776e–87e. doi:10.1097/PRS.0b013e31826d9c5e
5. Nie JY, Lu LJ, Gong X, Li Q, Nie JJ. Delineating the vascular territory (perforasome) of a perforator in the lower extremity of the rabbit with four-dimensional computed tomographic angiography. *Plast Reconstr Surg* (2013) **131**:565–71. doi:10.1097/PRS.0b013e31827c6e49
6. Gerstle TL, Ibrahim AM, Kim PS, Lee BT, Lin SJ. A plastic surgery application in evolution: three-dimensional printing. *Plast Reconstr Surg* (2014) **133**:446–51. doi:10.1097/01.prs.0000436844.92623.d3
7. Chae MP, Hunter-Smith DJ, Rozen WM. Image-guided 3D-printing and haptic modeling in plastic surgery. In: Saba L, Rozen WM, Alonso-Burgos A, Ribuffo

D, editors. *Imaging in Plastic Surgery*. London: CRC Taylor and Francis Press (2014). p. 819–30.
8. Goiato MC, Santos MR, Pesqueira AA, Moreno A, dos Santos DM, Haddad MF. Prototyping for surgical and prosthetic treatment. *J Craniofac Surg* (2011) **22**:914–7. doi:10.1097/SCS.0b013e31820f7f90
9. Levy GN, Schindel R, Kruth JP. Rapid manufacturing and rapid tooling with layer manufacturing (LM) technologies, state of the art and future perspectives. *CIRP Ann Manuf Technol* (2003) **52**:589–609. doi:10.1016/S0007-8506(07)60206-6
10. Sealy W. Additive manufacturing as a disruptive technology: how to avoid the pitfall. *Am J Eng Technol Res* (2011) **11**:86–93. doi:10.3727/19482413X3608676060655
11. Hoy MB. 3D printing: making things at the library. *Med Ref Serv Q* (2013) **32**:93–9. doi:10.1080/02763869.2013.749139
12. Srinivasan V, Bassan J. 3D printing and the future of manufacturing. *CSC Leading Edge Forum* (2012).
13. Schubert C, van Langeveld MC, Donoso LA. Innovations in 3D printing: a 3D overview from optics to organs. *Br J Ophthalmol* (2014) **98**:159–61. doi:10.1136/bjophthalmol-2013-304446
14. Klein GT, Lu Y, Wang MY. 3D printing and neurosurgery – ready for prime time? *World Neurosurg* (2013) **80**:233–5. doi:10.1016/j.wneu.2013.07.009
15. Hull CW. *Apparatus for Production of Three-Dimensional Objects by Stereolithography*. US Patent No. 4,575,330 (1986).
16. Hannen EJ. Recreating the original contour in tumor deformed mandibles for plate adapting. *Int J Oral Maxillofac Surg* (2006) **35**:183–5. doi:10.1016/j.ijom.2005.07.012
17. Rozen WM, Ting JW, Baillieu C, Leong J. Stereolithographic modeling of the deep circumflex iliac artery and its vascular branching: a further advance in computed tomography-guided flap planning. *Plast Reconstr Surg* (2012) **130**:380e–2e. doi:10.1097/PRS.0b013e31825903d1
18. Rozen WM, Ting JW, Leung M, Wu T, Ying D, Leong J. Advancing image-guided surgery in microvascular mandibular reconstruction: combining bony and vascular imaging with computed tomography-guided stereolithographic bone modeling. *Plast Reconstr Surg* (2012) **130**:227e–9e. doi:10.1097/PRS.0b013e318255028e
19. Ono I, Gunji H, Suda K, Kaneko F. Method for preparing an exact-size model using helical volume scan computed tomography. *Plast Reconstr Surg* (1994) **93**:1363–71. doi:10.1097/00006534-199406000-00005
20. Herlin C, Koppe M, Beziat JL, Gleizal A. Rapid prototyping in craniofacial surgery: using a positioning guide after zygomatic osteotomy – a case report. *J Craniomaxillofac Surg* (2011) **39**:376–9. doi:10.1016/j.jcms.2010.07.003
21. Cohen A, Laviv A, Berman P, Nashef R, Abu-Tair J. Mandibular reconstruction using stereolithographic 3-dimensional printing modeling technology. *Oral Surg Oral Med Oral Pathol Oral Radiol Endod* (2009) **108**:661–6. doi:10.1016/j.tripleo.2009.05.023
22. Tumbleston JR, Shirvanyants D, Ermoshkin N, Janusziewicz R, Johnson AR, Kelly D, et al. Additive manufacturing. Continuous liquid interface production of 3D objects. *Science* (2015) **347**:1349–52. doi:10.1126/science.aaa2397
23. Almquist TA, Smalley DR. *Thermal Stereolithography*. US Patent No. 5,141,680 (1992).
24. Deckard C. *Method and Apparatus for Producing Parts by Selective sintering*. US Patent No. 4,863,538 (1989).
25. Rengier F, Mehndiratta A, von Tengg-Kobligk H, Zechmann CM, Unterhinninghofen R, Kauczor HU, et al. 3D printing based on imaging data: review of medical applications. *Int J Comput Assist Radiol Surg* (2010) **5**:335–41. doi:10.1007/s11548-010-0476-x
26. Mottl-Link S, Hubler M, Kuhne T, Rietdorf U, Krueger JJ, Schnackenburg B, et al. Physical models aiding in complex congenital heart surgery. *Ann Thorac Surg* (2008) **86**:273–7. doi:10.1016/j.athoracsur.2007.06.001
27. McGurk M, Amis AA, Potamianos P, Goodger NM. Rapid prototyping techniques for anatomical modelling in medicine. *Ann R Coll Surg Engl* (1997) **79**:169–74.
28. Sachs EM, Haggerty JS, Cima MJ, Williams PA. *Three-Dimensional Printing Techniques*. US Patent No. 5,204,055 (1993).
29. Watson RA. A low-cost surgical application of additive fabrication. *J Surg Educ* (2014) **71**:14–7. doi:10.1016/j.jsurg.2013.10.012
30. Olszewski R, Szymor P, Kozakiewicz M. Accuracy of three-dimensional, paper-based models generated using a low-cost, three-dimensional printer. *J Craniomaxillofac Surg* (2014) **42**(8):1847–52. doi:10.1016/j.jcms.2014.07.002
31. Crump SS. *Apparatus and Method for Creating Three-Dimensional Objects*. US Patent No. 5,121,329 (1992).
32. Dikovsky D, Napadensky E. *Three-Dimensional Printing Process for Producing a Self-Destructible Temporary Structure*. US Patent No. 8,470,231 (2013)
33. Chen Y, Niu F, Yu B, Liu J, Wang M, Gui L. Three-dimensional preoperative design of distraction osteogenesis for hemifacial microsomia. *J Craniofac Surg* (2014) **25**:184–8. doi:10.1097/SCS.0000000000000391
34. Way TP, Barner KE. Automatic visual to tactile translation – part II: evaluation of the TACTile image creation system. *IEEE Trans Rehabil Eng* (1997) **5**:95–105. doi:10.1109/86.559354
35. D'Urso PS, Barker TM, Earwaker WJ, Bruce LJ, Atkinson RL, Lanigan MW, et al. Stereolithographic biomodelling in cranio-maxillofacial surgery: a prospective trial. *J Craniomaxillofac Surg* (1999) **27**:30–7. doi:10.1016/S1010-5182(99)80007-9
36. Guarino J, Tennyson S, McCain G, Bond L, Shea K, King H. Rapid prototyping technology for surgeries of the pediatric spine and pelvis: benefits analysis. *J Pediatr Orthop* (2007) **27**:955–60. doi:10.1097/bpo.0b013e3181594ced
37. Liu YF, Xu LW, Zhu HY, Liu SS. Technical procedures for template-guided surgery for mandibular reconstruction based on digital design and manufacturing. *Biomed Eng Online* (2014) **13**:63. doi:10.1186/1475-925X-13-63
38. Tsai MJ, Wu CT. Study of mandible reconstruction using a fibula flap with application of additive manufacturing technology. *Biomed Eng Online* (2014) **13**:57. doi:10.1186/1475-925X-13-57
39. Lim CG, Campbell DI, Clucas DM. Rapid prototyping technology in orbital floor reconstruction: application in three patients. *Craniomaxillofac Trauma Reconstr* (2014) **7**:143–6. doi:10.1055/s-0034-1371080
40. Engel M, Hoffmann J, Castrillon-Oberndorfer G, Freudlsperger C. The value of three-dimensional printing modelling for surgical correction of orbital hypertelorism. *Oral Maxillofac Surg* (2014). doi:10.1007/s10006-014-0466-1
41. Azuma M, Yanagawa T, Ishibashi-Kanno N, Uchida F, Ito T, Yamagata K, et al. Mandibular reconstruction using plates prebent to fit rapid prototyping 3-dimensional printing models ameliorates contour deformity. *Head Face Med* (2014) **10**:45. doi:10.1186/1746-160X-10-45
42. Jeong HS, Park KJ, Kil KM, Chong S, Eun HJ, Lee TS, et al. Minimally invasive plate osteosynthesis using 3D printing for shaft fractures of clavicles: technical note. *Arch Orthop Trauma Surg* (2014) **134**:1551–5. doi:10.1007/s00402-014-2075-8
43. Tam MD, Laycock SD, Bell D, Chojnowski A. 3-D printout of a DICOM file to aid surgical planning in a 6 year old patient with a large scapular osteochondroma complicating congenital diaphyseal aclasia. *J Radiol Case Rep* (2012) **6**:31–7. doi:10.3941/jrcr.v6i1.889
44. Schmauss D, Haeberle S, Hagl C, Sodian R. Three-dimensional printing in cardiac surgery and interventional cardiology: a single-centre experience. *Eur J Cardiothorac Surg* (2014). doi:10.1093/ejcts/ezu310
45. Witschey WR, Pouch AM, McGarvey JR, Ikeuchi K, Contijoch F, Levack MM, et al. Three-dimensional ultrasound-derived physical mitral valve modeling. *Ann Thorac Surg* (2014) **98**:691–4. doi:10.1016/j.athoracsur.2014.04.094
46. Schmauss D, Gerber N, Sodian R. Three-dimensional printing of models for surgical planning in patients with primary cardiac tumors. *J Thorac Cardiovasc Surg* (2013) **145**:1407–8. doi:10.1016/j.jtcvs.2012.12.030
47. Schmauss D, Schmitz C, Bigdeli AK, Weber S, Gerber N, Beiras-Fernandez A, et al. Three-dimensional printing of models for preoperative planning and simulation of transcatheter valve replacement. *Ann Thorac Surg* (2012) **93**:e31–3. doi:10.1016/j.athoracsur.2011.09.031
48. Sodian R, Weber S, Markert M, Loeff M, Lueth T, Weis FC, et al. Pediatric cardiac transplantation: three-dimensional printing of anatomic models for surgical planning of heart transplantation in patients with univentricular heart. *J Thorac Cardiovasc Surg* (2008) **136**:1098–9. doi:10.1016/j.jtcvs.2008.03.055
49. Sodian R, Schmauss D, Markert M, Weber S, Nikolaou K, Haeberle S, et al. Three-dimensional printing creates models for surgical planning of aortic valve replacement after previous coronary bypass grafting. *Ann Thorac Surg* (2008) **85**:2105–8. doi:10.1016/j.athoracsur.2007.12.033
50. Markert M, Weber S, Lueth TC. A beating heart model 3D printed from specific patient data. *Conf Proc IEEE Eng Med Biol Soc* (2007) **2007**:4472–5. doi:10.1109/IEMBS.2007.4353332
51. Nakada T, Akiba T, Inagaki T, Morikawa T. Thoracoscopic anatomical subsegmentectomy of the right S2b + S3 using a 3D printing model with rapid prototyping. *Interact Cardiovasc Thorac Surg* (2014) **19**(4):696–8. doi:10.1093/icvts/ivu174

52. Akiba T, Inagaki T, Nakada T. Three-dimensional printing model of anomalous bronchi before surgery. *Ann Thorac Cardiovasc Surg* (2014) **20**(Suppl):659–62. doi:10.5761/atcs.cr.13-00189
53. Tam MD, Laycock SD, Brown JR, Jakeways M. 3D printing of an aortic aneurysm to facilitate decision making and device selection for endovascular aneurysm repair in complex neck anatomy. *J Endovasc Ther* (2013) **20**:863–7. doi:10.1583/13-4450MR.1
54. Hakansson A, Rantatalo M, Hansen T, Wanhainen A. Patient specific biomodel of the whole aorta – the importance of calcified plaque removal. *Vasa* (2011) **40**:453–9. doi:10.1024/0301-1526/a000148
55. Sodian R, Schmauss D, Schmitz C, Bigdeli A, Haeberle S, Schmoeckel M, et al. 3-dimensional printing of models to create custom-made devices for coil embolization of an anastomotic leak after aortic arch replacement. *Ann Thorac Surg* (2009) **88**:974–8. doi:10.1016/j.athoracsur.2009.03.014
56. Silberstein JL, Maddox MM, Dorsey P, Feibus A, Thomas R, Lee BR. Physical models of renal malignancies using standard cross-sectional imaging and 3-dimensional printers: a pilot study. *Urology* (2014) **84**:268–72. doi:10.1016/j.urology.2014.03.042
57. Daniel M, Watson J, Hoskison E, Sama A. Frontal sinus models and onlay templates in osteoplastic flap surgery. *J Laryngol Otol* (2011) **125**:82–5. doi:10.1017/S0022215110001799
58. Suzuki M, Ogawa Y, Kawano A, Hagiwara A, Yamaguchi H, Ono H. Rapid prototyping of temporal bone for surgical training and medical education. *Acta Otolaryngol* (2004) **124**:400–2. doi:10.1080/00016480410016478
59. Igami T, Nakamura Y, Hirose T, Ebata T, Yokoyama Y, Sugawara G, et al. Application of a three-dimensional print of a liver in hepatectomy for small tumors invisible by intraoperative ultrasonography: preliminary experience. *World J Surg* (2014) **38**(12):3163–6. doi:10.1007/s00268-014-2740-7
60. Ikegami T, Maehara Y. Transplantation: 3D printing of the liver in living donor liver transplantation. *Nat Rev Gastroenterol Hepatol* (2013) **10**:697–8. doi:10.1038/nrgastro.2013.195
61. Zein NN, Hanouneh IA, Bishop PD, Samaan M, Eghtesad B, Quintini C, et al. Three-dimensional print of a liver for preoperative planning in living donor liver transplantation. *Liver Transpl* (2013) **19**:1304–10. doi:10.1002/lt.23729
62. Kang SH, Kim MK, Kim BC, Lee SH. Orthognathic Y-splint: a CAD/CAM-engineered maxillary repositioning wafer assembly. *Br J Oral Maxillofac Surg* (2014) **52**:667–9. doi:10.1016/j.bjoms.2014.01.023
63. Adolphs N, Liu W, Keeve E, Hoffmeister B. RapidSplint: virtual splint generation for orthognathic surgery – results of a pilot series. *Comput Aided Surg* (2014) **19**:20–8. doi:10.3109/10929088.2014.887778
64. Cousley RR, Turner MJ. Digital model planning and computerized fabrication of orthognathic surgery wafers. *J Orthod* (2014) **41**:38–45. doi:10.1179/1465313313Y.0000000075
65. Kim BC, Lee CE, Park W, Kim MK, Zhengguo P, Yu HS, et al. Clinical experiences of digital model surgery and the rapid-prototyped wafer for maxillary orthognathic surgery. *Oral Surg Oral Med Oral Pathol Oral Radiol Endod* (2011) **111**:278–85. doi:10.1016/j.tripleo.2010.04.038
66. Li B, Zhang L, Sun H, Yuan J, Shen SG, Wang X. A novel method of computer aided orthognathic surgery using individual CAD/CAM templates: a combination of osteotomy and repositioning guides. *Br J Oral Maxillofac Surg* (2013) **51**:e239–44. doi:10.1016/j.bjoms.2013.03.007
67. Metzger MC, Hohlweg-Majert B, Schwarz U, Teschner M, Hammer B, Schmelzeisen R. Manufacturing splints for orthognathic surgery using a three-dimensional printer. *Oral Surg Oral Med Oral Pathol Oral Radiol Endod* (2008) **105**:e1–7. doi:10.1016/j.tripleo.2007.07.040
68. D'Urso PS, Williamson OD, Thompson RG. Biomodeling as an aid to spinal instrumentation. *Spine (Phila Pa 1976)* (2005) **30**:2841–5. doi:10.1097/01.brs.0000190886.56895.3d
69. Spottiswoode BS, van den Heever DJ, Chang Y, Engelhardt S, Du Plessis S, Nicolls F, et al. Preoperative three-dimensional model creation of magnetic resonance brain images as a tool to assist neurosurgical planning. *Stereotact Funct Neurosurg* (2013) **91**:162–9. doi:10.1159/000345264
70. Fuller SM, Butz DR, Vevang CB, Makhlouf MV. Application of 3-dimensional printing in hand surgery for production of a novel bone reduction clamp. *J Hand Surg Am* (2014) **39**:1840–5. doi:10.1016/j.jhsa.2014.06.009
71. Rankin TM, Giovinco NA, Cucher DJ, Watts G, Hurwitz B, Armstrong DG. Three-dimensional printing surgical instruments: are we there yet? *J Surg Res* (2014) **189**:193–7. doi:10.1016/j.jss.2014.02.020
72. Waran V, Narayanan V, Karuppiah R, Owen SL, Aziz T. Utility of multimaterial 3D printers in creating models with pathological entities to enhance the training experience of neurosurgeons. *J Neurosurg* (2014) **120**:489–92. doi:10.3171/2013.11.JNS131066
73. Abla AA, Lawton MT. Three-dimensional hollow intracranial aneurysm models and their potential role for teaching, simulation, and training. *World Neurosurg* (2014). doi:10.1016/j.wneu.2014.01.015
74. Mashiko T, Otani K, Kawano R, Konno T, Kaneko N, Ito Y, et al. Development of three-dimensional hollow elastic model for cerebral aneurysm clipping simulation enabling rapid and low cost prototyping. *World Neurosurg* (2013). doi:10.1016/j.wneu.2013.10.032
75. Wurm G, Tomancok B, Pogady P, Holl K, Trenkler J. Cerebrovascular stereolithographic biomodeling for aneurysm surgery. Technical note. *J Neurosurg* (2004) **100**:139–45. doi:10.3171/jns.2004.100.1.0139
76. Wurm G, Lehner M, Tomancok B, Kleiser R, Nussbaumer K. Cerebrovascular biomodeling for aneurysm surgery: simulation-based training by means of rapid prototyping technologies. *Surg Innov* (2011) **18**:294–306. doi:10.1177/1553350610395031
77. Waran V, Narayanan V, Karuppiah R, Thambynayagam HC, Muthusamy KA, Rahman ZA, et al. Neurosurgical endoscopic training via a realistic 3-dimensional model with pathology. *Simul Healthc* (2014). doi:10.1097/SIH.0000000000000060
78. Costello JP, Olivieri LJ, Su L, Krieger A, Alfares F, Thabit O, et al. Incorporating three-dimensional printing into a simulation-based congenital heart disease and critical care training curriculum for resident physicians. *Congenit Heart Dis* (2014). doi:10.1111/chd.12238
79. Biglino G, Verschueren P, Zegels R, Taylor AM, Schievano S. Rapid prototyping compliant arterial phantoms for in-vitro studies and device testing. *J Cardiovasc Magn Reson* (2013) **15**:2. doi:10.1186/1532-429X-15-2
80. Bustamante S, Bose S, Bishop P, Klatte R, Norris F. Novel application of rapid prototyping for simulation of bronchoscopic anatomy. *J Cardiothorac Vasc Anesth* (2014) **28**:1134–7. doi:10.1053/j.jvca.2013.08.015
81. Cheung CL, Looi T, Lendvay TS, Drake JM, Farhat WA. Use of 3-dimensional printing technology and silicone modeling in surgical simulation: development and face validation in pediatric laparoscopic pyeloplasty. *J Surg Educ* (2014) **71**:762–7. doi:10.1016/j.jsurg.2014.03.001
82. Li J, Hsu Y, Luo E, Khadka A, Hu J. Computer-aided design and manufacturing and rapid prototyped nanoscale hydroxyapatite/polyamide (n-HA/PA) construction for condylar defect caused by mandibular angle ostectomy. *Aesthetic Plast Surg* (2011) **35**:636–40. doi:10.1007/s00266-010-9602-y
83. Klammert U, Gbureck U, Vorndran E, Rodiger J, Meyer-Marcotty P, Kubler AC. 3D powder printed calcium phosphate implants for reconstruction of cranial and maxillofacial defects. *J Craniomaxillofac Surg* (2010) **38**:565–70. doi:10.1016/j.jcms.2010.01.009
84. Saijo H, Igawa K, Kanno Y, Mori Y, Kondo K, Shimizu K, et al. Maxillofacial reconstruction using custom-made artificial bones fabricated by inkjet printing technology. *J Artif Organs* (2009) **12**:200–5. doi:10.1007/s10047-009-0462-7
85. Wurm G, Tomancok B, Holl K, Trenkler J. Prospective study on cranioplasty with individual carbon fiber reinforced polymer (CFRP) implants produced by means of stereolithography. *Surg Neurol* (2004) **62**:510–21. doi:10.1016/j.surneu.2004.01.025
86. D'Urso PS, Earwaker WJ, Barker TM, Redmond MJ, Thompson RG, Effeney DJ, et al. Custom cranioplasty using stereolithography and acrylic. *Br J Plast Surg* (2000) **53**:200–4. doi:10.1054/bjps.1999.3268
87. Bicanic G, Barbaric K, Bohacek I, Aljinovic A, Delimar D. Current concept in dysplastic hip arthroplasty: techniques for acetabular and femoral reconstruction. *World J Orthop* (2014) **5**:412–24. doi:10.5312/wjo.v5.i4.412
88. Koulouvaris P, Stafylas K, Sculco T, Xenakis T. Distal femoral shortening in total hip arthroplasty for complex primary hip reconstruction. A new surgical technique. *J Arthroplasty* (2008) **23**:992–8. doi:10.1016/j.arth.2007.09.013
89. Zopf DA, Hollister SJ, Nelson ME, Ohye RG, Green GE. Bioresorbable airway splint created with a three-dimensional printer. *N Engl J Med* (2013) **368**:2043–5. doi:10.1056/NEJMc1206319
90. Reeves P. Additive manufacturing & 3D printing medical & healthcare: a new industrial perspective. *The 3D Printing & Additive Manufacturing People*. Derbyshire (2014).
91. Wozniak K, Rzepecka-Wozniak E, Moskala A, Pohl J, Latacz K, Dybala B. Weapon identification using antemortem computed tomography with virtual 3D and rapid

prototype modeling – a report in a case of blunt force head injury. *Forensic Sci Int* (2012) **222**:e29–32. doi:10.1016/j.forsciint.2012.06.012

92. McMenamin PG, Quayle MR, McHenry CR, Adams JW. The production of anatomical teaching resources using three-dimensional (3D) printing technology. *Anat Sci Educ* (2014) **7**:479–86. doi:10.1002/ase.1475
93. Giovinco NA, Dunn SP, Dowling L, Smith C, Trowell L, Ruch JA, et al. A novel combination of printed 3-dimensional anatomic templates and computer-assisted surgical simulation for virtual preoperative planning in Charcot foot reconstruction. *J Foot Ankle Surg* (2012) **51**:387–93. doi:10.1053/j.jfas.2012.01.014
94. Groth C, Kravitz ND, Jones PE, Graham JW, Redmond WR. Three-dimensional printing technology. *J Clin Orthod* (2014) **48**:475–85.
95. Chen J, Zhang Z, Chen X, Zhang C, Zhang G, Xu Z. Design and manufacture of customized dental implants by using reverse engineering and selective laser melting technology. *J Prosthet Dent* (2014) **112**:1088–95. doi:10.1016/j.prosdent.2014.04.026
96. Flugge TV, Nelson K, Schmelzeisen R, Metzger MC. Three-dimensional plotting and printing of an implant drilling guide: simplifying guided implant surgery. *J Oral Maxillofac Surg* (2013) **71**:1340–6. doi:10.1016/j.joms.2013.04.010
97. Goyanes A, Buanz AB, Hatton GB, Gaisford S, Basit AW. 3D printing of modified-release aminosalicylate (4-ASA and 5-ASA) tablets. *Eur J Pharm Biopharm* (2014). doi:10.1016/j.ejpb.2014.12.003
98. Skowyra J, Pietrzak K, Alhnan MA. Fabrication of extended-release patient-tailored prednisolone tablets via fused deposition modelling (FDM) 3D printing. *Eur J Pharm Sci* (2014) **68C**:11–7. doi:10.1016/j.ejps.2014.11.009
99. Lueders C, Jastram B, Hetzer R, Schwandt H. Rapid manufacturing techniques for the tissue engineering of human heart valves. *Eur J Cardiothorac Surg* (2014) **46**:593–601. doi:10.1093/ejcts/ezt510
100. Chang JW, Park SA, Park JK, Choi JW, Kim YS, Shin YS, et al. Tissue-engineered tracheal reconstruction using three-dimensionally printed artificial tracheal graft: preliminary report. *Artif Organs* (2014) **38**:E95–105. doi:10.1111/aor.12310
101. Lee Ventola C. Medical applications for 3D printing: current and projected uses. *P T* (2014) **39**:704–11.
102. Fullerton JN, Frodsham GC, Day RM. 3D printing for the many, not the few. *Nat Biotechnol* (2014) **32**:1086–7. doi:10.1038/nbt.3056
103. Hieu LC, Zlatov N, Vander Sloten J, Bohez E, Khanh L, Binh PH, et al. Medical rapid prototyping applications and methods. *Assemb Autom* (2005) **25**:284–92. doi:10.1108/01445150510626415
104. Rosset A, Spadola L, Ratib O. OsiriX: an open-source software for navigating in multidimensional DICOM images. *J Digit Imaging* (2004) **17**:205–16. doi:10.1007/s10278-004-1014-6
105. Fedorov A, Beichel R, Kalpathy-Cramer J, Finet J, Fillion-Robin JC, Pujol S, et al. 3D slicer as an image computing platform for the quantitative imaging network. *Magn Reson Imaging* (2012) **30**:1323–41. doi:10.1016/j.mri.2012.05.001
106. Gering DT, Nabavi A, Kikinis R, Hata N, O'Donnell LJ, Grimson WE, et al. An integrated visualization system for surgical planning and guidance using image fusion and an open MR. *J Magn Reson Imaging* (2001) **13**:967–75. doi:10.1002/jmri.1139
107. Golby AJ, Kindlmann G, Norton I, Yarmarkovich A, Pieper S, Kikinis R. Interactive diffusion tensor tractography visualization for neurosurgical planning. *Neurosurgery* (2011) **68**:496–505. doi:10.1227/NEU.0b013e3182061ebb
108. Chae MP, Hunter-Smith DJ, Spychal RT, Rozen WM. 3D volumetric analysis for planning breast reconstructive surgery. *Breast Cancer Res Treat* (2014) **146**(2):457–60. doi:10.1007/s10549-014-3028-1
109. Chae MP, Lin F, Spychal RT, Hunter-Smith DJ, Rozen WM. 3D-printed haptic "reverse" models for preoperative planning in soft tissue reconstruction: a case report. *Microsurgery* (2014). doi:10.1002/micr.22293
110. Ibrahim D, Broilo TL, Heitz C, de Oliveira MG, de Oliveira HW, Nobre SM, et al. Dimensional error of selective laser sintering, three-dimensional printing and PolyJet models in the reproduction of mandibular anatomy. *J Craniomaxillofac Surg* (2009) **37**:167–73. doi:10.1016/j.jcms.2008.10.008
111. Silva DN, Gerhardt de Oliveira M, Meurer E, Meurer MI, Lopes da Silva JV, Santa-Barbara A. Dimensional error in selective laser sintering and 3D-printing of models for craniomaxillary anatomy reconstruction. *J Craniomaxillofac Surg* (2008) **36**:443–9. doi:10.1016/j.jcms.2008.04.003
112. Fitzwater KL, Marcellin-Little DJ, Harrysson OL, Osborne JA, Poindexter EC. Evaluation of the effect of computed tomography scan protocols and freeform fabrication methods on bone biomodel accuracy. *Am J Vet Res* (2011) **72**:1178–85. doi:10.2460/ajvr.72.9.1178
113. Bos EJ, Scholten T, Song Y, Verlinden JC, Wolff J, Forouzanfar T, et al. Developing a parametric ear model for auricular reconstruction: a new step towards patient-specific implants. *J Craniomaxillofac Surg* (2015) **43**:390–5. doi:10.1016/j.jcms.2014.12.016
114. Nishimoto S, Sotsuka Y, Kawai K, Fujita K, Kakibuchi M. Three-dimensional mock-up model for chondral framework in auricular reconstruction, built with a personal three-dimensional printer. *Plast Reconstr Surg* (2014) **134**:180e–1e. doi:10.1097/PRS.0000000000000263
115. Xu Y, Fan F, Kang N, Wang S, You J, Wang H, et al. Tissue engineering of human nasal alar cartilage precisely by using three-dimensional printing. *Plast Reconstr Surg* (2015) **135**:451–8. doi:10.1097/PRS.0000000000000856
116. Cabalag MS, Chae MP, Miller GS, Rozen WM, Hunter-Smith DJ. Use of three-dimensional printed 'haptic' models for preoperative planning in an Australian plastic surgery unit. *ANZ J Surg* (2015). doi:10.1111/ans.13168
117. Garcia Tutor E, Romeo M, Chae MP, Hunter-Smith DJ, Rozen WM. 3D volumetric modeling and microvascular reconstruction of irradiated lumbosacral defects after oncologic resection. *J Reconstr Microsurg* (2015).
118. Gillis JA, Morris SF. Three-dimensional printing of perforator vascular anatomy. *Plast Reconstr Surg* (2014) **133**:80e–2e. doi:10.1097/01.prs.0000436523.79293.64
119. Chae MP, Hunter-Smith DJ, De-Silva I, Tham S, Spychal RT, Rozen WM. Four-dimensional (4D) printing: a new evolution in computed tomography-guided stereolithographic modeling. Principles and application. *J Reconstr Microsurg* (2015). doi:10.1055/s-0035-1549006
120. Sutradhar A, Park J, Carrau D, Miller MJ. Experimental validation of 3D printed patient-specific implants using digital image correlation and finite element analysis. *Comput Biol Med* (2014) **52**:8–17. doi:10.1016/j.compbiomed.2014.06.002
121. Ciocca L, De Crescenzio F, Fantini M, Scotti R. Rehabilitation of the nose using CAD/CAM and rapid prototyping technology after ablative surgery of squamous cell carcinoma: a pilot clinical report. *Int J Oral Maxillofac Implants* (2010) **25**:808–12. doi:10.1080/10255840903251304
122. Ciocca L, De Crescenzio F, Fantini M, Scotti R. CAD/CAM bilateral ear prostheses construction for Treacher Collins syndrome patients using laser scanning and rapid prototyping. *Comput Methods Biomech Biomed Engin* (2010) **13**:379–86. doi:10.1080/10255840903251304
123. Rozen WM, Chubb D, Grinsell D, Ashton MW. Computed tomographic angiography: clinical applications. *Clin Plast Surg* (2011) **38**:229–39. doi:10.1016/j.cps.2011.03.007
124. Rozen WM, Garcia-Tutor E, Alonso-Burgos A, Acosta R, Stillaert F, Zubieta JL, et al. Planning and optimising DIEP flaps with virtual surgery: the Navarra experience. *J Plast Reconstr Aesthet Surg* (2010) **63**:289–97. doi:10.1016/j.bjps.2008.10.007
125. Donfrancesco A, Montemurro P, Heden P. Three-dimensional simulated images in breast augmentation surgery: an investigation of patients' satisfaction and the correlation between prediction and actual outcome. *Plast Reconstr Surg* (2013) **132**:810–22. doi:10.1097/PRS.0b013e3182a014cb
126. Rozen WM, Ashton MW. Modifying techniques in deep inferior epigastric artery perforator flap harvest with the use of preoperative imaging. *ANZ J Surg* (2009) **79**:598–603. doi:10.1111/j.1445-2197.2009.05013.x
127. Rozen WM, Ashton MW, Le Roux CM, Pan WR, Corlett RJ. The perforator angiosome: a new concept in the design of deep inferior epigastric artery perforator flaps for breast reconstruction. *Microsurgery* (2010) **30**:1–7. doi:10.1002/micr.20684
128. Lee JW, Fang JJ, Chang LR, Yu CK. Mandibular defect reconstruction with the help of mirror imaging coupled with laser stereolithographic modeling technique. *J Formos Med Assoc* (2007) **106**:244–50. doi:10.1016/S0929-6646(09)60247-3
129. Cao D, Yu Z, Chai G, Liu J, Mu X. Application of EH compound artificial bone material combined with computerized three-dimensional reconstruction in craniomaxillofacial surgery. *J Craniofac Surg* (2010) **21**:440–3. doi:10.1097/SCS.0b013e3181cfe9bc
130. Katsuragi Y, Kayano S, Akazawa S, Nagamatsu S, Koizumi T, Matsui T, et al. Mandible reconstruction using the calcium-sulphate three-dimensional model and rubber stick: a new method, 'mould technique', for more accurate, efficient and simplified fabrication. *J Plast Reconstr Aesthet Surg* (2011) **64**:614–22. doi:10.1016/j.bjps.2010.08.010
131. Hsieh MK, Chen AC, Cheng CY, Chou YC, Chan YS, Hsu KY. Repositioning osteotomy for intra-articular malunion of distal radius with radiocarpal and/or distal radioulnar joint subluxation. *J Trauma* (2010) **69**:418–22. doi:10.1097/TA.0b013e3181ca0834

132. Gan Y, Xu D, Lu S, Ding J. Novel patient-specific navigational template for total knee arthroplasty. *Comput Aided Surg* (2011) **16**:288–97. doi:10.3109/10929088.2011.621214
133. Kunz M, Ma B, Rudan JF, Ellis RE, Pichora DR. Image-guided distal radius osteotomy using patient-specific instrument guides. *J Hand Surg Am* (2013) **38**:1618–24. doi:10.1016/j.jhsa.2013.05.018
134. Kataoka T, Oka K, Miyake J, Omori S, Tanaka H, Murase T. 3-Dimensional prebent plate fixation in corrective osteotomy of malunited upper extremity fractures using a real-sized plastic bone model prepared by preoperative computer simulation. *J Hand Surg Am* (2013) **38**:909–19. doi:10.1016/j.jhsa.2013.02.024
135. Minns RJ, Bibb R, Banks R, Sutton RA. The use of a reconstructed three-dimensional solid model from CT to aid the surgical management of a total knee arthroplasty: a case study. *Med Eng Phys* (2003) **25**:523–6. doi:10.1016/S1350-4533(03)00050-X
136. Reinhardt JM, Ding K, Cao K, Christensen GE, Hoffman EA, Bodas SV. Registration-based estimates of local lung tissue expansion compared to xenon CT measures of specific ventilation. *Med Image Anal* (2008) **12**:752–63. doi:10.1016/j.media.2008.03.007
137. Chang JY, Li QQ, Xu QY, Allen PK, Rebueno N, Gomez DR, et al. Stereotactic ablative radiation therapy for centrally located early stage or isolated parenchymal recurrences of non-small cell lung cancer: how to fly in a "no fly zone". *Int J Radiat Oncol Biol Phys* (2014) **88**:1120–8. doi:10.1016/j.ijrobp.2014.01.022
138. Kontio R, Bjorkstrand R, Salmi M, Paloheimo M, Paloheimo KS, Tuomi J, et al. Designing and additive manufacturing a prototype for a novel instrument for mandible fracture reduction. *Surgery* (2012) **S1**:002. doi:10.4172/2161-1076.S1-002
139. Sugawara T, Higashiyama N, Kaneyama S, Takabatake M, Watanabe N, Uchida F, et al. Multistep pedicle screw insertion procedure with patient-specific lamina fit-and-lock templates for the thoracic spine: clinical article. *J Neurosurg Spine* (2013) **19**:185–90. doi:10.3171/2013.4.SPINE121059
140. Lambrecht JT, Berndt DC, Schumacher R, Zehnder M. Generation of three-dimensional prototype models based on cone beam computed tomography. *Int J Comput Assist Radiol Surg* (2009) **4**:175–80. doi:10.1007/s11548-008-0275-9
141. Kimura T, Morita A, Nishimura K, Aiyama H, Itoh H, Fukaya S, et al. Simulation of and training for cerebral aneurysm clipping with 3-dimensional models. *Neurosurgery* (2009) **65**:719–25. doi:10.1227/01.NEU.0000354350.88899.07
142. Chueh JY, Wakhloo AK, Gounis MJ. Neurovascular modeling: small-batch manufacturing of silicone vascular replicas. *AJNR Am J Neuroradiol* (2009) **30**:1159–64. doi:10.3174/ajnr.A1543
143. Sulaiman A, Boussel L, Taconnet F, Serfaty JM, Alsaid H, Attia C, et al. In vitro non-rigid life-size model of aortic arch aneurysm for endovascular prosthesis assessment. *Eur J Cardiothorac Surg* (2008) **33**:53–7. doi:10.1016/j.ejcts.2007.10.016
144. Kalejs M, von Segesser LK. Rapid prototyping of compliant human aortic roots for assessment of valved stents. *Interact Cardiovasc Thorac Surg* (2009) **8**:182–6. doi:10.1510/icvts.2008.194134
145. Armillotta A, Bonhoeffer P, Dubini G, Ferragina S, Migliavacca F, Sala G, et al. Use of rapid prototyping models in the planning of percutaneous pulmonary valved stent implantation. *Proc Inst Mech Eng H* (2007) **221**:407–16. doi:10.1243/09544119JEIM83
146. Bruyere F, Leroux C, Brunereau L, Lermusiaux P. Rapid prototyping model for percutaneous nephrolithotomy training. *J Endourol* (2008) **22**:91–6. doi:10.1089/end.2007.0025
147. Kim MS, Sbalchiero JC, Reece GP, Miller MJ, Beahm EK, Markey MK. Assessment of breast aesthetics. *Plast Reconstr Surg* (2008) **121**:186e–94e. doi:10.1097/01.prs.0000304593.74672.b8
148. Chan YC, Qing KX, Cheng SW. Custom-made fenestrated stent grafts to preserve accessory renal arteries in patients with abdominal aortic aneurysms. *Acta Chir Belg* (2014) **114**:183–8.
149. Hourfar J, Kanavakis G, Goellner P, Ludwig B. Fully customized placement of orthodontic miniplates: a novel clinical technique. *Head Face Med* (2014) **10**:14. doi:10.1186/1746-160X-10-14
150. Lee SJ, Lee HP, Tse KM, Cheong EC, Lim SP. Computer-aided design and rapid prototyping-assisted contouring of costal cartilage graft for facial reconstructive surgery. *Craniomaxillofac Trauma Reconstr* (2012) **5**:75–82. doi:10.1055/s-0031-1300964
151. Wu G, Zhou B, Bi Y, Zhao Y. Selective laser sintering technology for customized fabrication of facial prostheses. *J Prosthet Dent* (2008) **100**:56–60. doi:10.1016/S0022-3913(08)60138-9
152. Sykes LM, Parrott AM, Owen CP, Snaddon DR. Applications of rapid prototyping technology in maxillofacial prosthetics. *Int J Prosthodont* (2004) **17**:454–9.
153. Subburaj K, Nair C, Rajesh S, Meshram SM, Ravi B. Rapid development of auricular prosthesis using CAD and rapid prototyping technologies. *Int J Oral Maxillofac Surg* (2007) **36**:938–43. doi:10.1016/j.ijom.2007.07.013
154. Karayazgan-Saracoglu B, Gunay Y, Atay A. Fabrication of an auricular prosthesis using computed tomography and rapid prototyping technique. *J Craniofac Surg* (2009) **20**:1169–72. doi:10.1097/SCS.0b013e3181acdb95
155. De Crescenzio F, Fantini M, Ciocca L, Persiani F, Scotti R. Design and manufacturing of ear prosthesis by means of rapid prototyping technology. *Proc Inst Mech Eng H* (2011) **225**:296–302. doi:10.1243/09544119JEIM856
156. Ciocca L, Scotti R. Oculo-facial rehabilitation after facial cancer removal: updated CAD/CAM procedures. A pilot study. *Prosthet Orthot Int* (2013). doi:10.1177/0309364613512368
157. Xie P, Hu Z, Zhang X, Li X, Gao Z, Yuan D, et al. Application of 3-dimensional printing technology to construct an eye model for fundus viewing study. *PLoS One* (2014) **9**:e109373. doi:10.1371/journal.pone.0109373
158. Tsuji M, Noguchi N, Ihara K, Yamashita Y, Shikimori M, Goto M. Fabrication of a maxillofacial prosthesis using a computer-aided design and manufacturing system. *J Prosthodont* (2004) **13**:179–83. doi:10.1111/j.1532-849X.2004.04029.x
159. Fantini M, De Crescenzio F, Ciocca L. Design and rapid manufacturing of anatomical prosthesis for facial rehabilitation. *Int J Interact Des Manuf* (2013) **7**:51–62. doi:10.1007/s12008-012-0159-7
160. De Laurentis KJ, Mavroidis C. Mechanical design of a shape memory alloy actuated prosthetic hand. *Technol Health Care* (2002) **10**:91–106.
161. Eppley BL. Craniofacial reconstruction with computer-generated HTR patient-matched implants: use in primary bony tumor excision. *J Craniofac Surg* (2002) **13**:650–7. doi:10.1097/00001665-200209000-00011
162. Sammartino G, Della Valle A, Marenzi G, Gerbino S, Martorelli M, di Lauro AE, et al. Stereolithography in oral implantology: a comparison of surgical guides. *Implant Dent* (2004) **13**:133–9. doi:10.1097/01.ID.0000127526.36938.4C

2

# Comparison of an Innovative Rehabilitation, Combining Reduced Conventional Rehabilitation with Balneotherapy, and a Conventional Rehabilitation after Anterior Cruciate Ligament Reconstruction in Athletes

*Laetitia Peultier-Celli[1,2], Didier Mainard[3], Frank Wein[4], Nicolas Paris[4], Patrick Boisseau[5], Alexandre Ferry[5], René Gueguen[1], Isabelle Chary-Valckenaere[6,7], Jean Paysant[1,8] and Philippe Perrin[1,2]**

*[1] Faculty of Medicine and UFR STAPS, University of Lorraine, EA 3450, Development, Adaptation and Handicap, Villers-lès-Nancy, France, [2] Laboratory for the Analysis of Posture, Equilibrium and Motor Function (LAPEM), University Hospital of Nancy, Vandoeuvre-lès-Nancy, France, [3] Department of Orthopedics and Trauma Surgery, University Hospital of Nancy, Nancy, France, [4] Department of Orthopedics Surgery, Médipôle Gentilly-Saint-Jacques, Maxéville, France, [5] Institut de Formation en Masso-Kinésithérapie, Nancy, France, [6] Department of Rheumatology, University Hospital of Nancy, Vandoeuvre-lès-Nancy, France, [7] IMoPA, UMR 7365 CNRS, Vandoeuvre-lès-Nancy, France, [8] Regional Institute of Physical Medicine and Rehabilitation, Nancy Cedex, France*

**Edited by:**
*Vassilios S. Nikolaou, University General Hospital Attikon, Greece*

**Reviewed by:**
*Konstantinos Markatos, Biomedical Research Foundation of the Academy of Athens, Greece*
*Korres Stylianos Demetrios, Athens State University, United States*

***Correspondence:**
*Philippe Perrin*
*philippe.perrin@univ-lorraine.fr*

**Specialty section:**
*This article was submitted to Orthopedic Surgery, a section of the journal Frontiers in Surgery*

**Background:** Instability of the knee, related to anterior cruciate ligament injury, is treated by surgical reconstruction. During recovery, a loss of proprioceptive input can have a significant impact. Few studies have evaluated the benefits of rehabilitation of the knee in aquatic environment on functional outcomes.

**Objective:** This study aimed to compare an innovative rehabilitation protocol combining reduced conventional rehabilitation with aquatic rehabilitation, with a conventional rehabilitation, according to the National French Health Authority, in terms of kinetics, development of proprioceptive skills, and functional improvement of the knee.

**Methods:** 67 patients, who were amateur or professional athletes, were randomized into two groups: 35 patients followed the conventional rehabilitation protocol (Gr1) and 32 patients followed the innovative rehabilitation protocol (Gr2). Patients were evaluated before surgery, and at 2 weeks, 1, 2, and 6 months after surgery using posturography, and evaluation of muscular strength, walking performance and proprioception. This study is multicenter, prospective, randomized, and controlled with a group of patients following conventional rehabilitation (level of evidence I).

**Results:** For the same quality of postural control, Gr2 relied more on somesthesia than Gr1 at 6 months. The affected side had an impact on postural control and in particular on the preoperative lateralization, at 2 weeks and at 1 month. Lateralization depended on the affected knee, with less important lateralization in Gr2 preoperatively and at 1 month. The quadriceps muscular strength was higher in Gr2 than in Gr1 at 2 and 6 months and muscle strength of the external hamstring was greater in Gr2 than in Gr1 at 6 months. The isokinetic test showed a greater quadriceps muscular strength in Gr2. Gr2 showed a greater walking distance than Gr1 at one month. Gr2 showed an improvement in the proprioceptive capacities of the operated limb in flexion for the first 2 months.

**Conclusion:** The effectiveness of the innovative rehabilitation program permits faster recovery, allowing for an earlier return to social, sporting, and professional activities. Faster retrieval of knee function following aquatic rehabilitation would prevent both short-term risk of lesions of the contralateral limb due to overcompensation and long-term risk of surgery due to osteoarthritis.

**Registration of clinical trials:** NCT02225613.

**Keywords: anterior cruciate ligament injury, rehabilitation, balneotherapy, postural control, proprioception, sports injury**

## INTRODUCTION

Anterior cruciate ligament (ACL) injury is one of the main injuries in sporting activities with an incidence of nearly 32,000 victims per year in France (1), especially in young patients or athletes. This injury is rather unusual in the general population and can occur during most physical and sporting activities, particularly in activities which involve rotation constraints of the lower limbs such as football, rugby, handball, basketball, volleyball, and especially skiing (2). The ACL does not recover spontaneously due to its poor vascularity, and rupture of this ligament may result in short-term, medium-term, and long-term complications and poor functional prognosis. Instability of the knee and subsequent postural control impairments can occur in sporting activities, especially pivot sports, or during activities of daily living (3). This instability can affect other structures of the knee by damaging the meniscus which acts as a shock absorber. These events can also damage articular cartilage of the femur and the tibia leading to long-term osteoarthritis (4–7). Reconstruction of ACL by auto-graft tendon is the optimal treatment for these injuries, offering maximal joint stability with minimal surgical risk (3). Several studies have shown recovery of postural stability (8–10), which can be explained by the regeneration of sensory neurons after reconstruction of ACL (11). Among the reconstruction techniques, a hamstrings autograft uses the tendons of the gracilis and semitendinosus muscles. Once removed, these tendons are folded in half in order to obtain a new ligament with four strands. Among other techniques, a tape locking screw (TLS), developed by Collette in Brussels in 2001 (12), is nowadays used in France in 10% of cases (2). This technique uses only one fragment of the tendon of the semitendinosus muscle (the tendon of the gracilis may nevertheless sometimes be used). The graft is placed in small diameter bone tunnels with suspension strips and an interference screw. Finally, the Kenneth Jones (KJ) technique relies on the removal of the central third of the patellar tendon with a bone rod at each end, at the top of the femur and at the bottom on the tibia (13). Regardless of the technique, the graft taken is calibrated and then prepared before being inserted and fixed in both tibial and femoral bone tunnels. Surgery has to be followed by a long process of neuromotor reprograming through rehabilitation. Several rehabilitation techniques are used and studies have been carried out to compare the effects of rehabilitation in water versus more traditional rehabilitation on land. Tovin et al. (14) have shown that 2 months after surgery, aquatic exercises may not be as effective than on land for muscle strength but that water has a beneficial effect on edema and pain decrease. Zamarioli et al. (15) showed that during 9 weeks of rehabilitation, patients undergoing aquatic rehabilitation tended to recover faster than those who had undergone conventional land rehabilitation on clinical parameters such as pain, range of motion, muscle strength, swelling, and muscle mass circumference. Tovin et al. (14) suggested that future studies should analyze the effectiveness of a program that combines traditional and water-based exercises over a longer follow-up period.

The main objective of this study was to compare an innovative rehabilitation protocol with an "aquatic part" (balneotherapy) and a "dry part" and a conventional rehabilitation protocol (1) in terms of dynamics of recovery and development of the proprioceptive skills in athletes with ACL reconstruction. A secondary objective was to compare both groups in terms of functional improvement, i.e., pain, joint amplitude, muscular strength, and walking performance.

## PATIENTS AND METHODS

### Setting and Participants

Sixty-seven patients aged from 18 to 49 years participated in this study. The volunteers underwent surgery by orthopedic surgeons from the University Hospital of Nancy and private clinics around Nancy, East of France. Among the 67 patients, none have undergone surgical complications.

All subjects were leisure or competitive sportsmen (amateur or professional). All of them had chronic knee instability and the indication of a first-line ACL reconstruction using TLS, semitendinosus or gracilis tendons or KJ was given. Exclusion criteria were history of neurological disease (stroke, degenerative diseases of the central nervous system or the peripheral nervous system), medication for psychotropic or antihypertensive purposes, contraindications to aquatic activities (especially cutaneous), and recent sprains less than 3 months in the lower limbs that could interfere with postural control.

This study is multicenter, prospective, randomized, and controlled with a group of patients following conventional rehabilitation (level of evidence I). All participants gave written informed consent before the randomization. The study was approved by the French Medical Ethical Committee (Comité de Protection des Personnes de Lorraine), realized in structures (Nancy-Thermal) agreed for research (Agence Régionale de Santé), and registered in ClinicalTrials.gov with the identifier: NCT02225613.

## Randomization and Interventions

All patients began the same conventional rehabilitation protocol according to the recommendations of the National French Health Authority (HAS), until tissues healing (3). For 3 weeks, starting from the 15th postoperative day, subjects were randomized into two rehabilitation groups. To implement randomization, a statistician assigned numbers in two groups, each number corresponding to a patient. Sealed envelopes with the numbers were then prepared by the study Promotor (Direction for Research of the University Hospital who is not investigator of the study). No patient refused the group into which they were assigned. The first group (Gr1, $n$ = 35; mean age = 29.91 ± 7.70 years; 21 males) followed a conventional rehabilitation protocol (according to HAS recommendations) and the second group (Gr2; $n$ = 32; mean age = 28.22 ± 7.38; 26 males) followed an innovative rehabilitation protocol with a reduced conventional part and an aquatic part. The total duration of patient care was the same between the two groups regardless of the rehabilitation protocol followed: 45 min, once a day, five times a week, from Monday to Friday, for 3 weeks. After these 3 weeks, all patients returned to a conventional rehabilitation (according to HAS recommendations) (3) (**Figure 1**).

## Outcomes and Follow-up

### Postural Control Statement

Postural control tests, main endpoint, were carried out in a specially designed sound proof room devoted to posturography recordings. A vertical force platform, fitted with three strain-gauge force transducers (Medicapteurs, Balma, France) was used to perform posturography and to provide a measurement of the body sway in terms of displacement of the center of foot pressure (CoP) in a two-dimensional horizontal plane (recording time: 25.6 s, acquisition frequency: 40 Hz) (**Figure 2**). The signals from the transducers were amplified, converted from analog into digital form and then recorded on a computer. The sway path traveled and area covered by the CoP trajectory were used to quantify postural sway (**Figure 3**). The mean shift on the X-axis was also used to quantify the lateralization and its side. Each subject was asked to stand upright on the platform, barefoot, feet abducted at 30°, heels separated by 3 cm, arms along the body, remaining as stable as possible and breathing normally in six conditions (16–18) to test somatosensory cues (19) (**Table 1**).

In order to evaluate participants' ability to adapt and adjust balance control performance correctly and rapidly to change of external and internal constraints, a mean equilibrium score (MES) was calculated by adding the scores of each condition, and dividing that sum by six [MES = (sum C1–C6)/6], low values being representative of good postural control (20–22). Each score was adjusted to score area in C1 to identify the significance of each sensory system influencing postural control, ratio C2/C1 representing the somatosensory contribution to postural control ($R_{SOM}$), ratio C4/C1, the visual contribution ($R_{VIS}$) and ratio C5/C1, the vestibular contribution ($R_{VEST}$) (23, 24) (**Table 1**). A lower ratio of a sensory input is representative of a better use of this sensory input.

All patients were submitted to postural control tests before surgery (Ev1), and four times after the beginning of rehabilitation; at 2 weeks (Ev2) (corresponding to the beginning of the specific rehabilitation to the study), at 1 month (Ev3) (corresponding to the end of the specific rehabilitation to the study), at 2 months (Ev4) and at 6 months (Ev5) (**Figure 3**).

### Clinical Parameters Statement

The functional improvement, secondary endpoints, was evaluated by different clinical assessments:

(1) The intensity of affected knee joint pain was assessed with the Visual Analog Scale (VAS) for pain. The VAS consisted of a 100 mm line whose endpoints were designated as "no pain" (at 0 mm) and "unbearable pain" (at 100 mm), respectively. Patients were requested to locate the level of knee pain on the line with a small vertical mark (25, 26).

(2) The proprioception test was carried out in a sitting position, on an examination table, without contact with the base of

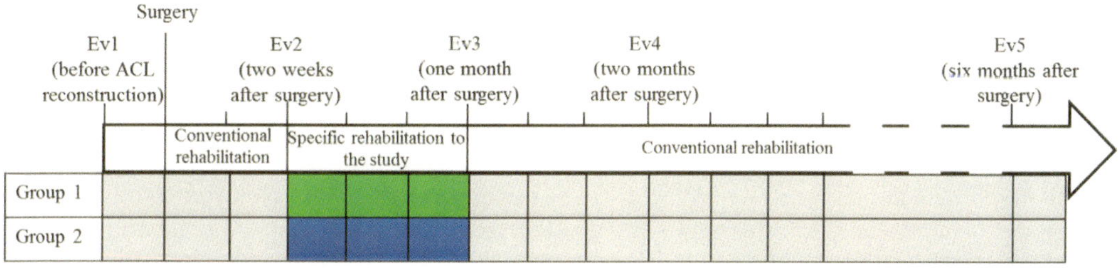


**FIGURE 1** | Timeline of the rehabilitation protocol. Phases of conventional rehabilitation and specific rehabilitation to the study. Group 1: conventional rehabilitation group; Group 2: innovative rehabilitation protocol with a conventional part and an aquatic part.

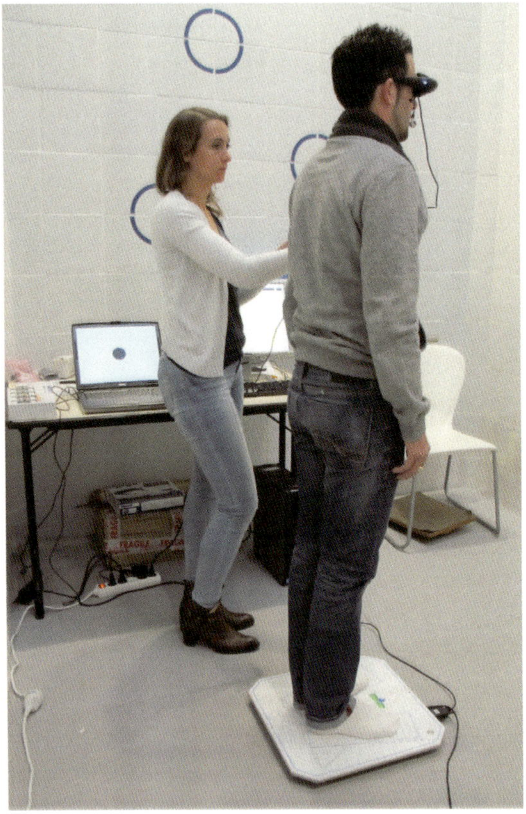

**FIGURE 2** | Postural control analysis on a posturography platform (Medicapteurs, Balma, France). Virtual reality goggles (RM Ingénierie, Rodez, France).

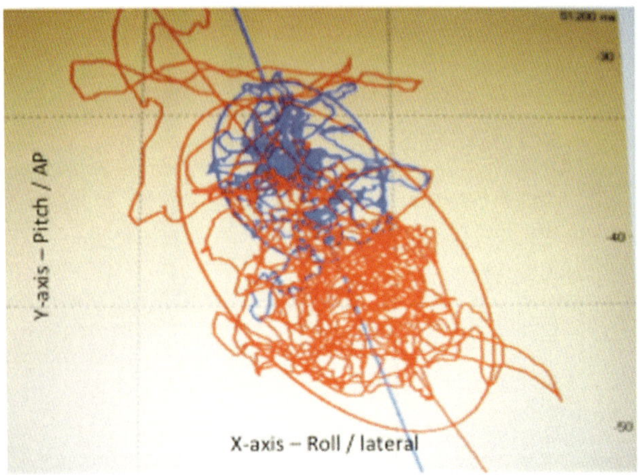


**FIGURE 3** | Posturography: statokinesigram, sway path traveled and area covered (confidence ellipse covering 90% of the points) by the center of foot pressure, in eyes open (blue) and eyes closed (red) conditions.

the lower half of the posterior part of the thigh. The tested member was placed on a skateboard. Flexion and extension movements were realized with the patients' eyes closed. The lower limb was passively flexed or extended by the physiotherapist at an arbitrary angle before being returned passively to the neutral position. Patients were instructed to flex actively the tested limb to the same angle than the passive position determined by the physiotherapist (27–31). The error was measured in degrees by an inclinometer placed on the proximal part of the tibia below the anterior tuberosity.

(3) Joint amplitudes were evaluated in flexion and extension, active and passive (28, 32, 33).

(4) Trophicity refers to all the mechanisms and processes involved in the nutrition of organs and tissues. This test consisted of digital pressure on the edema after which it was observed whether the imprint left by the finger disappeared rapidly or not. This test was positive if the impression disappeared slowly (28).

(5) Muscle strength testing was performed in knee extension to evaluate the strength of the femoral quadriceps, and then in knee flexion to assess strength of the hamstrings. A score ranging from 0 (no contraction) to 5 (normal contraction) was attributed to muscle strength (28). An isokinetic test allowed evaluating parameters such as strength, muscle deficit, and hamstring/quadriceps ratio. The evaluation was performed on the contralateral and ipsilateral limbs in order to establish a comparison of the muscle strength of the two limbs at speeds of $60°s^{-1}$ and then $180°s^{-1}$.

(6) The 6 min walk test consisted of measuring the greatest possible distance that a patient could walk at their own pace in 6 min (34).

(7) Patients had to respond to the Lysholm-Tegner (35), International Knee Documentation Committee (IKDC) (36), and Knee injury and Osteoarthritis Outcome Score (KOOS) (37) questionnaires.

For each of the five evaluation times, the clinical tests performed are presented in **Table 2**.

## Statistical Analysis

Qualitative data were expressed in terms of number ($n$) and percentage (%). Quantitative data were expressed as mean and SD.

A cross-sectional analysis was used to compare the two rehabilitation groups at each evaluation time. Frequency comparisons in independent series were performed with the Chi squared test. Comparisons of means between the two rehabilitation groups were done using the Student's $t$ test for independent series. The ANOVA variance analysis was used to study the relationships between a quantitative dependent variable and several independent explanatory variables. Due to the small sample size tested on the isokinetic test, a nonparametric Mann–Whitney test was used to make comparisons between the two groups. A probability level $p \leq 0.05$ was considered significant.

A longitudinal analysis was used to assess the progression of patients in a given group between two evaluations. Comparisons of mean values between the different evaluations in the same group were made by the Student's $t$ test for paired series. The ANOVA variance analysis was used to study the relationships between the difference between two evaluations and an independent explanatory variable. The McNemar analysis was used with

**TABLE 1** | Postural control test.

| Postural control test | | |
|---|---|---|
| **Name** | **Situation** | **Sensory consequences** |
| ***Conditions*** | | |
| Condition 1 (C1) | Eyes open on firm support | – |
| Condition 2 (C2) | Eyes closed on firm support | Vision absent |
| Condition 3 (C3) | Vision altered (virtual reality goggles), on firm support | Altered vision |
| Condition 4 (C4) | Eyes open on foam support | Altered proprioception |
| Condition 5 (C5) | Eyes closed on foam support | Vision absent, altered proprioception |
| Condition 6 (C6) | Vision altered (virtual reality goggles) on foam support | Altered vision and proprioception |
| **Name** | **Pair** | **Significance** |
| ***Ratios*** | | |
| Somatosensory ($R_{SOM}$) | C2/C1 | Question: does sway increase when visual cues are removed? Lower scores: better use of somatosensory references |
| Visual ($R_{VIS}$) | C4/C1 | Question: does sway increase when somatosensory cues are inaccurate? Lower scores: better use of visual references |
| Vestibular ($R_{VEST}$) | C5/C1 | Question: does sway increase when visual cues are removed and somatosensory cues are inaccurate? Lower scores: better use of vestibular cues |

*Determination of the six conditions and significance of sensory ratios.*

**TABLE 2** | Tests schedule.

| | Ev1 | Ev2 | Ev3 | Ev4 | Ev5 |
|---|---|---|---|---|---|
| Posturography | x | x | x | x | x |
| Visual Analog Scale (VAS) pain | x | x | x | x | x |
| Proprioception test | x | | | x | |
| Joint amplitudes | | x | x | x | x |
| Trophicity | | x | x | x | x |
| Muscular strenght | | x | x | x | x |
| Isokinetic test | | | | | x |
| 6 min walk test | | | x | | x |
| Questionnaires (Lysholm-Tegner, International Knee Documentation Committee, Knee injury and Osteoarthritis Outcome Score) | x | | | | x |

*Ev1: evaluation before anterior cruciate ligament reconstruction; Ev2: 2 weeks after surgery; Ev3: 1 month; Ev4: 2 months; Ev5: 6 months.*

ordinal variable to compare frequencies across time in each group. A probability level $p \leq 0.05$ was considered significant except for the results of the posturography test. To take into account multiple comparisons, the Bonferroni procedure was applied to

**TABLE 3** | Baseline anthropometric characteristics of patients with conventional rehabilitation (Group 1) protocol and innovative rehabilitation protocol (Group 2).

| | Group 1 (*n* = 35) | Group 2 (*n* = 32) | *p*-value |
|---|---|---|---|
| | **Mean ± SD** | **Mean ± SD** | **Student's *t* test** |
| Age (years) | 29.91 ± 7.70 | 28.22 ± 7.38 | 0.364 |
| Height (m) | 1.72 ± 0.08 | 1.76 ± 0.10 | 0.064 |
| Weight (kg) | 69.59 ± 11.55 | 73.34 ± 13.54 | 0.225 |
| BMI (kg.m$^{-2}$) | 23.46 ± 2.70 | 23.44 ± 2.57 | 0.971 |
| | ***n* (%)** | ***n* (%)** | **Chi2** |
| Sex, males | 21 (60.00) | 26 (80.25) | 0.058 |

*SD, standard deviation; BMI, body mass index.*

pairwise comparisons with a significant $p < 0.05/5 = 0.01$ adjustment due to the five evaluations.

The SPSS Statistics software (IBM, Armonk, NY, USA) version 23.0 was used for all analyzes.

# RESULTS

## Participants

No statistically significant difference was observed for anthropometric variables (age, sex, height, weight, body max index) between the two groups of patients at baseline (**Table 3**). No significant difference was observed between the two rehabilitation groups regarding the surgical techniques used ($p = 0.427$).

## Postural Control

No statistically significant differences of the MES of the sway path traveled and the area covered by the center of foot pressure were observed between the two rehabilitation groups at the five evaluations. No statistically significant differences of $R_{VIS}$ and $R_{VEST}$ were observed between the two rehabilitation groups at the five evaluations whereas $R_{SOM}$ score was significantly lower in Gr2 than in Gr1 ($p = 0.008$) at Ev5, reflecting a greater use of somesthesia in balance control (**Table 4**). Patients of the two groups rely on the contralateral limb to the surgery to the evaluation at Ev1 ($p = 0.002$), Ev2 ($p < 0.001$) and Ev3 ($p = 0.001$). Gr1 rely more than Gr2 on the contralateral limb to the surgery at Ev1 ($p = 0.037$) and Ev3 ($p = 0.039$).

Significant differences were showed between Ev1 and Ev2 for $R_{VIS}$ and $R_{VEST}$ in both groups. Patients used more visual and the vestibular input at Ev2 to maintain their balance control (Gr1: $R_{VIS}$, $p = 0.004$; $R_{VEST}$, $p < 0.001$; Gr2: $R_{VIS}$, $p = 0.001$; $R_{VEST}$, $p < 0.001$). In Gr1, the area decreased between Ev2 and Ev3 ($p = 0.004$) and between Ev3 and Ev4 ($p = 0.001$), and the sway path decreased between Ev3 and Ev4 ($p = 0.001$). In Gr2, the sway path increased between Ev1 and Ev2 ($p = 0.003$) and decreased between Ev2 and Ev3 ($p = 0.001$). Gr1 relied more on the limb contralateral to the operated limb between Ev1 and Ev2 ($p < 0.001$), whereas they relied less on the contralateral limb between Ev2 and Ev3 ($p < 0.001$) and Ev1 and Ev5 ($p = 0.010$). Gr2 relied more on the limb contralateral to the surgery between Ev1 and Ev2 ($p < 0.001$), whereas they relied less on the contralateral limb between Ev2 and Ev3 ($p < 0.001$).

**TABLE 4** | Comparison of the postural control between the two groups of rehabilitation.

| | Group 1 (*n* = 35) | Group 2 (*n* = 32) | Student's *t* test |
|---|---|---|---|
| | Mean ± SD | Mean ± SD | *p*-value |
| **Evaluation 1** | | | |
| Area (mm²) | 633.78 ± 229.36 | 767.64 ± 459.74 | 0.131 |
| Sway path (mm) | 660.53 ± 215.01 | 649.83 ± 235.13 | 0.846 |
| $R_{SOM}$ | 1.46 ± 0.80 | 1.60 ± 0.98 | 0.506 |
| $R_{VIS}$ | 3.69 ± 2.42 | 3.81 ± 1.59 | 0.812 |
| $R_{VEST}$ | 12.11 ± 5.73 | 16.09 ± 11.36 | 0.081 |
| **Evaluation 2** | | | |
| Area (mm²) | 696.13 ± 251.07 | 740.90 ± 348.25 | 0.546 |
| Sway path (mm) | 729.58 ± 187.42 | 732.20 ± 231.81 | 0.959 |
| $R_{SOM}$ | 1.35 ± 0.54 | 1.63 ± 1.06 | 0.176 |
| $R_{VIS}$ | 2.44 ± 1.32 | 2.51 ± 1.26 | 0.825 |
| $R_{VEST}$ | 7.88 ± 5.08 | 8.22 ± 4.95 | 0.784 |
| **Evaluation 3** | | | |
| Area (mm²) | 610.53 ± 205.35 | 656.21 ± 213.39 | 0.375 |
| Sway path (mm) | 676.18 ± 183.81 | 631.80 ± 187.17 | 0.331 |
| $R_{SOM}$ | 1.46 ± 1.02 | 1.54 ± 1.15 | 0.746 |
| $R_{VIS}$ | 2.83 ± 1.86 | 2.59 ± 1.42 | 0.548 |
| $R_{VEST}$ | 8.17 ± 3.81 | 7.52 ± 3.51 | 0.478 |
| **Evaluation 4** | | | |
| Area (mm²) | 556.13 ± 173.78 | 595.04 ± 205.83 | 0.243 |
| Sway path (mm) | 612.64 ± 165.88 | 589.98 ± 176.82 | 0.590 |
| $R_{SOM}$ | 1.45 ± 0.67 | 1.31 ± 0.61 | 0.356 |
| $R_{VIS}$ | 3.27 ± 1.63 | 2.95 ± 1.44 | 0.404 |
| $R_{VEST}$ | 8.07 ± 3.88 | 7.92 ± 4.14 | 0.880 |
| **Evaluation 5** | | | |
| Area (mm²) | 583.72 ± 196.31 | 639.65 ± 286.87 | 0.352 |
| Sway path (mm) | 629.10 ± 220.00 | 603.67 ± 198.25 | 0.622 |
| $R_{SOM}$ | 1.62 ± 0.87 | 1.14 ± 0.50 | **0.008** |
| $R_{VIS}$ | 4.32 ± 3.25 | 3.09 ± 2.27 | 0.080 |
| $R_{VEST}$ | 11.51 ± 7.26 | 9.57 ± 7.86 | 0.297 |

*SD, standard deviation.*

## Clinical Parameters

(1) No statistically significant difference in pain was observed between the two rehabilitation groups over time. In Gr1, pain decreased between Ev2 and Ev3 ($p = 0.007$) and Ev1 and Ev5 ($p = 0.039$). In Gr2, pain increased between Ev1 and Ev2 ($p = 0.027$), then decreased between Ev2 and Ev3 ($p < 0.001$), Ev4 and Ev5 ($p = 0.030$), and Ev1 and Ev5 ($p = 0.012$).

(2) No statistically significant difference in proprioception was observed between the two groups over time. In Gr2, an improvement of proprioception in flexion was observed at Ev4 ($p = 0.002$).

(3) No statistically significant difference in joint amplitude was observed between the two groups over time. In the two groups, an improvement in active and passive flexion was observed between Ev2 and Ev3 ($p < 0.001$), Ev3 and Ev4 ($p < 0.001$), Ev4 and Ev5 ($p < 0.001$). In Gr1, an improvement in passive extension was observed between Ev2 and Ev3 ($p = 0.015$) and Ev3 and Ev4 ($p = 0.006$), and an improvement in active extension was observed between Ev4 and Ev5 ($p < 0.001$). In Gr2, an improvement in active extension was observed between Ev2 and Ev3 ($p = 0.008$), Ev3 and Ev4 ($p = 0.038$), and Ev4 and Ev5 ($p = 0.002$). An improvement in passive extension was observed between Ev2 and Ev3 ($p = 0.021$) and Ev4 and Ev5 ($p = 0.006$) in Gr2.

(4) No statistically significant difference in trophicity was observed between the two groups over time. An improvement in trophicity was observed in the two groups between Ev2 and Ev3 (Gr1: $p = 0.039$; Gr2: $p = 0.006$) and Ev4 and Ev5 (Gr1: $p = 0.004$; Gr2: $p = 0.035$).

(5) Statistically significant differences in quadriceps muscle strength were observed at Ev4 ($p = 0.015$) and Ev5 ($p = 0.027$) between the two groups. At Ev4 in Gr2, 14 patients obtained a score of 5 (43.75%), 17 a score of 4 (53.13%) and 1 a score of 3 (3.12%) versus 5 a score of 5 (14.29%), 25 a score of 4 (71.43%) and 1 a score of 3 (2.85%) in Gr1. At Ev5 in Gr2, 24 patients obtained a score of 5 (75%) and 8 a score of 4 (25%) versus 17 a score of 5 (48.57%) and 18 a score of 4 (51.43%) in Gr1. Statistically significant differences in internal hamstring muscle strength were observed at Ev2 ($p = 0.026$). In Gr2, 13 patients obtained a score of 4 (40.63%), 14 a score of 3 (43.75%), and 5 a score between 0 and 2 (15.62%) versus 8 a score of 4 (22.86%), 26 a score of 3 (74.29%) and 1 a score between 0 and 2 (2.85%) in Gr1. Statistically significant differences in external hamstring muscle strength were observed at Ev5 ($p = 0.019$) between the two groups. In Gr2, 22 patients obtained a score of 5 (68.75%), 9 a score of 4 (28.13%) and 1 a score of 3 (3.12%) versus 12 a score of 5 (34.29%), 21 a score of 4 (60.00%) and 2 a score of 3 (5.71%) in Gr1. The statistical analysis showed an increase in the muscle strength of the quadriceps between Ev2 and Ev3 ($p = 0.006$) and Ev3 and Ev4 ($p = 0.039$) in Gr1. The muscle strength of the hamstring increased between Ev2 and Ev3 ($p = 0.001$) and Ev4 and Ev5 ($p = 0.031$). In Gr2, the muscle strength of the quadriceps increased between Ev2 and Ev3 ($p < 0.001$), and the muscle strength of the hamstring increased between Ev2 and Ev3 ($p < 0.001$). At Ev5, the muscle strength of the quadriceps developed in isokinetic testing was significantly greater in Gr2 at either $60°s^{-1}$ ($p = 0.027$) or $180°s^{-1}$ ($p = 0.047$). Moreover, muscle deficit of the quadriceps of the ipsilateral limb compared to the contralateral limb was lower in Gr2 ($p = 0.020$).

(6) A statistically significant difference in the 6 min walk test was observed between the two groups at Ev3 ($p = 0.025$). Gr1 traveled 425.27 ± 158.45 m against 506.59 ± 127.70 m for the Gr2. 6 min walking performance significantly increased at Ev5 compared to Ev3 in the two groups ($p < 0.001$) and there was no significant difference at Ev5.

(7) No statistically significant difference for questionnaires was observed between the two groups. An improvement in the functional Lysholm-Tegner score was observed between Ev1 and Ev5 in Gr1 ($p < 0.001$) and Gr2 ($p = 0.004$). Statistical analysis showed an improvement in the IKDC functional score in both groups ($p < 0.001$). Significant improvement in knee function after injury was observed in both groups ($p < 0.001$). In both groups an improvement was observed for pain (Gr1, $p = 0.001$; Gr2, $p = 0.016$), daily life (Gr1, $p < 0.001$; Gr2, $p < 0.001$), quality of life (Gr1, $p < 0.001$;

Gr2, $p < 0.001$) and an increase in sports and leisure activities (Gr1, $p < 0.001$; Gr2, $p < 0.001$).

## DISCUSSION

This study aimed to compare an innovative rehabilitation protocol combining a dry and an aquatic part with a conventional rehabilitation protocol with the same total duration of patient care, in terms of dynamics of recovery, development of proprioceptive skills and functional improvement in athletes with ACL reconstruction. The main results of this study showed that for the same quality of postural control, patients who followed the innovative rehabilitation protocol had less lateralization at the side contralateral to the surgery than patients who followed the conventional rehabilitation protocol after the specific period of rehabilitation. The innovative group also relied more on somesthesia 6 months after surgery. Secondary results showed that, although muscle strength increased in both rehabilitation groups during follow-up, patients who followed the innovative rehabilitation protocol had greater muscle strength of the external hamstring 6 months after surgery and greater muscle strength of the quadriceps 2 months and 6 months after surgery. This difference in muscle strength of the quadriceps 6 months after surgery was confirmed by the isokinetic test. This test confirmed a difference in muscle strength between the two groups at the rate of $60°s^{-1}$ as well as at the rate of $180°s^{-1}$ and a lower deficit of the quadriceps in the innovative rehabilitation protocol group. On the other hand, although walking distance in 6 min increased in both groups between the 1st month and the 6th months after surgery, patients who followed the innovative rehabilitation protocol walked a greater distance 1 month after surgery. Finally, although both rehabilitation groups had similar proprioceptive performances before and 2 months after surgery, patients who followed the innovative rehabilitation protocol showed an improvement of proprioception at the ipsilateral limb 2 months after surgery compared to before surgery.

The main endpoint showed that for the same quality of postural control 6 months after surgery, patients who followed the innovative rehabilitation protocol increased the weight of somesthesia more than the conventional rehabilitation protocol group. The conventional group did not increase somesthesia in the course of evaluations. This means that patients who followed innovative rehabilitation had developed more proprioceptive capacities during rehabilitation. On the other hand, in agreement with the study of Dauty et al. (38), 15 days after surgery, patients of both groups relied more heavily on the contralateral limb as demonstrated by the posturography test. This compensation necessity decreased in both groups one month after surgery and was less needed in patients receiving the aquatic rehabilitation protocol than in patients who had followed the conventional rehabilitation protocol. Reduced gravity and water buoyancy decrease the detrimental effects of weight bearing and impact forces on joint structure (39) and the Archimedes' principle allows an early and progressive loading by lowering the immersion level (40). This progressive loading can explain the reduced lateralization in the patients who followed the protocol of innovative rehabilitation one month after surgery.

In this study, measurements of joint amplitudes, trophicity, pain assessment, and Lysholm-Tegner, IKDC and KOOS questionnaires did not show any significant difference between the two groups. The evolution of these parameters during the 6 months of follow-up showed similarities in the two groups. First, an improvement in the flexion and extension of the knee joint was observed in the two rehabilitation groups between the 15th day and the 1st postoperative month, between the 1st month and the 2nd postoperative month, and between the 2nd month and the 6th postoperative month. In rehabilitation, the gain in joint amplitude is obtained initially by soft techniques of recovery of the mobility. Then, massages of all the planes of articular sliding with kneading, frictions, and deep transverse massages make possible to avoid retractions. Passive and active mobilization allows for an increase in flexion by the use of supra-patellar supports, contraction-relaxation and the search for lateral sliding by manual support or contraction of the hamstrings.

We also compared pain reduction in the two groups. A reduction in pain was observed between the 15th day and the 1st postoperative month, and between the 2nd month and the 6th postoperative month in the group following the innovative rehabilitation protocol. The analgesic means used in rehabilitation such as circulatory massages, cryotherapy, or scar massages to avoid the formation of tissue adhesions, all participate to this reduction of pain. This is supported by the fact that pain 6 months after surgery is lower than the pain experienced before surgery.

An improvement in trophicity was found between the 15th day and the first postoperative month, as well as between the 2nd month and the 6th postoperative month in both groups. Massages allowed lymphatic drainage and decreased edema. Finally, the Lysholm-Tegner, IKDC, and KOOS questionnaires showed an increase in scores between preoperative evaluation and evaluation 6 months after surgery in both rehabilitation groups (41). Thus, patients judged the functionality of their knee to be better 6 months after surgery than before surgery. They also have less pain, improve their daily life and quality of life, and take up recreational activities and sports activities.

Patients who followed the innovative rehabilitation protocol had significantly greater muscular strength than patients who followed the conventional rehabilitation protocol 2 months and 6 months after surgery. Several properties of the aquatic environment can explain this difference. First, a body immersed in water is subjected to a resistance effect called drag force and turbulence (40). This resistance to advancement increases with the square of the speed: the faster the body or part of the body moves, the greater the driving strength (42). In an aquatic environment, when a patient feels pain, he can stop his movement; the force then falls precipitously because the viscosity of the water dampens the movement almost instantaneously. This allows better control of muscle building (40). Second, after any intra-articular injury of the knee, resting of the quadriceps is observed. The Archimedes' principle allows the quadriceps to be stressed in discharge, and therefore, a soft muscle building. Third, lowering the body's apparent weight allows early loading, and therefore, progressive muscular strengthening by lowering the immersion level (40, 42). In addition, water temperature causes a muscular heating which can favor the mobilization of the operated member and thus allow indirectly a muscular building. Hydrostatic pressure also plays an indirect role in muscle strengthening by promoting venous and lymphatic return. As a result of this, contractures (i.e., the defense mechanism that takes place after a trauma to block the traumatized zone) will disappear and thus allow a progressive mobilization, and therefore, a muscular effort of the initially contracted area. However, it was reported that electromyographic activity of under water exercises was decreased as compared to similar exercises performed on dry land (44–46). Moreover, in 1994, Tovin et al. (14) had already compared rehabilitation exercises in the aquatic environment with dry rehabilitation exercises in patients having surgery of the ACL injury and showed that aquatic exercises were not as effective as dry exercises for strength gain and muscle trophicity. Nevertheless, the studies on the subject are contradictory since Zamarioli et al. (15) showed that patients following an aquatic rehabilitation had a better recovery of the muscular strength. Our study had the specificity of combining dry aquatic rehabilitation and aquatic rehabilitation. Dry exercises and exercises in the aquatic environment differ in nature and this could explain this difference in muscular strength in favor of patients who have followed the protocol of innovative rehabilitation. The Archimedes' principle allows standing exercises with a normal motor pattern for the patient, which is directly transferable on the land and which allows a better dry muscle strengthening than exercises that would be made in seated or lying down positions. Despite this difference in muscle strength between the two rehabilitation groups, a progressive improvement was observed in both groups during the 6 months of follow-up. Our study is in agreement with other studies that have shown an improvement in muscle strength and a reduction in the difference in muscle strength between the operated limb and the contralateral limb after different rehabilitation programs (41, 47–49). This progressive improvement can be explained by a muscular building process. On the one hand, muscular rehabilitation aims at combating muscular amyotrophy. On the other hand, the hamstrings play the role of braking the last degrees of extension and also stabilizing the joint when the knee is bent under load. At the end of rehabilitation, muscular building favors exercises derived from sporting activities.

This study showed that patients who followed the innovative rehabilitation protocol walked a greater distance in 6 min than patients who followed the conventional rehabilitation protocol 1 month after surgery. With water immersion, gravitational forces can be partially or completely compensated so that only the forces of the couple act on the injured site. For example, for an immersion up to the shoulders, the body's apparent weight is 15–20 kg and only a few active motor units are needed to make the movement possible. Due to the apparent decrease in body weight, progressive loading is made possible by lowering the immersion level (40, 43). Immersion thus allows active movements, which are automatically transferred to walking pattern in land conditions. In addition, 6 months after surgery, there was no significant difference between the two rehabilitation groups, suggesting that patients who followed the innovative rehabilitation protocol recovered capacities faster than the group following the conventional rehabilitation protocol but patients who followed conventional protocol did catch up by 6 months.

The proprioception test revealed no significant difference between the two rehabilitation groups before surgery and 2 months after surgery. Nevertheless, after comparing the results obtained before and 2 months after surgery, this study showed that patients who followed the innovative rehabilitation protocol significantly reduced the proprioceptive deficit in flexion of the operated knee after surgery. The aquatic environment forces the patient to maintain balance under new conditions. These conditions allow the stimulation of the proprioceptive pathway by creating situations of imbalance that the patient must gradually control. For example, a patient standing with a swimming board placed under the foot develops proprioceptive information. As the swimming board tends to rise to the surface, the patient has to demonstrate good coordination to maintain it, strengthening his neuromuscular vigilance and work in balance (40). Moreover, hydrostatic pressure associated with the environment viscosity is the source of external sensory stimuli. Immersing part of the body results in developing a better perception of the position of the limbs. Similarly, the resistance to displacement created swirling sensations, which enhances exteroceptive or even proprioceptive information, and thus, allows a better awareness of the body pattern (40).

This work has several limitations. This study required 14 physiotherapists but to avoid variations by ensuring repeatability, harmonization of practices was carried out before the first patient was enrolled. Another limitation of this study was due to auto-questionnaires. This always results in subjectivity of responses and it is possible that some patients may overestimate or underestimate the functional capacity of the knee. The duration of management in aquatic rehabilitation specific to the study was short. Nevertheless, this duration had been chosen to align with the model of spa treatment in France, which lasts an average of 3 weeks.

## CONCLUSION

This study shows that the innovative rehabilitation protocol (therapy incorporating both a dry and aquatic segment) improves proprioception and limits overcompensation on the limb contralateral to the operated limb. Even if patients undergoing a conventional rehabilitation protocol recover the delay after 6 months of surgery, faster and better recovery of knee functionality, following aquatic rehabilitation would in the short-term prevent injury to the contralateral limb as a result of overcompensation, and serve in the longer term to reduce the risk of osteoarthritis. The effectiveness of such rehabilitation could also enable patients to recover social, physical and professional activities earlier, which would also be of economic benefit, in particular with a reduction in work absence.

## AUTHOR CONTRIBUTIONS

All authors listed have made substantial, direct, and intellectual contribution to the work and approved it for publication.

## ACKNOWLEDGMENTS

The authors thank the orthopedics surgeons of the Médipôle Gentilly: Dr. Nicolas Hummer, Dr. Nicolas Paris, Dr. Frank Wein; of Louis Pasteur Clinic: Dr. Benoît Goudot, Dr. Frank Wein; of Saint-André Clinic: Dr. Maurice Morel; of the University Hospital: Dr. Manuela Barla, Dr. Rémi Belleville, Dr. Jean-Baptiste Gross, Prof. Didier Mainard, Dr. Michael Mangin, Dr. Vincent Seivert. The authors thank the physiotherapists: Mr., Ms. Johnny Afonso, Patrick Boisseau, Xavier Celli, Jessy Courtier, Suzy Diller, Jean-Philippe De Jesus Goncalves, Antoine Fourcaulx, Alexandre Ferry, Laureline Grajon, Elodie Jussy, Angélique Labeys, Thibaut Lombardet, Aurélie Muller, Camille Pons, Thomas Wysocki. The authors acknowledge Prof. Michel Boulangé, Dr. Jean-Marc Geoffroy, and Prof. Gisèle Kanny for their advices and help in this study. This study was promoted by the Nancy University Hospital, France, with a grant from the Métropole du Grand Nancy, France. In the Métropole du Grand Nancy, the authors would like to thank especially Dr. André Rossinot, president, former minister, and Ms. Marie-Catherine Tallot. The authors acknowledge Dr. Art Mallinson (Vancouver, BC, Canada) for its helpful advice in the final read-through of the manuscript.

## REFERENCES

1. Haute Autorité de Santé (HAS). Prise en charge thérapeutique des lésions méniscales et des lésions isolées du ligament croisé antérieur du genou chez l'adulte. *Service des bonnes pratiques professionnelles*. La Plaine – Saint-Denis: Haute Autorité de Santé (HAS) (2008). 105 p.
2. Alidrissi N, Elyaacoubi M, Berrada MS, Elbardouni A, Mahfoud M, Dahmani O, et al. Ligamentoplastie du LCA aux ischiojambiers sous arthroscopie avec fixation de l'implant par le système TLS. Principes et résultats de 38 cas. *J Traumatol Sport* (2011) 28:159–64. doi:10.1016/j.jts.2011.07.003
3. Haute Autorité de Santé (HAS). Critères de suivi en rééducation et d'orientation en ambulatoire ou en SSR après ligamentoplastie du croisé antérieur du genou. *Service recommandations professionnelles, Service Evaluation médico-économique*. La Plaine – Saint-Denis: Haute Autorité de Santé (HAS) (2008). 85 p.
4. Blalock D, Miller A, Tilley M, Wang J. Joint instability and osteoarthritis. *Clin Med Insights Arthritis Musculoskelet Disord* (2015) 18(8):15–23. doi:10.4137/CMAMD.S22147
5. Keays SL, Newcombe PA, Bullock-Saxton JE, Bullock MI, Keays AC. Factors involved in the development of osteoarthritis after anterior cruciate ligament injury. *Am J Sports Med* (2010) 38(3):455–63. doi:10.1177/0363546509350914
6. Li RT, Lorenz S, Xu Y, Harner CD, Fu FH, Irrgang JJ. Predictors of radiographic knee osteoarthritis after anterior cruciate ligament reconstruction. *Am J Sports Med* (2011) 39(12):2595–603. doi:10.1177/0363546511424720
7. Meunier A, Odensten M, Good L. Long-term results after primary repair or non-surgical treatment of anterior cruciate ligament rupture: a randomized study with a 15-year follow-up. *Scand J Med Sci Sports* (2007) 17(3):230–7. doi:10.1111/j.1600-0838.2006.00547.x
8. Harrison EL, Duenkel N, Dunlop R, Russell G. Evaluation of single-leg standing following anterior cruciate ligament surgery and rehabilitation. *Phys Ther* (1994) 74(3):245–52. doi:10.1093/ptj/74.3.245
9. Shiraishi M, Mizuta H, Kubota K, Otsuka Y, Nagamoto N, Takagi K. Stabilometric assessment in the ACL reconstructed knee. *Clin J Sport Med* (1996) 6(1):32–9. doi:10.1097/00042752-199601000-00008
10. Henriksson M, Ledin T, Good L. Postural control after ACL reconstruction and functional rehabilitation. *Am J Sports Med* (2001) 29(3):359–66. doi:10.1177/03635465010290031801
11. Ochi M, Iwasa I, Uchio Y, Adachi N, Sumen Y. The regeneration of sensory neurones in the reconstruction of the anterior cruciate ligament. *J Bone Joint Surg Br* (1999) 81-B(5):902–6. doi:10.1302/0301-620X.81B5.9202
12. Collette M, Cassard X. The tape locking screw technique (TLS): a new ACL reconstruction method using a short hamstring graft. *Orthop Traumatol Surg Res* (2011) 97:555–9. doi:10.1016/j.otsr.2011.03.016
13. Jones KG. Reconstruction of the anterior cruciate ligament. A technique using the central one-third of the patellar ligament. *J Bone Joint Surg Am* (1963) 45:925–32. doi:10.2106/00004623-196345050-00003
14. Tovin BJ, Wolf SL, Greenfield BH, Crouse J, Woodfin BA. Comparison of the effects of exercise in water and on land on the rehabilitation of patients with intra-articular anterior cruciate ligament reconstructions. *Phys Ther* (1994) 74(8):710–9. doi:10.1093/ptj/74.8.710
15. Zamarioli A, Pezolato A, Mieli E, Shimano AC. The significance of water rehabilitation in patients with anterior cruciate ligament reconstruction. *Fizjoterapia* (2008) 16(2):3–6. doi:10.2478/v10109-009-0013-z
16. Lion A, Spada RS, Bosser G, Gauchard GC, Anello G, Bosco P, et al. Biological determinants of postural disorders in elderly women. *Int J Neurosci* (2013) 123(1):24–30. doi:10.3109/00207454.2012.722570
17. Perrin P, Jeandel C, Perrin CA, Béné MC. Influence of visual control, conduction, and central integration on static and dynamic balance in healthy older adults. *Gerontology* (1997) 43(4):223–31. doi:10.1159/000213854
18. Kingma H, Gauchard GC, de Waele C, van Nechel C, Bisdorff A, Yelnick A, et al. Stocktaking on the development of posturography for clinical use. *J Vestib Res* (2011) 21(3):117–25. doi:10.3233/VES-2011-0397
19. Shumway-Cook A, Horak F. Assessing the influence of sensory interaction on balance. *Phys Ther* (1986) 66(10):1548–50. doi:10.1093/ptj/66.10.1548
20. Peultier L, Lion A, Chary-Valckenaere I, Loeuille D, Zhang Z, Ray AC, et al. Influence of meteorological elements on balance control and pain in patients with symptomatic knee osteoarthritis. *Int J Biometeorol* (2017) 61:903. doi:10.1007/s00484-016-1269-x
21. Tarantola J, Nardone A, Tacchini E, Schieppati M. Human stability improves with the repetition of the task: effect of foot position and visual condition. *Neurosci Lett* (1997) 228(2):75–8. doi:10.1016/S0304-3940(97)00370-4
22. Vouriot A, Hannhart B, Gauchard G, Barot A, Ledin T, Mur JM, et al. Long-term exposure to solvents impairs vigilance and postural control in serigraphy workers. *Int Arch Occup Environ Health* (2005) 78:510–5. doi:10.1007/s00420-005-0609-7
23. Gauchard GC, Vançon G, Meyer P, Mainard D, Perrin P. On the role of knee joint in balance control and posture strategies: effects of total knee replacement in elderly subjects with knee osteoarthrisis. *Gait Posture* (2010) 32(2):155–60. doi:10.1016/j.gaitpost.2010.04.002
24. Lion A, Bosser G, Gauchard GC, Djaballah K, Mallié JP, Perrin P. Exercise and dehydration: a possible role of inner ear in balance control disorder. *J Electromyogr Kinesiol* (2010) 20:1196–202. doi:10.1016/j.jelekin.2010.07.016
25. Boureau F, Luu M. Les méthodes d'évaluation de la douleur clinique. *Doul Analg* (1988) 1(2):65–73. doi:10.1007/BF03006125
26. Huskisson EC. Measurement of pain. *Lancet* (1974) 2(7889):1127–31. doi:10.1016/S0140-6736(74)90884-8
27. Carter ND, Jenkinson TR, Wilson D, Jones DW, Torode AS. Joint position sense and rehabilitation in the anterior cruciate ligament deficient knee. *Br J Sports Med* (1997) 31:209–12. doi:10.1136/bjsm.31.3.209
28. Chatrenet Y. Evaluations Clinique et fonctionnelle du genou. *EMC Kinésithérapie Médecine physique Réadaptation* (2013) 9(1):1–17. doi:10.1016/S1283-0887(12)43932-9
29. Fischer-Rasmussen T, Jensen PE. Proprioceptive sensitivity and performance in anterior cruciate ligament-deficient knee joints. *Scand J Med Sci Sports* (2000) 10:85–9. doi:10.1034/j.1600-0838.2000.010002085.x

30. Good L, Roos H, Gottlied DJ, Rentröm PA, Beynnon BD. Joint position sense is not changed after acute disruption of the anterior cruciate ligament. *Acta Orthop Scand* (1999) 70(2):194–8. doi:10.3109/17453679909011261
31. Missaoui B, Portero P, Bendaya S, Hanktie O, Thoumie P. Posture and equilibrium in orthopedic and rheumatologic diseases. *Neurophysiol Clin* (2008) 38:447–57. doi:10.1016/j.neucli.2008.09.004
32. Neiger H, Genot C. Goniométrie articulaire, recherche des amplitudes articulaires et transcription des résultats. *Ann Kinesither* (1983) 10(6): 215–9.
33. Royer A, Cecconello R. Bilans articulaires cliniques et goniométriques. Généralités. *EMC Podologie Kinésithérapie* (2004) 1(2):82–91. doi:10.1016/j.emck.2004.02.001
34. Abdel Kafi S, Deboeck G. Le test de marche de six minutes en réhabilitation respiratoire. *Rev Mal Respi* (2005) 22:5. doi:10.1016/S0761-8425(05)85692-X
35. Tegner Y, Lysholm J. Rating systems in the evaluation of knee ligament injuries. *Clin Orthop Relat Res* (1985) 198:43–9.
36. Hefti F, Müller W, Jakob RP, Stäubli HU. Evaluation of knee ligament injuries with IKDC form. *Knee Surg Sports Traumatol Arthrosc* (1993) 1(3–4): 226–34. doi:10.1007/BF01560215
37. Roos EM, Roos HP, Lohmander LS, Ekdahl C, Beynnon BD. Knee injury and osteoarthritis outcome score (KOOS) – development of a self-administered outcome measure. *J Orthop Sports Phys Ther* (1998) 28(2):88–96. doi:10.2519/jospt.1998.28.2.88
38. Dauty M, Collon S, Dubois C. Change in posture control after recent knee anterior cruciate ligament reconstruction? *Clin Physiol Funct Imaging* (2010) 30:187–91. doi:10.1111/j.1475-097X.2010.00926.x
39. Harrison R, Bulstrode S. Percentage of weight bearing during partial immersion in the hydrotherapy pool. *Physiother Pract* (1987) 3:60–3. doi:10.3109/09593988709087741
40. Kemoun G, Watelain E, Carette P. Hydrokinésithérapie. *EMC Kinésithérapie-Médecine physique-Réadaptation* (2006) 2(3):1–28. doi:10.1016/S1283-0887(06)43711-7
41. Dragicevic-Cvjetkovic D, Jandric S, Bijeljac S, Palija S, Manojlovic S, Talic G. The effects of rehabilitation protocol on functional recovery after anterior cruciate ligament reconstruction. *Med Arch* (2014) 68(5):350–2. doi:10.5455/medarh.2014.68.350-352
42. Chevutschi A, Dengremont B, Lensel G, Thevenon A. La balnéothérapie au sein de la littérature: propriété de l'eau. *Kinesither Rev* (2007) 7:14–20. doi:10.1016/S1779-0123(07)70482-5
43. Becker BE. Aquatic therapy: scientific foundations and clinical rehabilitation applications. *PM R* (2009) 1:859–72. doi:10.1016/j.pmrj.2009.05.017
44. Fugisawa H, Suenaga N, Minami A. Electromyographic study during isometric exercise of the shoulder in head-out water immersion. *J Shoulder Elbow Surg* (1998) 7:491–4. doi:10.1016/S1058-2746(98)90200-2
45. Kelly BT, Roskin LA, Kirkendall DT, Speer KP. Shoulder muscle activation during aquatic and dry land exercise in nonimpaired subjects. *J Orthop Sports Phys Therapy* (2000) 30:204–10. doi:10.2519/jospt.2000.30.4.204
46. Pöyhönen T, Keskinen KL, Hautala A, Savolainen J, Mälkiä E. Human isometric force production and eletromyogram activity of knee extensor muscles in water and on dry land. *Eur J Appl Phys* (1999) 80:52–6. doi:10.1007/s004210050557
47. Beard DJ, Dodd CA. Home or supervised rehabilitation following anterior cruciate ligament reconstruction: a randomized controlled trial. *J Orthop Sports Phys Ther* (1998) 27(2):134–43. doi:10.2519/jospt.1998.27.2.134
48. Shelbourne KD, Gray T. Anterior cruciate ligament reconstruction with autogeous patellar tendon graft followed by accelerated rehabilitation. A two- to nine-year followup. *Am J Sports Med* (1997) 25(6):786–95. doi:10.1177/036354659702500610
49. Timm KE. The clinical and cost-effectiveness of two different programs for rehabilitation following ACL reconstruction. *J Orthop Sports Phys Ther* (1997) 25(1):43–8. doi:10.2519/jospt.1997.25.1.43

3

# Breast Reconstruction after Mastectomy

*Daniel Schmauss[1], Hans-Günther Machens[1] and Yves Harder[1,2]**

[1] *Department of Plastic Surgery and Hand Surgery, Klinikum rechts der Isar, Technische Universität München, Munich, Germany,* [2] *Department of Plastic, Reconstructive and Aesthetic Surgery, Ospedale Regionale di Lugano, Ente Ospedaliero Cantonale, Lugano, Switzerland*

Breast cancer is the leading cause of cancer death in women worldwide. Its surgical approach has become less and less mutilating in the last decades. However, the overall number of breast reconstructions has significantly increased lately. Nowadays, breast reconstruction should be individualized at its best, first of all taking into consideration not only the oncological aspects of the tumor, neo-/adjuvant treatment, and genetic predisposition, but also its timing (immediate versus delayed breast reconstruction), as well as the patient's condition and wish. This article gives an overview over the various possibilities of breast reconstruction, including implant- and expander-based reconstruction, flap-based reconstruction (vascularized autologous tissue), the combination of implant and flap, reconstruction using non-vascularized autologous fat, as well as refinement surgery after breast reconstruction.

**Keywords: breast reconstruction, breast cancer, mastectomy, DIEP flap, breast implants, autologous fat grafting**

***Edited by:***
*Adrien Daigeler, BG-University Hospital Bergmannsheil, Germany*

***Reviewed by:***
*Andreas Arkudas, University Hospital of Erlangen, Germany*
*Marcus Lehnhardt, BG-University Hospital Bergmannsheil, Germany*

***Correspondence:**
*Yves Harder*
*yves.harder@eoc.ch*

***Specialty section:***
*This article was submitted to Surgical Oncology, a section of the journal Frontiers in Surgery*

## INTRODUCTION

Breast cancer is the leading cause of cancer death among women worldwide with ~1.7 million new diagnoses and 521.900 deaths in 2012 (1). One important modality of breast cancer therapy is surgical treatment, which has become increasingly less mutilating over the last century.

William Halsted introduced radical mastectomy including resection of the breast and its underlying pectoralis major muscle in order to cure all stages of breast cancer at the end of the nineteenth century (2). Approximately 40 years later, Patey described a less radical modified type of mastectomy with preservation of the pectoralis major muscle yielding comparable local control and overall survival compared to Halsted (3). In 1985, Fisher et al. introduced the concept of breast conserving therapy (BCT), demonstrating that lumpectomy – by that time regarded as segmental mastectomy – followed by adjuvant radiotherapy of the remnant breast in patients with stage I and II breast cancer was indeed associated with an increased local recurrence rate, yet resulted in equal survival rates compared to mastectomy (4). Oncoplastic breast surgery, i.e., reshaping of the breast after local tumor resection, has shown to allow larger tumor excision, yet conserving large parts of the breast, maintaining shape (5) and resulting in improved quality of life and self-esteem (6). While surgical breast cancer treatment decreased in radicalness and invasiveness, breast cancer guidelines were defined, breast cancer screening programs were initiated, and breast centers offering an interdisciplinary and comprehensive therapeutical approach for breast cancer were established. This resulted in an increased detection and treatment of predominantly early breast cancers with improved survival rates and consequently superior esthetic outcome. Nowadays, BCT is a safe treatment for most women with early-stage breast cancers and can be safely applied in 70–80% of the cases requiring surgical tumor removal (7). Though, the primary goal of BCT is to preserve shape and, to a lesser extent, size of the breast in order to best match the contralateral breast. Thereby, one should take into account that postoperative radiotherapy may result in some extent of tissue shrinkage (8). Although decreasing in number over the last two decades, the rate of mastectomy has again increased lately due to the detection of multifocal tumors, tumors with an extended *in situ* proportion that is difficult to delimit and due to an unfavorable breast-to-tumor size ratio in rather thin patients with small-to-intermediate sized breasts. Furthermore, the awareness of the disease itself in the female population and the relatively frequent detection of a genetic predisposition to breast cancer (i.e., BRCA-1, BRCA-2, p53) have confirmed this trend toward an increased rate of mastectomy, be it curative or prophylactic (9).

Although BCT remains the absolute gold standard for surgical breast cancer treatment, many women must or wish to undergo mastectomy. Consequently, reconstruction of the breast must be offered, particularly in young patients. This article provides an overview of various reconstruction techniques of the female breast after both, breast cancer-related and prophylactic mastectomy. This article does not cover partial breast reconstruction after extensive breast conservative therapy.

## MASTECTOMY

Mastectomy aims at resecting as much breast tissue as possible, knowing that glandular tissue will almost always remain in the region of the inframammary fold (10). Nowadays, basically two ways of mastectomy are performed, including skin-sparing mastectomy and total ablation of the breast. The latter consists of complete removal of both, breast skin and glandular breast tissue (**Figure 1**), whereas skin-sparing mastectomy preserves as much of the breast's skin envelope as possible, including the areola and the nipple (skin-sparing mastectomy, areola-sparing mastectomy, nipple-sparing mastectomy, skin-reducing mastectomy) and the inframammary fold. Furthermore, biopsy scars and skin overlying a tumor or even infiltrated by the tumor are excised in order to reduce the risk of local recurrence (11). Provided that the oncological indication is correct, skin-sparing mastectomy has been associated with equal oncological local safety and improved esthetic outcome compared to modified radical mastectomy (10). Furthermore, the need for secondary surgery to adjust the contralateral breast in order to achieve symmetry is reduced after skin-sparing mastectomy, particularly if autologous reconstruction with flaps is used (12).

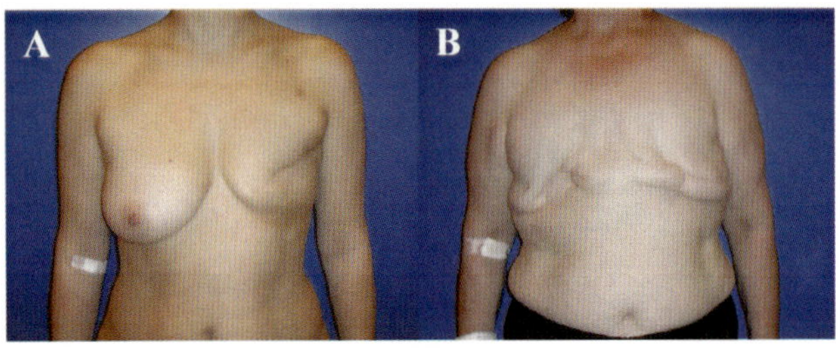


**FIGURE 1 | The 43- and 63-year-old patients after modified radical mastectomy of the left breast (A), respectively, of both breasts (B).** Indication for autologous reconstruction with a microvascular flap, particularly if skin and fat excess is available and adjuvant radiotherapy has been performed.

Lately, prophylactic bilateral mastectomy has to be offered more and more frequently due to the increased detection of patients carrying a genetic mutation or predisposition to develop breast cancer (e.g., BRCA-1, BRCA-2, p53). Understandably, these women have high demands to the esthetic outcome that can be overcome with nipple-sparing mastectomy being accepted as the gold standard in patients with prophylactic mastectomies (13).

Noteworthy, skin- and nipple-sparing mastectomies are associated with a high rate of ischemia-related wound breakdown and necrosis of up to 54%, which is a consequence of a critically impaired blood supply of the distant areas of the often very thin skin flap. Meanwhile, various approaches have been described to decrease ischemia-associated complications of the mastectomy skin flap, including surgical skin reduction of the mastectomy flap, temporary insertion of an expandable implant, and local application of vasodilators. Interestingly, first clinical data have shown that local heat preconditioning was able to safely and significantly reduce ischemia-related mastectomy skin flap complications in patients with skin-sparing mastectomy and immediate breast reconstruction (14).

## RECONSTRUCTION TECHNIQUES OF THE BREAST

Breast reconstruction depends primarily on the type of mastectomy and may be classified in various ways, such as reconstruction type and reconstruction time point. The latter includes delayed breast reconstruction (DBR; secondary breast reconstruction) and immediate breast reconstruction during the same surgery (IBR; primary breast reconstruction). IBR has the advantage of reducing the total number of surgical procedures. Since breast reconstruction *per se* represents an additional procedure to mastectomy, the potential surgery-related complications of both mastectomy and reconstruction accumulate due to prolonged surgery time, particularly if mastectomy is performed using a skin reducing or skin-sparing approach (hematoma due to bleeding of the mastectomy flap, ischemic complications of the mastectomy flap, infection, etc.), respectively, reconstruction is performed with implants. This has to be taken into consideration in order not to postpone adjuvant therapy, i.e., foremost chemotherapy, to the disadvantage of the patient (15). Despite very effective diagnostic work-up of breast cancer and highly standardized neo- and adjuvant treatment regimes, IBR bears the risk that unforeseen adjuvant radiotherapy may compromise the final result of the reconstructed breast, such as capsular contracture in implant-based reconstructions, respectively flap shrinkage in autologous reconstructions. Therefore, many surgeons may tend to a DBR when using free (microvascular) flaps in cases of an invasive tumor requiring adjuvant radiotherapy. In order not to lose the skin envelope after skin-sparing mastectomy, one can place a spacer until completion of adjuvant therapy. Nonetheless, IBR is advantageously associated with a reduced recovery time, a better esthetic outcome, an improved quality of life, and, finally, lower surgery- and recovery-related costs (16–18).

Nowadays, the seek for bilateral prophylactic mastectomy particularly in women with a genetic predisposition for breast cancer (e.g. BRCA-1, BRCA-2, p53) increases and accordingly represents an ideal indication for IBR of any type, knowing that neither adjuvant chemotherapy nor adjuvant radiotherapy will be required (19).

Generally, three different approaches of breast reconstruction may be considered: (1) breast reconstruction using implants and skin expanders, (2) breast reconstruction using flaps (vascularized autologous tissue), and (3) breast reconstruction using non-vascularized lipoaspirate autologous fat. In the following, the different approaches will be briefly highlighted, including the advantages and disadvantages of each approach.

## Breast Reconstruction Using Implants and Skin Expanders

The use of implants and skin expanders is not only the oldest way to reconstruct a breast but also the quickest and presumably easiest method of breast reconstruction. Accordingly, implant-based breast reconstruction is by far the most often used technique worldwide (9, 20). The prerequisite for implant-based breast reconstruction is an adequate skin envelope that allows covering the implant that is usually introduced in a submuscular plane detaching the medial insertions of the pectoralis major muscle from the ribs.

### Implant-Based Breast Reconstruction

Basically, the first "implant"-based breast reconstruction was performed 1895 by Vincenz Czerny, who used a patient's lipoma from the lumbar region to reconstruct a post-surgical asymmetry after tumor removal (21).

Cronin and Gerow fathered the modern era of silicone gel-filled breast implants and so allowed DBR (22, 23). Nowadays, fifth generation silicone gel-filled breast implants that contain a highly viscous and more or less form-stable gel are usually used. The implants are available in both, round and anatomical shape and vary in width, height, and projection (profile). Implant-based breast reconstruction is used in women who do not want any additional scars (flap harvesting) (**Figure 2**) or do not have any adequate flap donor site (e.g., lean patient, pre-existing scars, and medical conditions).

Implant-based breast reconstructions prone to develop implant-related local complications during the subsequent 10 years with a risk for a reoperation of 70% (24). Approximately 25 and 35% of the patients are being diagnosed with severe capsular contracture and, respectively, implant rupture (25). This high complication rate results from the thin skin envelope remaining after mastectomy, which does not provide any robust coverage of the implant. This complication rate does neither consider breast shape deformity and asymmetry in the context of mild to moderate capsular contracture nor does it consider an even worse outcome in implant-based breast reconstruction with irradiated skin. *De facto*, breast reconstruction using implants may yield very nice long-term results that suffice many patients, yet the implant will always remain more or less fixed to the thoracic wall and consequently the breast maintains a unique shape, independently from the patient's posture. Finally, implant-based breast reconstruction will not allow recreating a naturally shaped ptotic breast in most patients, and therefore often requires adaptive surgery of the contralateral breast to achieve symmetry. Though, implant-based breast reconstruction prevents from "collateral damage," such as scars, contour deformity, and muscular weakness, as it might be seen after flap harvesting for flap-based breast reconstruction (**Figure 3**).

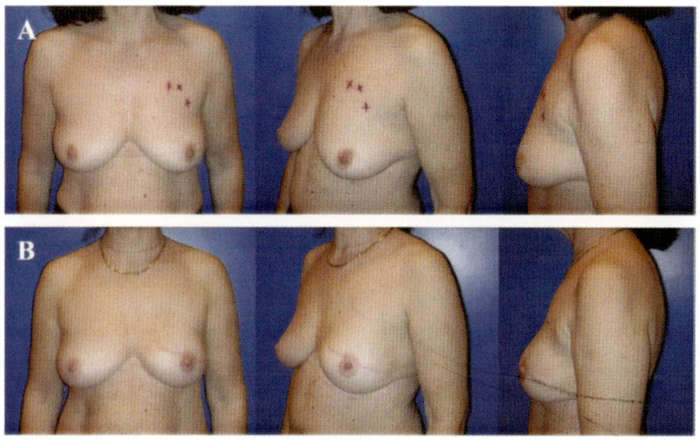


**FIGURE 2 | A 58-year-old patient before skin-sparing mastectomy for multifocal cancer of the left breast (A)**. Four years after primary reconstruction of the left breast using an implant in a subpectoral plane to cover the upper half of the implant and a resorbable mesh to prevent cranialization of the partially detached pectoralis major muscle, as well as reconstruction of the nipple–areolar complex (star flap for the nipple and tatoo of the nipple and neo-areola). Note the almost symmetric size and contour of both breasts **(B)**.

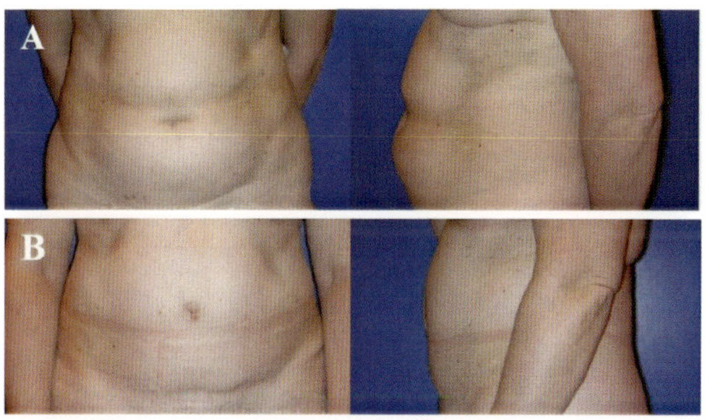


**FIGURE 3 | Typical donor site for abdominal flap-based breast reconstruction**. A 57-year-old patient before **(A)** and 4 years after **(B)** harvesting a microvascular deep inferior epigastric perforator (DIEP) artery flap from the abdominal region. Note the adipocutaneous excess cranially and distally of the umbilicus, the almost invisible scar at the umbilicus and the suprapubic region, as well as the significantly improved abdominal contour [profile view **(A,B)**]. The reconstructed breast of this patient is shown in **Figure 6**.

### Expander-Based Breast Reconstruction

The technique of tissue expansion has first been described by Radovan in 1976, and since then, it has been used on a regular base in order to recreate the amount of lost skin after mastectomy through stepwise expansion of the remaining chest skin (26). Ideally, the contralateral breast volume should not exceed a volume of 300–400 g. Typically, patients with pre-expansion of the breast skin undergo secondary breast reconstruction with implants. In selected cases, especially in young and skinny patients with insufficient skin laxity, yet enough adipose tissue to reconstruct a breast mound of ~300–350 g, one might pre-expand the breast skin after mastectomy in order to substitute the expander with an autologous flap.

The main drawback of skin expansion are the frequent outpatient visits to gradually fill the expander, the need for an additional procedure (i.e., expander removal for permanent implant or flap) and the relatively high rate of complications, such as infection, capsular contracture, and skin perforation (27).

Alternatively, skin expanders can be used as "spacers" after skin-sparing mastectomy in order not to lose the skin pocket. This approach is particularly helpful in patients who are sure to get adjuvant radiotherapy of the skin and/or the thoracic wall. Indeed, postoperative radiotherapy will not significantly increase the rate of flap-related complications (28). Yet, IBR is more and more frequently performed using microvascular (free) flaps despite postoperative radiotherapy. However, we currently do not know at what extent the flap will indurate and shrink at long-term follow-up.

### Breast Reconstruction with Acellular Dermis

The use of acellular dermal matrices in implant- and expander-based breast reconstruction has lately become more and more popular. Matrices are usually of human, porcine, or bovine origin. They have shown to improve esthetic outcome and reduce implant-related morbidity (29), such as a decreased rate of capsular contracture (30–32), an improved tolerance to radiotherapy, and a more natural anatomical reconstruction of the inframammary fold and final breast contour (33).

Nahabedian demonstrated a high safety and excellent results using acellular dermis in a 12-year follow-up, even in the setting of reconstruction after infection or radiotherapy. However, other authors reported several matrix-related complications, such as hematoma, infection, and foremost late seromas (29). The use of matrices is again and again associated with a rather high rate of early complications. Lardi et al. have demonstrated that these complications were mostly related to patient characteristics and a learning curve, highlighting the importance of patient selection and technical principles (34).

## Breast Reconstruction Using Flaps (Vascularized Autologous Tissue)

The myocutaneous flaps that are being used for breast reconstruction have a long history, although the techniques of today are much more sophisticated than those of the past. Louis Ombredanne from France was the first to use a pedicled pectoralis muscle flap for IBR in 1906. Differently as his colleagues, Ombredanne was the first who wittingly tried to reconstruct not only the skin defect after mastectomy but also the breast mound that was considered at that time a "luxury" procedure with limited indications (35). Almost simultaneously, Tanzani from Italy used the pedicled myocutaneous latissimus dorsi flap to close mastectomy defects for the first time.

Flap surgery for breast reconstruction has been performed on a regular base, since the mid 70s, initially using both, tubed flaps from the abdomen (36) and thoraco-epigastric, necessitating several surgical stages (23). The initial attempts were still not able to really reconstruct the breast mound and therefore primarily aimed at resurfacing the thoracic wall's defects after radical mastectomy. Finally, it was the introduction of the myocutaneous latissimus dorsi flap with its overlying skin island, as described by Tanzani 70 years earlier, which allowed to restore mastectomy-induced skin loss and to a lesser extent also volume loss (37–39).

Almost at the same time, Bostwick described the combined use of the myocutaneous latissimus dorsi flap and a silicone implant to consistently provide adequate skin coverage, respectively, to restore the breast mound in postmastectomy reconstruction (40).

The advantage of the latissimus dorsi flap is its rather consistent anatomy and therefore easy flap harvest. However, flap transfer from the back can be associated with highly visible scars, contour deformity of the thorax ventrally and the back dorsally as well as animation of the skin/muscle-implant complex of the pectoralis major respectively latissimus dorsi muscle due to innervation of the latter one (**Figure 4**). Otherwise, the muscle undergoes atrophy of 50–75% of its volume unconditionally, almost always requiring an implant to restore volume, unless the patient is rather thin (**Figure 5**).

Since this reconstructive approach combines two basic techniques of reconstructive surgery, i.e., skin replacement with the flap and volume restoration with the implant, the patients are subject to an accumulation of the two technique's morbidities, which might be significant, particularly years after reconstruction. Tarantino et al. demonstrated that 57% of the patients treated with a latissimus dorsi flap and implants had revisional surgery for implant replacement or implant removal after a mean follow-up of 10 years, and concluded that the indication for this

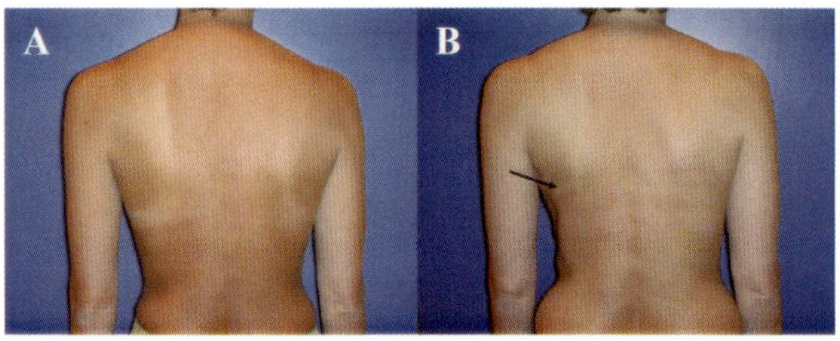


**FIGURE 4 | Typical donor site for myocutaneous latissimus dorsi flap-based breast reconstruction**. A 36-year-old patient before **(A)** and 2 years after secondary reconstruction of the left breast using a pedicled myocutaneous latissimus dorsi flap **(B)**. The skin island is harvested along the posterior axillary line. Note the well concealed scar (usually in the bra-line) that does not interfere with the back of the patient, yet skin and muscle harvesting result in a slight contour deformity of the periscapular region [arrow; **(B)**]. The reconstructed breast of this patient is shown in **Figure 5**.

procedure should be restricted to patients who do not qualify for either implant-based or flap-based breast reconstruction (41).

In 1987, Hokin and Silfverskiold described the use of an extended latissimus dorsi flap to avoid the use of an implant. The flap's volume was significantly increased by dissecting the subcutaneous fat surrounding the skin island (42). Unfortunately, donor site morbidity increased dramatically, including prolonged seroma respectively wound dehiscence rate, and contour deformity (43).

The true progress in flap-based breast reconstruction occurred in 1982 when Hartrampf and colleagues used the cranially pedicled rectus abdominis muscle flap with a horizontally oriented adipocutaneous skin island (TRAM flap) supplied by the deep superior epigastric artery to anatomically reconstruct volume and shape of the breast in one single stage without using implants (44).

Although this procedure was able to both, restore the ablated breast and improve abdominal contour despite scars at the umbilicus and the waistline, following significant disadvantages have to be taken into consideration: a high tissue-to-blood supply ratio of the flap, protracted recovery of the patient and abdominal wall weakness, including bulging and herniation due to sacrifice of the rectus abdominis muscle and large part of its anterior fascia.

To overcome these drawbacks of the donor site of the pedicled TRAM flap, Arnez and colleagues and Grotting et al. popularized the free TRAM flap, i.e., the microvascular anastomosis of at least one artery and one vein of the flap to recipient vessels. In doing so, the authors were able to demonstrate a more limited harvest of the rectus abdominis muscle, a safer transfer due to improved perfusion originating from the larger caudal pedicle (deep inferior epigastric artery instead of deep superior epigastric artery), and an improved medial breast contour due to the lack of tunneling of the flap's cranial pedicle (45, 46). Further refinement of the surgical technique over time aimed at decreasing as much as possible the weakening of the abdominal wall despite transferring most of the abdominal skin and its underlying subcutaneous tissue, including muscle sparing free TRAM flap (47), fascia sparing free TRAM flap (48), to finally achieve complete muscle preservation. The latter was obtained by dissecting the vascular pedicle of the adipocutaneous abdominal flap perforating the rectus abdominis muscle (deep inferior epigastric perforator (DIEP) artery flap) as described by Allen and Treece (49) and Blondeel and Boeckx (50) (**Figure 6**). The concept of this so-called "perforator flap" or DIEP flap has somehow revolutionized breast reconstruction by maximizing the amount of safe tissue transfer, yet minimizing donor site morbidity. Abdominal tissue is very suitable for breast reconstruction, since many patients have a certain abdominal excess of skin and fat. Consequently, autologous breast reconstruction using a DIEP flap nowadays represents the gold standard. In case of concomitant chronic lymphedema of the arm after sentinel lymph node biopsy, axillary lymph node dissection and or/radiotherapy of the lymph node basins, one can surgically address this problem using lymphaticovenous anastomosis or microvascular lymph node transfer. The latter can easily be combined with a DIEP flap, since the flap mostly consists of the lymph nodes in the groin area lateral to the femoral vessels and depends on the pedicle originating from the superficial inferior epigastric vessels (51). Given that not every women is suitable for breast reconstruction using abdominal skin and fat, many more donor sites were described in the following years, aiming at harvesting the most suitable microvascular flap to best personalize breast reconstruction. This included, among others, the superior gluteal artery perforator (sGAP) flap (52), the inferior gluteal artery perforator (iGAP) flap (53) from the gluteal region, the fasciocutaneous infragluteal (FCI) flap (54), the profunda femoral artery perforator (PAP) flap (55) from the infragluteal region, and the transverse myocutaneous gracilis (TMG) flap from the inner thigh region (56).

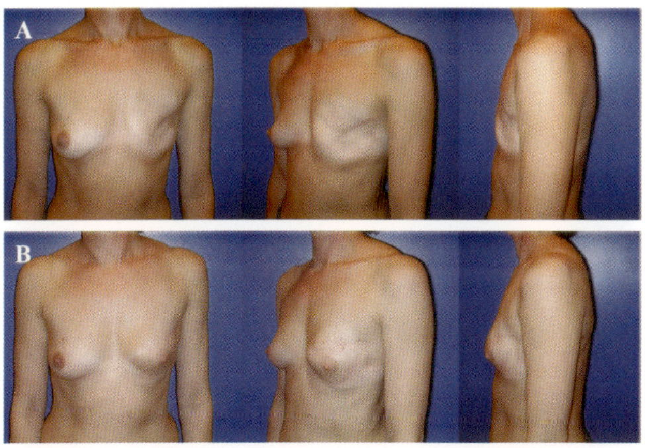


**FIGURE 5 | A 36-year-old patient 3 years after modified radical mastectomy of the left breast and adjuvant radio-chemotherapy**. Note the oblique scar and rather large skin envelope in a thin patient **(A)**. Two years after secondary reconstruction of the left breast using a pedicled myocutaneous latissimus dorsi flap without implant and reconstruction of the nipple–areolar complex (star flap for the nipple and tatoo of the nipple and neo-areola). Note the almost symmetric neckline and the slight volume loss of the lower pole of the breast resulting in contour deformity **(B)**. The donor site of this patient is shown in **Figure 4**.

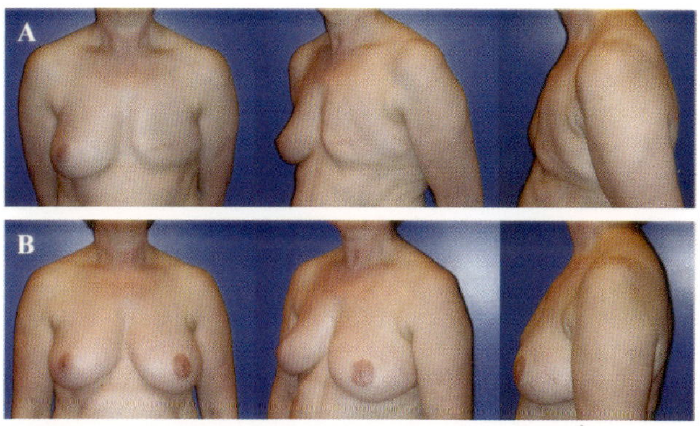


**FIGURE 6 | A 57-year-old patient 2 years after modified radical mastectomy of the left breast and adjuvant radio-chemotherapy**. Note the lack of skin and volume **(A)**. Four years after secondary reconstruction of the left breast using a microvascular deep inferior epigastric perforator (DIEP) artery flap from the abdominal region and reconstruction of the nipple–areolar complex (star flap for the nipple and tatoo of the nipple and neo-areola). Note the almost symmetric size and contour of both breasts without corrective surgery of the non operated contralateral breast **(B)**. The donor site of this patient is shown in **Figure 3**.

Nowadays, the internal mammary artery and its concomitant vein are predominantly used as the recipient vessels. Alternatively, the arterial branches originating from the subscapular artery (e.g., thoracodorsal artery, circumflex scapulae artery) or sternal perforators arising through the pectoral muscle are used.

Although breast reconstruction using autologous flap tissue allows a natural and durable result, flap harvest will cause a "collateral damage" at the flap's donor site, including potential surgery-related complications, scars, contour deformity, and functional impairment. Furthermore, microvascular flap-based breast reconstruction is not only technically more demanding, but also requires more infrastructures within a breast reconstruction unit, as compared to implant-based breast reconstruction (**Table 1**).

## Fat Graft-Based Breast Reconstruction Using Non-Vascularized Lipoaspirate Fat

Autologous fat grafting (AFG; lipografting, lipofilling) describes the harvesting of the patient's fat using liposuction followed by its reinjection into the tissue to be corrected or augmented. Fat grafting to the breast is more than 100 years old since Holländer corrected a retracted scar after mastectomy by injecting parceled fat into the scar (57). AFG to the breast has become a popular tool over the last 20 years, both in esthetic and reconstructive surgery. Regarding the breast, AFG has proven to be particularly effective to correct post-surgical irregularities, such as contour deformities and volume asymmetries after BCT, "rippling" after implant-based reconstruction and improvement of the transition zone between flap and skin in the neckline (58–60), as well as the preparation of the postmastectomy irradiated chest wall prior to implant placement (61). In selected cases, *de novo* reconstruction of the breast by means of AFG has shown very promising results. The patient must have several donor sites equipped with fat, because the reconstructive procedure usually takes four to six stages of fat grafting, each separated by 3 months at least (62). Irradiated skin does almost preclude this approach, since injected fat is not engrafted as desired (63).

**TABLE 1 | Advantages and disadvantages of implant-based versus autologous tissue-based techniques of breast reconstruction.**

| | Implant-based breast reconstruction | Autologous tissue-based breast reconstruction |
|---|---|---|
| Duration of surgery (h) | 1–2 | 4–6 |
| Infrastructural effort | Low | High[a] |
| Surgical complexity | Low | High |
| Donor site | None | Depending on flap[b] (abdominal, thigh, gluteal, dorsal region) |
| Complication rate (30 days) (implant-, respectively, flap-related) (%) | 2–4 | 2–4 |
| Complication rate (long-term) | Higher (due to capsular contracture) | Lower |
| Long-term reoperation rate | More likely | Less likely |
| Patient satisfaction | Short-term | Long-term |

[a]*Microscope, specific instruments, trained personnel (nurses in OR).*
[b]*Discomfort, pain, scars, abdominal bulging, hernia, asymmetry, and contour deformity.*

Autologous fat grafting is a "natural" filler, and unlike synthetic fillers will neither induce any foreign body reaction nor be resorbed completely. Today, harvesting of the fat is discussed, among others, with regard to composition of the infiltration solution, to diameter and shape of the harvesting cannula and to suction forces. In order to be structural, injection of the fat should be performed in small aliquots using blunt cannulas in multiple directions and multiple layers. This multi-planar approach maximizes the fat-to-tissue contact, thereby the exposition of non-vascularized fat to vascularized host tissue (64). Consensus exists on the fact that fat may not be injected into the glandular tissue of the breast. Commonly, 60–70% of the injected fat is engrafted to the host tissue. Fat necrosis and oil cysts are common complications after AFG and occur in ~5% (65). Unfortunately, necrosis of the grafted fat might also be associated with microcalcifications, which sometimes may be difficult to distinguish from malignant breast cancer-associated microcalcifications (66). Presumably, the radiologist is an expert, fat grafting-induced microcalcifications do no impact on the radiological follow-up (67). Yet, this fact may unsettle the patient who has to appear for regular follow-up imaging and eventually undergo diagnostic biopsy to exclude malignancy.

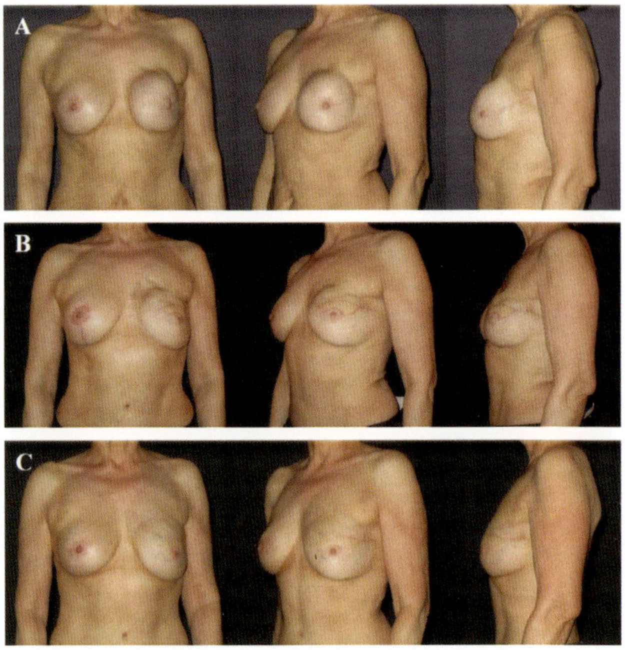


**FIGURE 7 | A 58-year-old patient 2 years after modified radical mastectomy of the left breast, adjuvant radio-chemotherapy, and secondary expander–implant-based reconstruction**. The patient developed a capsular contracture Baker grade IV with a hard, deformed, and painful breast fixed to the thoracic wall **(A)**. One year after implant removal, radical capsulectomy and secondary reconstruction of the left breast using a microvascular deep inferior epigastric perforator (DIEP) artery flap from the abdominal region. Note the contour deformity in the neckline and upper pole region of the breast resulting from partial fat necrosis of the flap **(B)**. Approximately 1.5 years after refinement of the contour deformity using two sessions of autologous fat grafting. Note the almost symmetric size and contour of both breasts **(C)**.

Currently, fat grafting to the breast is controversially discussed, particularly in the presence of remaining glandular breast tissue, as, for example, after BCT. Grafted fat that naturally contains progenitor and stem cells has lately been associated with breast cancer progression and metastasic spread in an experimental setting (68, 69). Despite the lack of prospective follow-up studies, fat grafting to reconstruct or to refine a breast after mastectomy and/or after breast reconstruction – BCT not included – is nowadays considered safe (70–72).

## REFINEMENT SURGERY AFTER BREAST RECONSTRUCTION

After breast reconstruction, particularly if breast reconstruction is performed unilaterally, refinement surgery may be necessary to reach symmetry of the breasts with regard to shape, contour, and size. The procedures usually consist of mastopexy, breast reduction, or breast augmentation using implants. Nowadays, AFG is often used to correct small volume asymmetries and contour deformities. The latter may occur after implant-based breast reconstruction (e.g., "rippling"), as well as after flap-based breast reconstruction (e.g., partial fat necrosis of the flap, transition zone between flap and neckline cranially). Refinement surgery is usually offered not earlier than 3 months after reconstruction or 6 months after completion of adjuvant radiotherapy. Fat grafting has often to be repeated. Its engraftment rate is ~60% (~40% fat resorption) (**Figure 7**). Last but not least, mastectomy is associated with the loss of the nipple–areolar complex (except for nipple-sparing mastectomy), requiring its reconstruction. Many techniques of reconstruction are available, including local flaps of the adjacent skin, skin grafts, tattoo, and a combination of all techniques.

## CONCLUSION

Breast cancer is the leading cause of cancer death in women. Its surgical approach has become less and less mutilating, allowing for 70–80% of the operated cases to undergo (BCT) that has proven to be as safe as mastectomy with regard to overall survival. In other words, 20–30% of the operated women are subjected to mastectomy. Since ~25 years, the skin-sparing mastectomy approach is an alternative to ablation of the breast allowing for better esthetic results due to preservation of the breast's skin envelope, yet from an oncological point of view as safe as mastectomy. Other than mastectomy, skin-sparing mastectomy needs immediate reconstruction in order not to lose the skin envelope that unreconstructed will inevitably retract and shrink to the level of the thoracic wall. Nowadays, breast reconstruction should be personalized at its best, first of all taking into consideration not only the oncological aspects of the tumor, neo-/adjuvant treatment and genetic predisposition, but also its timing (IBR versus DBR), as well as the patient's condition and wish. Despite this complex decision-making including many aspects, the overall number of breast reconstruction has lately considerably increased. Breast reconstruction itself can basically be classified into three categories, including (1) implant- and expander-based breast reconstruction, (2) flap-based breast reconstruction (vascularized autologous tissue), a combination of both (flap and implant), and (3) breast reconstruction using fat grafting (non-vascularized autologous lipoaspirate fat). However, fat grafting is predominantly used to refine post-reconstructive asymmetries. Nowadays, it is of importance that every woman having a high risk constellation (family history), being diagnosed with a genetic mutation and/or being affected with breast cancer gets the possibility to be presented to a multidisciplinary board of a certified breast center prior to surgery in order to be informed about all treatment modalities, including the various modalities of breast reconstruction. The goal of this multidisciplinary board is to best personalize breast reconstruction, of course putting to the fore the adequate oncological treatment. The patients also need to know the advantages and disadvantages of any reconstructive option, including the presumably less complex implant-based techniques that may result in high temporary satisfaction without any donor site morbidity and likelihood of reoperation due to capsular contracture and the clearly more complex flap-based techniques that will yield in high long-term satisfaction with the risk of donor site-associated complications.

## REFERENCES

1. Torre LA, Bray F, Siegel RL, Ferlay J, Lortet-Tieulent J, Jemal A. Global cancer statistics, 2012. *CA Cancer J Clin* (2015) **65**(2):87–108. doi:10.3322/caac.21262
2. Sakorafas GH, Safioleas M. Breast cancer surgery: an historical narrative. Part II. 18th and 19th centuries. *Eur J Cancer Care (Engl)* (2010) **19**(1):6–29. doi:10.1111/j.1365-2354.2008.01060.x
3. Patey DH. A review of 146 cases of carcinoma of the breast operated on between 1930 and 1943. *Br J Cancer* (1967) **21**(2):260–9. doi:10.1038/bjc.1967.28
4. Fisher B, Bauer M, Margolese R, Poisson R, Pilch Y, Redmond C, et al. Five-year results of a randomized clinical trial comparing total mastectomy and segmental mastectomy with or without radiation in the treatment of breast cancer. *N Engl J Med* (1985) **312**(11):665–73. doi:10.1056/NEJM198503143121102
5. Malhaire C, Hequet D, Falcou MC, Feron JG, Tardivon A, Leduey A, et al. Outcome of oncoplastic breast-conserving surgery following bracketing wire localization for large breast cancer. *Breast* (2015) **24**(4):370–5. doi:10.1016/j.breast.2015.02.037
6. Veiga DF, Veiga-Filho J, Ribeiro LM, Archangelo I Jr, Balbino PF, Caetano LV, et al. Quality-of-life and self-esteem outcomes after oncoplastic breast-conserving surgery. *Plast Reconstr Surg* (2010) **125**(3):811–7. doi:10.1097/PRS.0b013e3181ccdac5
7. Early Breast Cancer Trialists' Collaborative Group (EBCTCG), Darby S, McGale P, Correa C, Taylor C, Arriagada R, et al. Effect of radiotherapy after breast-conserving surgery on 10-year recurrence and 15-year breast cancer death: meta-analysis of individual patient data for 10,801 women in 17 randomised trials. *Lancet* (2011) **378**(9804):1707–16. doi:10.1016/S0140-6736(11)61629-2
8. Haviland JS, Owen JR, Dewar JA, Agrawal RK, Barrett J, Barrett-Lee PJ, et al. The UK Standardisation of Breast Radiotherapy (START) trials of radiotherapy hypofractionation for treatment of early breast cancer: 10-year follow-up results of two randomised controlled trials. *Lancet Oncol* (2013) **14**(11):1086–94. doi:10.1016/S1470-2045(13)70386-3
9. Albornoz CR, Bach PB, Mehrara BJ, Disa JJ, Pusic AL, McCarthy CM, et al. A paradigm shift in U.S. breast reconstruction: increasing implant rates. *Plast Reconstr Surg* (2013) **131**(1):15–23. doi:10.1097/PRS.0b013e3182729cde
10. Barton FE Jr, English JM, Kingsley WB, Fietz M. Glandular excision in total glandular mastectomy and modified radical mastectomy: a comparison. *Plast Reconstr Surg* (1991) **88**(3):389–92; discussion 393–4. doi:10.1097/00006534-199109000-00001
11. Singletary SE, Robb GL. Oncologic safety of skin-sparing mastectomy. *Ann Surg Oncol* (2003) **10**(2):95–7. doi:10.1245/ASO.2003.01.910
12. Simmons RM, Adamovich TL. Skin-sparing mastectomy. *Surg Clin North Am* (2003) **83**(4):885–99. doi:10.1016/S0039-6109(03)00035-5

13. Hartmann LC, Schaid DJ, Woods JE, Crotty TP, Myers JL, Arnold PG, et al. Efficacy of bilateral prophylactic mastectomy in women with a family history of breast cancer. *N Engl J Med* (1999) **340**(2):77–84. doi:10.1056/NEJM199901143400201
14. Mehta S, Rolph R, Cornelius V, Harder Y, Farhadi J. Local heat preconditioning in skin sparing mastectomy: a pilot study. *J Plast Reconstr Aesthet Surg* (2013) **66**(12):1676–82. doi:10.1016/j.bjps.2013.07.034
15. Johnson A. The timing of treatment in breast cancer: gaps and delays in treatment can be harmful. *Breast Cancer Res Treat* (2000) **60**(3):201–9. doi:10.1023/A:1006441018271
16. Joslyn SA. Patterns of care for immediate and early delayed breast reconstruction following mastectomy. *Plast Reconstr Surg* (2005) **115**(5):1289–96. doi:10.1097/01.PRS.0000156974.69184.5E
17. Neyt MJ, Blondeel PN, Morrison CM, Albrecht JA. Comparing the cost of delayed and immediate autologous breast reconstruction in Belgium. *Br J Plast Surg* (2005) **58**(4):493–7. doi:10.1016/j.bjps.2004.12.002
18. Yang X, Zhu C, Gu Y. The prognosis of breast cancer patients after mastectomy and immediate breast reconstruction: a meta-analysis. *PLoS One* (2015) **10**(5):e0125655. doi:10.1371/journal.pone.0125655
19. Gurunluoglu R, Gurunluoglu A, Williams SA, Tebockhorst S. Current trends in breast reconstruction: survey of American Society of Plastic Surgeons 2010. *Ann Plast Surg* (2013) **70**(1):103–10. doi:10.1097/SAP.0b013e31822ed5ce
20. Kwok AC, Goodwin IA, Ying J, Agarwal JP. National trends and complication rates after bilateral mastectomy and immediate breast reconstruction from 2005 to 2012. *Am J Surg* (2015) **210**(3):512–6. doi:10.1016/j.amjsurg.2015.03.019
21. Champaneria MC, Wong WW, Hill ME, Gupta SC. The evolution of breast reconstruction: a historical perspective. *World J Surg* (2012) **36**(4):730–42. doi:10.1007/s00268-012-1450-2
22. Cronin TD, Greenberg RL. Our experiences with the silastic gel breast prosthesis. *Plast Reconstr Surg* (1970) **46**(1):1–7. doi:10.1097/00006534-197046010-00001
23. Cronin TD, Upton J, McDonough JM. Reconstruction of the breast after mastectomy. *Plast Reconstr Surg* (1977) **59**(1):1–14. doi:10.1097/00006534-197701000-00001
24. Gabriel SE, Woods JE, O'Fallon WM, Beard CM, Kurland LT, Melton LJ III. Complications leading to surgery after breast implantation. *N Engl J Med* (1997) **336**(10):677–82. doi:10.1056/NEJM199703063361001
25. Spear SL, Murphy DK; Allergan Silicone Breast Implant U.S. Core Clinical Study Group. Natrelle round silicone breast implants: core study results at 10 years. *Plast Reconstr Surg* (2014) **133**(6):1354–61. doi:10.1097/PRS.0000000000000021
26. Radovan C. Breast reconstruction after mastectomy using the temporary expander. *Plast Reconstr Surg* (1982) **69**(2):195–208. doi:10.1097/00006534-198202000-00001
27. Anker CJ, Hymas RV, Ahluwalia R, Kokeny KE, Avizonis V, Boucher KM, et al. The effect of radiation on complication rates and patient satisfaction in breast reconstruction using temporary tissue expanders and permanent implants. *Breast J* (2015) **21**(3):233–40. doi:10.1111/tbj.12395
28. Patel KM, Albino F, Fan KL, Liao E, Nahabedian MY. Microvascular autologous breast reconstruction in the context of radiation therapy: comparing two reconstructive algorithms. *Plast Reconstr Surg* (2013) **132**(2):251–7. doi:10.1097/PRS.0b013e31829586e2
29. Sbitany H, Serletti JM. Acellular dermis-assisted prosthetic breast reconstruction: a systematic and critical review of efficacy and associated morbidity. *Plast Reconstr Surg* (2011) **128**(6):1162–9. doi:10.1097/PRS.0b013e318230c29e
30. Spear SL, Howard MA, Boehmler JH, Ducic I, Low M, Abbruzzesse MR. The infected or exposed breast implant: management and treatment strategies. *Plast Reconstr Surg* (2004) **113**:1634–44. doi:10.1097/01.PRS.0000117194.21748.02
31. Stump A, Holton LH III, Connor J, Harper JR, Slezak S, Silverman RP. The use of acellular dermal matrix to prevent capsule formation around implants in a primate model. *Plast Reconstr Surg* (2009) **124**:82–91. doi:10.1097/PRS.0b013e3181ab112d
32. Komorowska-Timek E, Oberg KC, Timek TA, Gridley DS, Miles DA. The effect of AlloDerm envelopes on periprosthetic capsule formation with and without radiation. *Plast Reconstr Surg* (2009) **123**:807–16. doi:10.1097/PRS.0b013e318199eef3
33. Spear SL, Pelletiere CV, Lockwood M. Immediate breast reconstruction with tissue expanders and AlloDerm. In: Spear SL, Wiley SC, Robb GL, Hammond DC, Nahabedian MY, editors. *Surgery of the Breast: Principles and Art*. Philadelphia, PA: Lippincott Williams & Wilkins (2006). p. 484–8.
34. Lardi AM, Ho-Asjoe M, Mohanna PN, Farhadi J. Immediate breast reconstruction with acellular dermal matrix: factors affecting outcome. *J Plast Reconstr Aesthet Surg* (2014) **67**(8):1098–105. doi:10.1016/j.bjps.2014.05.020
35. Teimourian B, Adham MN. Louis Ombredanne and the origin of muscle flap use for immediate breast mound reconstruction. *Plast Reconstr Surg* (1983) **72**(6):905–10. doi:10.1097/00006534-198312000-00037
36. Millard DR Jr. Breast reconstruction after a radical mastectomy. *Plast Reconstr Surg* (1976) **58**(3):283–91. doi:10.1097/00006534-197609000-00004
37. McCraw JB, Dibbell DG, Carraway JH. Clinical definition of independent myocutaneous vascular territories. *Plast Reconstr Surg* (1977) **60**(3):341–52. doi:10.1097/00006534-197760030-00003
38. Schneider WJ, Hill HL Jr, Brown RG. Latissimus dorsi myocutaneous flap for breast reconstruction. *Br J Plast Surg* (1977) **30**(4):277–81. doi:10.1016/0007-1226(77)90117-5
39. Olivari N. The latissimus flap. *Br J Plast Surg* (1976) **29**(2):126–8. doi:10.1016/0007-1226(76)90036-9
40. Bostwick J. Reconstruction of the breast. *Acta Chir Belg* (1980) **79**(2):125–9.
41. Tarantino I, Banic A, Fischer T. Evaluation of late results in breast reconstruction by latissimus dorsi flap and prosthesis implantation. *Plast Reconstr Surg* (2006) **117**(5):1387–94. doi:10.1097/01.prs.0000207396.22527.68
42. Hokin JA, Silfverskiold KL. Breast reconstruction without an implant: results and complications using an extended latissimus dorsi flap. *Plast Reconstr Surg* (1987) **79**(1):58–66. doi:10.1097/00006534-198701000-00010
43. Chang DW, Youssef A, Cha S, Reece GP. Autologous breast reconstruction with the extended latissimus dorsi flap. *Plast Reconstr Surg* (2002) **110**(3):751–9; discussion 760–1. doi:10.1097/00006534-200209010-00005
44. Hartrampf CR, Scheflan M, Black PW. Breast reconstruction with a transverse abdominal island flap. *Plast Reconstr Surg* (1982) **69**(2):216–25. doi:10.1097/00006534-198202000-00006
45. Arnez ZM, Smith RW, Eder E, Solinc M, Kersnic M. Breast reconstruction by the free lower transverse rectus abdominis musculocutaneous flap. *Br J Plast Surg* (1988) **41**(5):500–5. doi:10.1016/0007-1226(88)90007-0
46. Grotting JC, Urist MM, Maddox WA, Vasconez LO. Conventional TRAM flap versus free microsurgical TRAM flap for immediate breast reconstruction. *Plast Reconstr Surg* (1989) **83**(5):828–41; discussion 842–4. doi:10.1097/00006534-198905000-00009
47. Feller AM. Free TRAM. Results and abdominal wall function. *Clin Plast Surg* (1994) **21**(2):223–32.
48. Erni D, Harder YD. The dissection of the rectus abdominis myocutaneous flap with complete preservation of the anterior rectus sheath. *Br J Plast Surg* (2003) **56**(4):395–400. doi:10.1016/S0007-1226(03)00132-2
49. Allen RJ, Treece P. Deep inferior epigastric perforator flap for breast reconstruction. *Ann Plast Surg* (1994) **32**(1):32–8. doi:10.1097/00000637-199401000-00007
50. Blondeel PN, Boeckx WD. Refinements in free flap breast reconstruction: the free bilateral deep inferior epigastric perforator flap anastomosed to the internal mammary artery. *Br J Plast Surg* (1994) **47**(7):495–501. doi:10.1016/0007-1226(94)90033-7
51. Saaristo AM, Niemi TS, Viitanen TP, Tervala TV, Hartiala P, Suominen EA. Microvascular breast reconstruction and lymph node transfer for postmastectomy lymphedema patients. *Ann Surg* (2012) **255**(3):468–73. doi:10.1097/SLA.0b013e3182426757
52. Gurunluoglu R, Spanio S, Rainer C, Ninkovic M. Skin expansion before breast reconstruction with the superior gluteal artery perforator flap improves aesthetic outcome. *Ann Plast Surg* (2003) **50**(5):475–9. doi:10.1097/01.SAP.0000041489.11933.03
53. Granzow JW, Levine JL, Chiu ES, Allen RJ. Breast reconstruction with gluteal artery perforator flaps. *J Plast Reconstr Aesthet Surg* (2006) **59**(6):614–21. doi:10.1016/j.bjps.2006.01.005
54. Papp C, Windhofer C, Gruber S. Breast reconstruction with the fasciocutaneous infragluteal free flap (FCI). *Ann Plast Surg* (2007) **58**(2):131–6. doi:10.1097/01.sap.0000237635.05337.a1
55. Saad A, Sadeghi A, Allen RJ. The anatomic basis of the profunda femoris artery perforator flap: a new option for autologous breast reconstruction – a cadaveric and computer tomography angiogram study. *J Reconstr Microsurg* (2012) **28**(6):381–6. doi:10.1055/s-0032-1313773
56. Schoeller T, Huemer GM, Wechselberger G. The transverse musculocutaneous gracilis flap for breast reconstruction: guidelines for flap and patient selection. *Plast Reconstr Surg* (2008) **122**(1):29–38. doi:10.1097/PRS.0b013e318177436c

57. Holländer. Die kosmetische Chirurgie. In: Joseph M, editor. *Handbuch der Kosmetik*. Leipzig: Veit & Comp (1912). p. 669–712; 673.
58. Delay E, Gosset J, Toussoun G, Delaporte T, Delbaere M. [Efficacy of lipomodelling for the management of sequelae of breast cancer conservative treatment]. *Ann Chir Plast Esthet* (2008) **53**(2):153–68. doi:10.1016/j.anplas.2007.09.005
59. Kanchwala SK, Glatt BS, Conant EF, Bucky LP. Autologous fat grafting to the reconstructed breast: the management of acquired contour deformities. *Plast Reconstr Surg* (2009) **124**(2):409–18. doi:10.1097/PRS.0b013e3181aeeadd
60. Weichman KE, Broer PN, Tanna N, Wilson SC, Allan A, Levine JP, et al. The role of autologous fat grafting in secondary microsurgical breast reconstruction. *Ann Plast Surg* (2013) **71**(1):24–30. doi:10.1097/SAP.0b013e3182920ad0
61. Sarfati I, Ihrai T, Duvernay A, Nos C, Clough K. [Autologous fat grafting to the postmastectomy irradiated chest wall prior to breast implant reconstruction: a series of 68 patients]. *Ann Chir Plast Esthet* (2013) **58**(1):35–40. doi:10.1016/j.anplas.2012.10.007
62. Hoppe DL, Ueberreiter K, Surlemont Y, Peltoniemi H, Stabile M, Kauhanen S. Breast reconstruction de novo by water-jet assisted autologous fat grafting – a retrospective study. *Ger Med Sci* (2013) **12**(11):Doc17. doi:10.3205/000185
63. Longo B, Laporta R, Sorotos M, Pagnoni M, Gentilucci M, Santanelli di Pompeo F. Total breast reconstruction using autologous fat grafting following nipple-sparing mastectomy in irradiated and non-irradiated patients. *Aesthetic Plast Surg* (2014) **38**(6):1101–8. doi:10.1007/s00266-014-0406-3
64. Coleman SR. Structural fat grafting: more than a permanent filler. *Plast Reconstr Surg* (2006) **118**(3 Suppl):108S–20S. doi:10.1097/01.prs.0000234610.81672.e7
65. Kaoutzanis C, Xin M, Ballard TN, Welch KB, Momoh AO, Kozlow JH, et al. Autologous fat grafting after breast reconstruction in postmastectomy patients: complications, biopsy rates, and locoregional cancer recurrence rates. *Ann Plast Surg* (2015). doi:10.1097/SAP.0000000000000561
66. Rubin JP, Coon D, Zuley M, Toy J, Asano Y, Kurita M, et al. Mammographic changes after fat transfer to the breast compared with changes after breast reduction: a blinded study. *Plast Reconstr Surg* (2012) **129**(5):1029–38. doi:10.1097/PRS.0b013e31824a2a8e
67. Gosset J, Guerin N, Toussoun G, Delaporte T, Delay E. [Radiological evaluation after lipomodelling for correction of breast conservative treatment sequelae]. *Ann Chir Plast Esthet* (2008) **53**(2):178–89. doi:10.1016/j.anplas.2007.09.003
68. Schweizer R, Tsuji W, Gorantla VS, Marra KG, Rubin JP, Plock JA. The role of adipose-derived stem cells in breast cancer progression and metastasis. *Stem Cells Int* (2015) **2015**:120949. doi:10.1155/2015/120949
69. Kamat P, Schweizer R, Kaenel P, Salemi S, Calcagni M, Giovanoli P, et al. Human adipose-derived mesenchymal stromal cells may promote breast cancer progression and metastatic spread. *Plast Reconstr Surg* (2015) **136**(1):76–84. doi:10.1097/PRS.0000000000001321
70. Lohsiriwat V, Curigliano G, Rietjens M, Goldhirsch A, Petit JY. Autologous fat transplantation in patients with breast cancer: "silencing" or "fueling" cancer recurrence? *Breast* (2011) **20**(4):351–7. doi:10.1016/j.breast.2011.01.003
71. Claro F Jr, Figueiredo JC, Zampar AG, Pinto-Neto AM. Applicability and safety of autologous fat for reconstruction of the breast. *Br J Surg* (2012) **99**(6):768–80. doi:10.1002/bjs.8722
72. Petit JY, Botteri E, Lohsiriwat V, Rietjens M, De Lorenzi F, Garusi C, et al. Locoregional recurrence risk after lipofilling in breast cancer patients. *Ann Oncol* (2012) **23**(3):582–8. doi:10.1093/annonc/mdr158

4

# Reconstruction of Soft-Tissue Defects at the Foot and Ankle after Oncological Resection

*Andrej Ring*†, Pascal Kirchhoff, Ole Goertz, Bjorn Behr, Adrien Daigeler, Marcus Lehnhardt and Kamran Harati*

*Department for Plastic and Hand Surgery, Burn Center/Sarcoma Reference Center, Ruhr-University Bochum, Bochum, Germany*

**Introduction:** Solid malignancies at the foot and ankle region are rare and include mainly soft-tissue sarcomas, bone sarcomas, and skin malignancies. Complete surgical resection with clear margins still remains the mainstay of therapy in these malignancies. However, attainment of negative surgical margins in patients with locally advanced tumors of the foot and ankle region may require extensive surgery and could result in loss of extremity function. In these circumstances, plastic surgical techniques can frequently reduce functional impairment and cover soft-tissue defects, particularly in cases of large tumor size or localization adjacent to critical anatomic structures, thereby improving the quality of life for these patients. The aim of this article is to illustrate the various treatment options of plastic surgery in the multimodal therapy of patients with malignant tumors of the foot and ankle region.

**Materials and methods:** This article is based on the review of the current literature and the evaluation of the author's own patient database.

**Results:** The local treatment of malignant extremity tumors has undergone major changes over the last few decades. Primary amputations have been increasingly replaced by limb-sparing techniques, preserving extremity function as much as possible. Although defect coverage at the foot and ankle region is demanding due to complex anatomical features and functional requirements, several plastic surgical treatment options can be implemented in the curative treatment of patients with malignant solid tumors in this area. Soft-tissue defects after tumor resection can be covered by a variety of local flaps. If local flaps are not applicable, free flap transfers, such as the anterolateral thigh flap, parascapular flap, or latissimus dorsi flap, can be utilized to cover nearly all kinds of defects in the foot and ankle region.

**Conclusion:** Soft-tissue reconstruction in the foot and ankle region is a vital component of limb-sparing surgery. It enables complete resection of locally advanced tumors and subsequent adjuvant radiotherapy. Modern plastic surgical techniques should, therefore, be integrated in the multimodal treatment concept of malignancies in the foot and ankle region.

**Keywords: sarcoma, reconstructive surgical procedures, lower extremity, microsurgery, flap**

***Edited by:***
*Gyu Seog Choi, Kyungpook National University Medical Center, South Korea*

***Reviewed by:***
*Andreas Arkudas, University Hospital of Erlangen, Germany*
*Osama Hussein, Mansoura University, Egypt*

***Correspondence:***
*Andrej Ring*
*a.ring@lukas-gesellschaft.de*

***†Present address:***
*Andrej Ring, Department of Plastic Surgery, St. Rochus Hospital, Castrop-Rauxel, Germany*

***Specialty section:***
*This article was submitted to Surgical Oncology, a section of the journal Frontiers in Surgery*

## TUMORS OF THE FOOT AND ANKLE REGION

Malignant neoplasms on the foot and ankle make up about 4% of all bone and soft-tissue tumors of the body (1–3). Soft-tissue sarcomas, as rare tumors of mesenchymal origin, account for about 1% of all adult malignancies but are located in the extremities in about 60% of all cases (4). Regarding the content of soft tissues, the lower extremities are affected more frequently than the upper extremities, with a ratio of 3:1. Other rare malignancies with localization at the foot are, for example, tumors of the skin, such as melanoma, and giant cell tumors of the tendon-sheath, vascular sarcomas, and carcinoma metastases. The local treatment of soft-tissue sarcomas has undergone major changes over the last few decades. Primary amputations have been increasingly replaced by limb-sparing techniques, preserving extremity function as much as possible (3, 5). Interestingly, a recently published meta-analysis revealed that the width of negative surgical margins has no significant impact on overall survival (6). The data within the latter suggested that patients with clear margins had a better prognosis, but surgery to preserve functionality may result in very close margins without impairing survival. However, in patients with locally advanced soft-tissue sarcomas of the extremities, attainment of negative surgical margins may require extensive surgery and could result in a loss of extremity function. In these circumstances, plastic surgical techniques can frequently reduce functional impairment and cover soft-tissue defects, particularly in cases of large tumor size or localization adjacent to critical anatomic structures, thereby improving the quality of life for these patients. Whether limb preservation or ablative procedures are applied is also determined by the location of the tumor and the expectations and the functional demands of the patient.

## ONCOLOGICAL TREATMENT STRATEGIES AND CONCEPTS

Contemporary treatment strategies should include concepts of complete resection with negative surgical margins in combination with plastic reconstructive surgery, especially considering the postoperative functional aspects. The factors that determine the resectability of sarcomas are mainly the tumor size and localization. Regarding surgical resectability, the localization of the tumor is of great relevance. Deep or subfascial localization is associated with a higher risk of local recurrence or distant metastasis when compared with superficial or epifascial localization (7–9). Regarding tumor size, large soft-tissue sarcomas are shown to have a diminished survival when compared with small tumors. However, large tumor size is found more frequently in high-grade tumors. Most survival studies have revealed that the tumor grade is the most significant prognostic factor (9, 10). Dedifferentiated and high tumor grade is also associated with higher invasiveness, resulting in extensive infiltration of the surrounding tissues.

In cases with extensive infiltration of functional structures, amputation still has to be considered as a treatment option in order to obtain clear margins (7, 11, 12). However, the fact that amputation as a curative treatment strategy for sarcomas in the extremities has no survival benefit when compared to limb-preserving surgical procedures should be taken into account. It has been shown that amputation, especially in combination with radiotherapy, has no advantage compared to resection (6). The use of reconstructive surgery and adjuvant radiation since the 1980s has been able to reduce the amputation rate to less than 20% (13–16). The incidence of local recurrences under limb preservation therapy has decreased to 10–15% in recent years; however, no change in terms of overall survival has been shown (17, 18). Local control rates for high-grade tumors amounted to about 90% and to 90–100% for low-grade sarcomas. Notably, high-grade tumors are associated with a higher risk of local recurrence (19, 20). Subsequently, local recurrence has been found to be associated with a diminished survival when compared with the primary disease (7, 21, 22). Nowadays, primary indications for amputations are fortunately rare. Primary amputations are indicated when negative margins are not otherwise attainable. However, whenever an amputation is deemed necessary to obtain local control of an extremity soft-tissue sarcoma, isolated limb perfusion should be considered. Tumor necrosis factor alpha-based isolated limb perfusion has been demonstrated to result in a limb salvage rate of 81% in patients with locally advanced extremity soft-tissue sarcoma who would have otherwise undergone amputation (23, 24). The second indication for primary amputation is the palliation of extensive ulcerative, bleeding, or odor-intensive tumors with complete loss of extremity function. A primary amputation must also be drawn early into consideration when satisfactory functional results cannot be expected from reconstructive techniques after extensive or disabling limb-sparing resections. In such cases, timely recovery and mobilization might be achieved earlier after primary amputation.

## PRINCIPLES OF TUMOR RESECTION AT THE FOOT AND ANKLE

The implementation of a radical surgical procedure in the distal region of the limb is often difficult due to a limited soft-tissue situation. Attainment of clear margins becomes much more difficult in distal tumors and can result in soft-tissue defects. Plastic surgical techniques remain particularly indispensable in the treatment of such distal tumors. The extent of resection after histological confirmation depends on the size, grading, and local relationship to functional structures. Decisions regarding further leading reconstructive procedures also depend on it. Negative margins should be the goal of surgical therapy. Performance of the appropriate margins in soft-tissue sarcomas is often complicated by the extended growth of the tumor. Margins to adjacent functional structures should be taken into account in the oncosurgical considerations. These functional structures are fascia, synovia, periosteum, and perivascular and perineural tissue. When there is tumor infiltration of such structures, en-block resection should be performed. The course of vascular structures should be taken into account during the resection to allow planning of reconstructive procedures by using pedicled or free tissue transplantation.

## ANATOMICAL AND SURGICAL FEATURES

Whereas limb salvage has become the standard of care in the treatment of tumor in an extremity, the unique anatomy of the foot presents challenges in reconstructing a viable and functional limb. The defect coverage in the area of the foot and ankle region is demanding due to complex anatomical features and functional requirements. The skeletal stability of the foot and ankle region, the resilience of the soft tissues, and the preservation of sensation are at the forefront of reconstructive considerations. Here, profound knowledge of the anatomy of the foot and ankle area is essential for the development of a rational treatment algorithm for covering soft-tissue defects. Hidalgo and Shaw studied the arterial anatomy and the cutaneous nerve supply of the plantar skin extensively in the 1980s, providing guidelines of safe plantar incisions and flap design (25, 26). Prior to their work, flap designs on the plantar aspect of the foot were based on the concept that blood supply proceeds from the deep to the superficial tissue. Therefore, plantar flaps were usually raised subfascially requiring extensive dissection of the plantar soft tissue and, thus, resulting in severe foot and donor site morbidities (27). However, Hidalgo and Shaw demonstrated that local flaps at the plantar aspect could be designed with preserved sensitivity and abundant blood supply as reliable and safe alternatives without the need of subfascial dissection. Based on their findings, they further divided the foot into four major areas based on different requirements for reconstruction and the types of flaps available (28, 29). These are the proximal and distal weight-bearing plantar areas, the dorsum and the ankle region including the malleoli, the Achilles tendon, and the non-weight-bearing heel area. Furthermore, they provided a classification of foot defects and an algorithm of their coverage whose principles are still relevant. They preferred to cover soft-tissue losses less than 3 $cm^2$ with local flaps in weight-bearing areas and with skin grafts in non-weight-bearing areas (Type I). Local flaps are more durable than skin grafts and allow normal weight-bearing on the reconstructed surface. Plain local flaps, such as V-Y flaps and transposition flaps, should be preferred to avoid a soft-tissue surplus, which could enhance strains on the scar at walking and, thus, increasing the risk of ulceration. Skin grafting represents a simple and safe procedure to cover small defects with a well-vascularized wound bed. However, skin grafts are usually suitable for smaller defects at the dorsum and non-weight-bearing areas at the instep but are fragile and can generate painful scars and ulcerations when transplanted on tenuous soft tissue. Therefore, Hidalgo and Shaw do not recommend skin grafting alone for larger defects. Such Type II defects, which are defined to be larger than 3 $cm^2$ without bone involvement were preferred to be covered by free fasciocutaneous, free musculocutaneous flaps, or local flaps to ensure a durable soft-tissue coverage preventing recurrent ulcerations, improving the scar qualities, and reducing strains on the scars. Large tissue losses with bone involvement (Type III) were recommended to be reconstructed with free flaps or free osteocutaneous transfers if necessary. Here, adequate soft-tissue coverage also provides an essential base for following necessary surgical bone procedures. Bulky soft-tissue surpluses can be thinned out easily in future procedures after healing.

The reconstruction of the highly specific, thick, load-capable, and stress-resistant skin of the weight-bearing proximal and distal plantar area is more difficult, because the patient's own tissue from other donor regions of the body does not often meet the requirements with regard to tissue quality and functional needs. By contrast, soft-tissue coverage of the dorsum of the foot and the ankle region is of thin and pliable skin with a delicate subcutaneous adipose tissue layer. This feature is often severe in surgical interventions, for example, in osteosynthetic care of ankle fractures. In this case, due to the peculiarity of the soft-tissue cover, wound complications with exposure of structures, such as tendons, joint capsule, bone, and hardware, can occur. Furthermore, the mobility of the soft tissue covering the foot and ankle is due to quite limited multiple zones of adherence. Consequently, defects in serving areas can rarely be treated by local tissue displacement. In such cases, tissue from other parts of the body must be free transplanted. However, the tissue units used for microvascularized transfer are often bulky and have to be thinned out and adapted in the course of correction operations for subsequent shoe care and esthetic perception. Furthermore, the fact that the free transplanted tissue is not innervated must be considered. This fact may stimulate the formation of pressure ulcers. The reconstruction of complex defects of the foot has experienced a steady improvement in recent decades. Achievements in the therapy have been kept particularly for innovative surgical techniques and a better understanding of the specific tissue situation and functional requirements of the foot and ankle area.

## PLASTIC SURGICAL RECONSTRUCTION OPTIONS

Tumor removal is often accompanied by major tissue defects. Furthermore, there might be an exposure of functional structures, such as bones, tendons, nerves, and blood vessels. Therefore, plastic surgical reconstruction methods must be an integral part of oncosurgical treatment concepts. Moreover, transfer of healthy tissue with adequate blood supply enables adjuvant radiation and chemotherapy, and might improve the effectiveness by improving oxygen nourishment in the tumor bed. A simple reconstructive procedure, such as skin grafting, is, therefore, not usual, since the resulting soft-tissue coverage is often insufficient for adjuvant radiotherapy. However, the reconstructive ladder should still be addressed when considering soft-tissue coverage at the foot and ankle area. Some local flaps have proven to be very efficacious in the treatment of foot and ankle defects. Small defects at the non-weight-bearing sole can be covered by simple cutaneous or myocutaneous V-Y flaps. Due to its reliable vascular supply, its proportions and the moderate donor site defect, the distally based sural flap has proven itself in the coverage of smaller defects at the hind foot and malleolar region (30–33). The dominant pedicle of the distally based sural artery flap is a branch arising from the popliteal artery descending from the popliteal fossa between the heads of the gastrocnemius muscle. It is accompanied by the medial sural cutaneous nerve from the tibial nerve and small venae comitantes. The sural artery flap is a fasciocutaneous flap located at the proximal dorsal area of the lower leg. Elevation of the flap proceeds proximally after visualization of the entrance of the dominant pedicle into the deep fascia in a subfascial plane until an adequate arc of rotation is achieved. Notably, the pivot point of the pedicle should be at least 5 cm proximal of the lateral malleolus in order to preserve the anastomoses with the peroneal artery. The maximum size of the distally based sural flap is limited because of its slight perfusion provided by the arterial network surrounding the sensory medial sural cutaneous nerve. Delayed distally based sural flaps can be raised larger and present an improved reliability but require a two-step surgical approach (34). Such delayed reverse sural flaps are particularly suited for small hind foot defects (35, 36). However, defects at the weight-bearing hind foot should ideally be reconstructed with sensible local flaps to avoid ulcerations. Mendieta et al. reported a case of a heel defect in which they connected the severed nerve end of a distally based sural flap with the intermediate dorsal cutaneous branch of the superficial peroneal nerve to give sensibility to the flap (37). Tan et al. recently reported a case series of such neurotized distally based sural flaps in 14 patients where all flaps survived and two-point discrimination achieved at least 14 mm after 6 months (38). The neurotized sural flap represents an interesting modification for the sensory reconstruction of weight-bearing hind foot defects and upcoming studies deserve attention. In the armamentarium of local flaps, the instep-island flap based on the medial plantar neurovascular pedicle provides another option for the sensory soft-tissue reconstruction of small hind foot defects (39, 40). The instep-island flap occupies the skin of the non-weight-bearing instep between the first metatarsal head and the distal portion of the heel. The flap is elevated distally deep to the plantar fasica and dissection continues proximally toward the medial plantar artery and nerve. Here, the medial plantar nerve can be split from distal to proximal in order to preserve the sensitivity of the flap and the medial foot (41, 42). The instep-island flap is suited for smaller defects, and the donor site must usually be transplanted with a skin graft.

If local flaps are not applicable for soft-tissue coverage, free tissue transfers can be utilized. Following the resection of a malignant tumor in the foot, the use of microvascularized tissue has been proven to be a successful surgical technique, offering an alternative to ablative surgery with functional restoration of the salvaged limb. Large defects of the foot can be treated by free microvascular myocutaneous or fasciocutaneous tissue transfer. If small defects, exposing bones or tendons, are not eligible for local flaps, small free microvascular flaps can be applied. These flaps cause a very low donor site morbidity. Myocutaneous and fasciocutaneous flaps have the advantage of replacing the missing tissue volume. Osseous surfaces can also be adequately covered and padded. If local flaps are not available, the implementation of a free tissue transfer should be taken into consideration. Such flaps provide adequate soft-tissue coverage for adjuvant radiation. A new group of propeller perforator flaps based on perforators from the anterior and posterior tibial artery and from the peroneal artery has been established in recent years, which also allows good defect management. In the Tokyo consensus, a propeller flap is defined as an island flap that reaches the recipient site through an axial rotation. The classification is based on the nourishing pedicle (subcutaneous pedicled propeller flap, perforator pedicled propeller flap, and supercharged propeller flap), the degrees of skin island rotation (from 90 to 180°), and, when possible, the artery of origin of the perforator (43, 44). Dong et al. recently reported a series of 20 patients with soft-tissue defects of the lower leg and foot that were covered by perforator pedicled propeller flaps (45). All flaps survived and the areas of soft-tissue defect ranged from 2 cm × 8cm to 10 cm × 20 cm. The donor sites could be closed primarily in 12 patients and skin grafted in 8 patients. Georgescu et al. reported another retrospectively analyzed series using perforator pedicled propeller flaps in 24 diabetic patients with acute and chronic wounds at the foot (46). A primary healing rate (96%) was obtained in 72% of all cases, whereas flap necrosis occurred in 24% and complete flap loss in 4%. Specific data after oncological resection and adjuvant therapy are still missing to date, but in experienced hands and in well selected cases, propeller perforator flaps can cover defects at the foot and ankle region reliably and provide an alternative to free flaps. In our experience, plastic reconstructive procedures after tumor resection in the foot and ankle area are required in about 50% of cases and are associated with a high success rate. Free transplants, such as fasciocutaneous flaps from the anterolateral thigh (ALT) and parascapular region, and also myocutaneous flaps, such as latissimus flap with or without a skin island, dominate. The ALT flap represents a versatile fasciocutaneous flap and is located at the anterolateral surface of the thigh (**Figures 1** and **2**). Its dominant pedicle proceeds from the septocutaneous or myocutaneous perforators of the descending branch of the lateral circumflex femoral artery. Primary closure of the donor site is usually possible when the flap width is 10 cm or less. Larger flaps need skin grafting of the donor site. Depending on the distribution of the subcutaneous fat in corpulent patients, the ALT flap might be less bulky than the parascapular flap in some cases and, thus, should be preferred in the soft-tissue reconstruction of the foot. The parascapular flap is a fasciocutaneous flap of the posterior trunk and is nourished by the descending branch of the circumflex scapular artery, which emerges from the triangular space between teres major, teres minor, and the long head of the triceps brachii muscle (**Figures 3** and **4**). The parascapular flap can be harvested up to 12 cm in width and 25 cm in length with primary closure. Similar to the parascapular flap, the latissimus dorsi muscle flap is also one of the most versatile flaps available to soft-tissue reconstruction (**Figure 5**). The expendable muscle with its reliable pedicle (thoracodorsal artery) can be harvested with or without a skin island from the posterior trunk and is excellently suited for widespread defects. The donor site morbidity of most free flaps is moderate and well tolerated by most of the patients, especially if the donor site can be closed primarily (47–49). Despite the adjuvant radiotherapy applied, the postoperative complications are tolerable and do not limit the use of microvascular tissue transfer.

As a reconstructive option after tumor resection, local flaps represent a reliable tool and can cover a wide range of smaller defects. Nevertheless, concerns over distant iatrogenic implantation of tumor cells at the donor site of local flaps exist when tumor resection and flap coverage were performed in the same surgical procedure. Reviewing the literature, there has, unfortunately, been no systematic analysis on this issue. However, iatrogenic

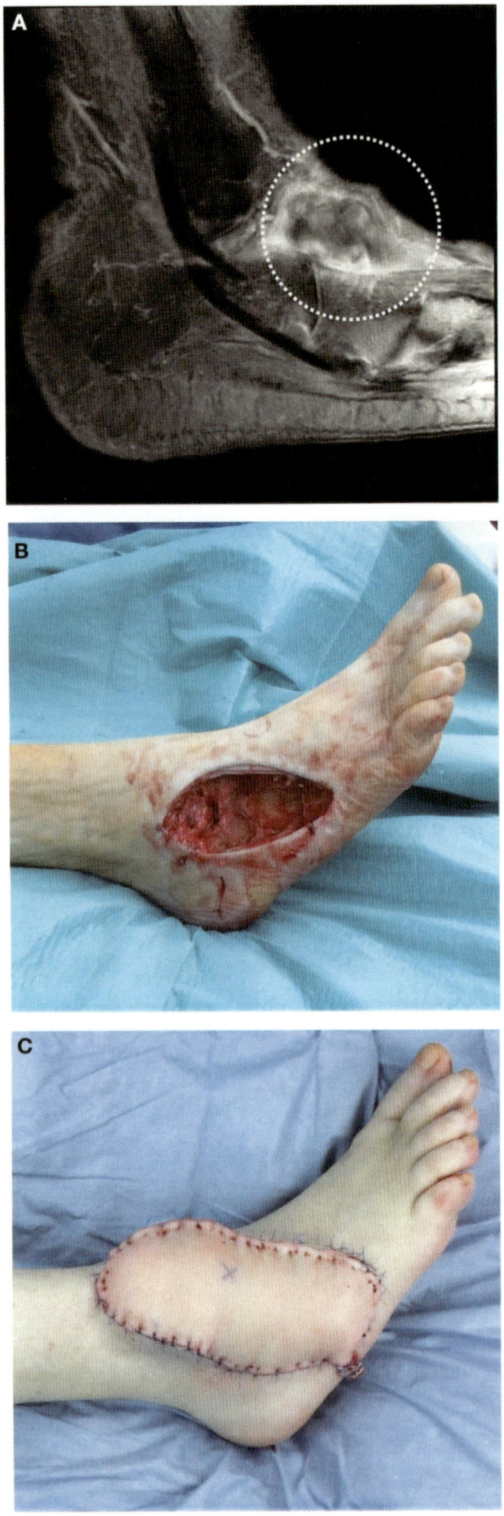

**FIGURE 1 | A 77-year-old female was presented after incomplete resection of a liposarcoma G2 on the lateral ankle of her right foot.** The initial tumor localization is shown by MRI image **(A)**. A two-stage reconstruction of the defect after extensive resection **(B)** was done by free transplantation of an adipocutaneous flap **(C)** from the anterolateral region of the thigh (ALT flap).

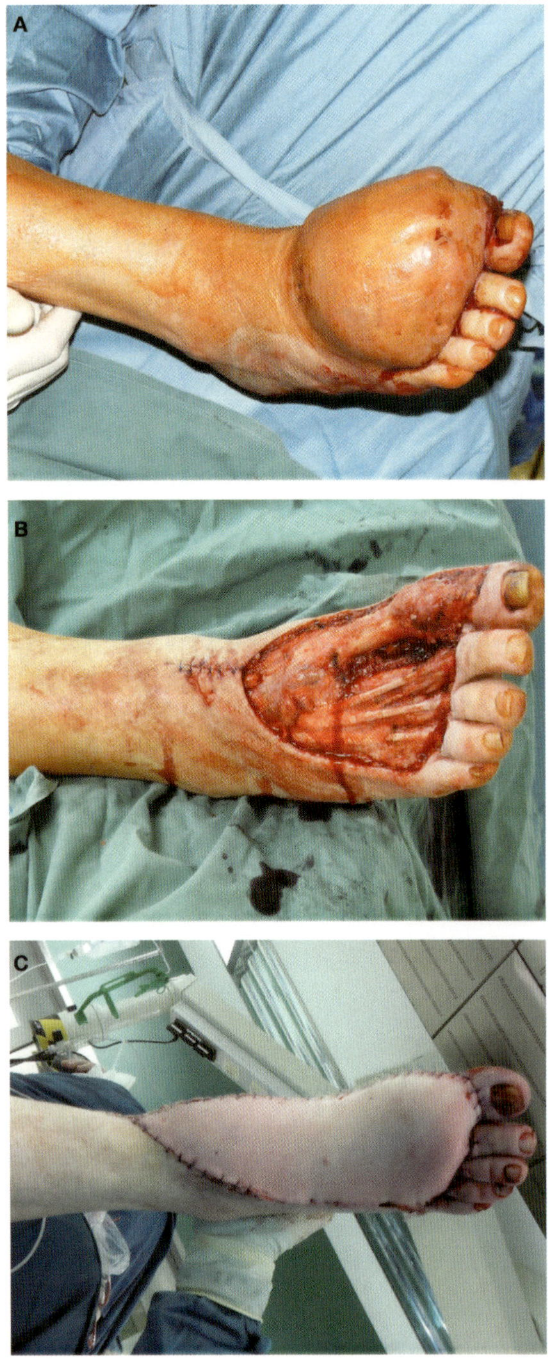

**FIGURE 2 | A 62-year-old male presented with first diagnosis of a myxoid fibrosacoma G2 at the dorsum of his right foot (A).** After oncological tumor resection, the defect was reconstructed with a free fasciocutaneous ALT flap from the thigh **(B,C)**.

tumor metastases at donor tissue sites after local flap reconstruction are a rare occurrence and should not preclude the use of local flap reconstruction (50). They have been described only in selected case reports (51). Furthermore, the effect of donor site radiation on the incidence of iatrogenic tumor metastases

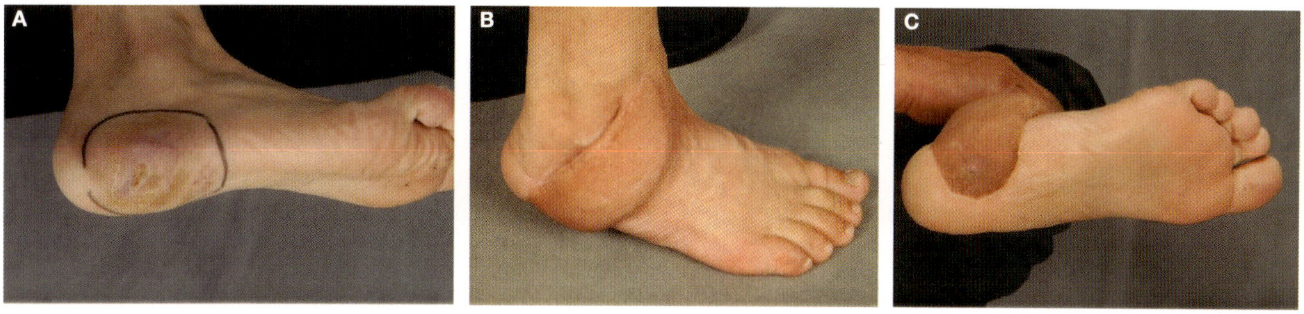


**FIGURE 3 | A 49-year-old male with a clear cell sarcoma G2 localized on his right foot (A).** The patient was transferred to our department for oncological resection and plastic reconstruction after an incomplete tumor resection. The coverage of the soft-tissue defect about the load-exposed part of the sole was performed by a free fasciocutaneous flap **(B,C)** from the parascapular area.

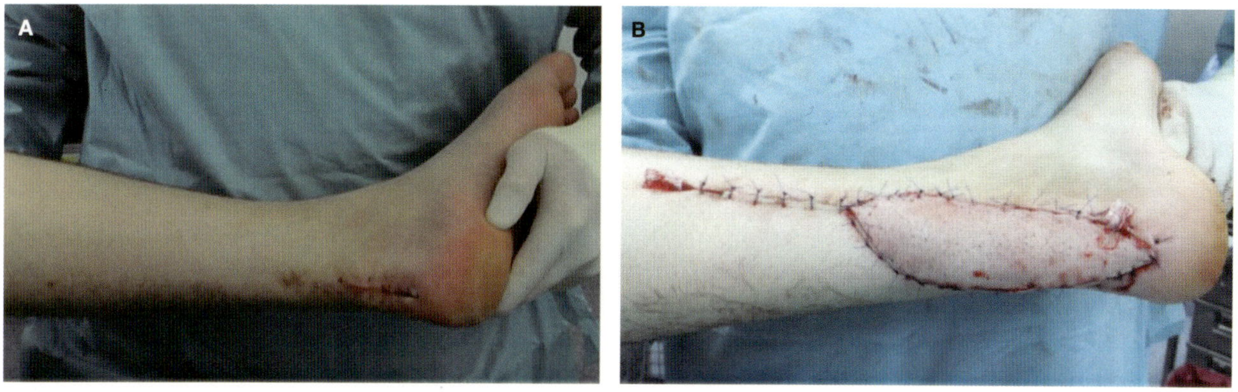


**FIGURE 4 | A 54-year-old male with infiltrative myxoid fibrosarcoma G2 of the Achilles' tendon of his left leg and R2 status after foreign surgery (A).** Reconstructive procedure after oncological resection was performed by use of a free parascapular flap **(B)**.

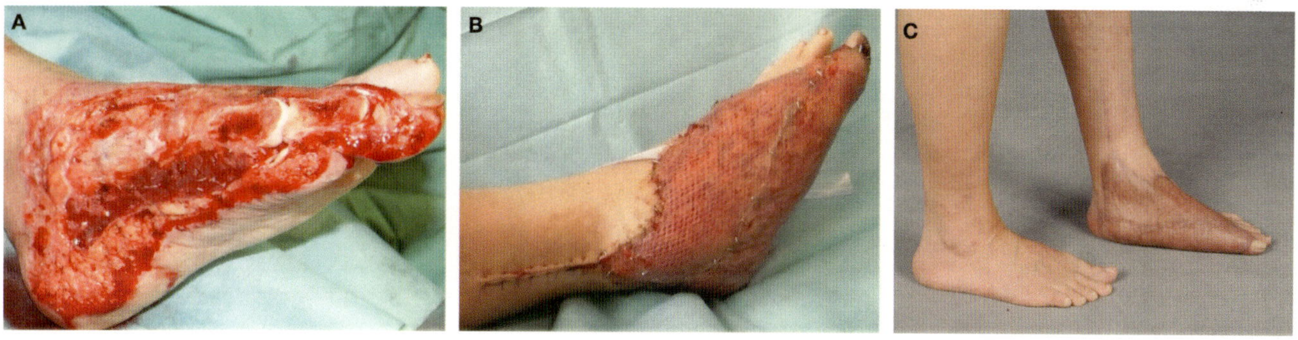


**FIGURE 5 | A 46-year-old female with soft-tissue defect on her left foot after tumor resection (A).** The reconstruction was carried out by free transplantation of a latissimus dorsi muscle with split skin **(A,B).** Image of the foot after healing **(C)**.

still remains unclear and should be examined (50). Beside the aforementioned concerns, local flaps can offer some slight but noteworthy advantages. In contrast to free flaps, local flaps do not require intensive postoperative flap inspections. Postoperative positioning protocols and anticoagulation regimens are less stringent. However, there has been a paradigm shift in the last few decades. Free tissue transfers can be performed with the same or even higher degree of safety than local flap transfer as a result of the improvements in microsurgical techniques nowadays. Safe dissection and positioning of a local flap at the hind foot can be technically more demanding, risky, and time-consuming when compared to a free flap transfer in a two-team approach. Due to the microsurgical and anesthesiological improvements, free flap transfers have become physically less demanding surgical procedures and have also become suitable for patients with vascular comorbidities.

Unfortunately, not all postoperative wound complications can be anticipated. For defects that extend to the tendons or joints, flap reconstruction is always required for adequate closure. A forced wound closure and "unexpected" wound complications can be slow to heal, devastating for the patient, and delay adjuvant radiotherapy. In this instance, early referral to a plastic surgeon is necessary in these cases to prevent devitalized superficial tissue from becoming infected and generating a deep infection that involves tendon, bone, or hardware. The use of free tissue transfer remains at the highest level on the reconstructive ladder. Although it is more complex, free tissue transfer may be necessary as a first choice. Our experience indicates that microvascularized tissue transfer is often the most suitable first option in accordance with established reconstructive principles. Furthermore, wound complications can occur more often after adjuvant radiation. Although defects, at first appearance, may be closed primarily or by using simple methods, such as split-thickness skin grafts, one must take the possibility of postoperative and postradiogenic wound complication into consideration. In those cases where there is an increased risk of exposure of tendons, bones or osteosynthetic material, a prophylactic use of an effective free flap for reconstruction should be considered. In the presence of avascular scar tissue, it should be removed before reconstruction. The use of prophylactic flaps in foot and ankle reconstruction is of great interest in patients with a high risk of wound healing disorders.

In addition to transplantation of tissue to cover the defects, the replacement of functional structures, such as tendons, vessels, and nerves, are at the forefront. Common peroneal nerve lesions or extensive loss of the anterior tibialis muscle might be an inevitable part of oncological resection and lead to a drop foot deformity. Primary transfer of the posterior tibialis tendon to the anterior tibialis tendon can restore the active extension of the foot (52, 53). There have been several technical modifications of this procedure to date and most of them improve the extremity function notably (54, 55). Indications for the oncological resection of the tibial or peroneal nerve are fortunately rare, but, if necessary, nerve grafting using the sural nerve can restore some protective touch sensibility at the plantar foot even after nerve defects of several centimeters (56, 57). However, there are still controversies about the timing of nerve grafting, especially when adjuvant radiation treatment is planned. There are missing specific data for peroneal and tibial nerve reconstructions to date, but a very recent study that analyzed the functional outcome of multiple sural nerve grafts for facial nerve defects after oncological resection could not detect any adverse effects of adjuvant radiation treatment on the outcome of the nerve grafts and endorsed an immediate nerve grafting after primary tumor resection (58).

## CONCLUSION

Surgical therapy provides the basis for local tumor control in soft-tissue sarcoma. The goal defined is the resection of the tumor with clear surgical margins, followed by adjuvant radiotherapy in highly malignant tumors. In many cases, more complex plastic surgical reconstructions, such as the replacement of nerves, blood vessels, and bone, or transfer of muscles or tendons, are required due to the close proximity to functionally relevant anatomical structures. Defects can be covered by means of plastic surgery techniques so that the foremost unresectable tumors become curable. In our institution, we use the treatment algorithm depicted in **Figure 6** in order to cover most of the defects resulting after tumor resection.

At the present time, due to efforts in reconstructive plastic surgery, complex tumor resection with clear margins can be performed while still preserving the function that once may have been considered unsalvageable, particularly in the case of advanced tumors.

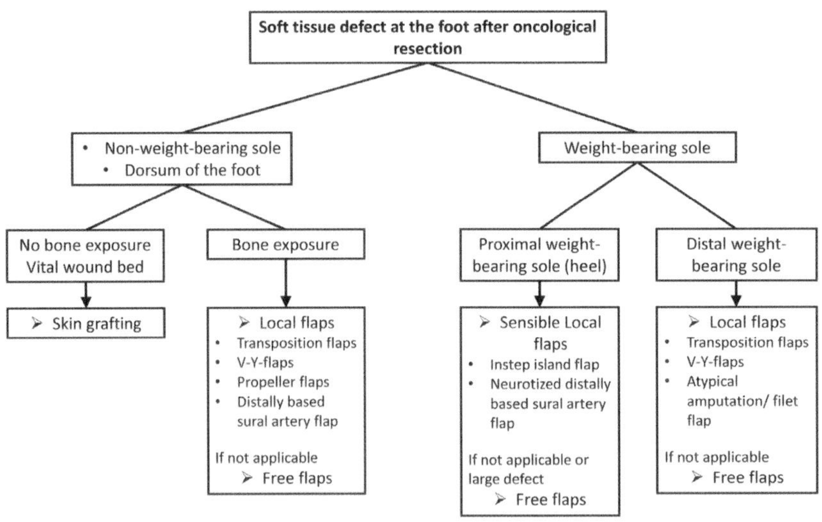


**FIGURE 6 | Treatment algorithm for soft-tissue reconstructions at the foot after oncological resection.**

Patients are frequently presented with incompletely resected tumors. In such situations, the resection required is usually far more complex and extensive than the primary intervention. Due to this fact and the rarity and wide heterogeneity of soft-tissue sarcomas, they should be treated in specialized centers with plastic surgery as part of an interdisciplinary and multimodal treatment concept.

Our experience shows that reconstructive plastic surgery can play an integral role in the multimodal treatment concept including radiation and chemotherapy. The current plastic surgery techniques allow for the preservation and reconstruction of function after the resection of malignant tumors. The quality of life of the oncologic patient can be significantly improved by knowing and applying the opportunities of plastic reconstructive surgery.

## AUTHOR CONTRIBUTIONS

AR and KH have written and prepared the manuscript. AD and ML reviewed and edited the manuscript. OG, PK, and BB helped to prepare the manuscript and the figures.

## REFERENCES


1. Weiss SW, Goldblum JR, Folpe AL. *Enzinger and Weiss's Soft Tissue Tumors*. Philadelphia, USA: Elsevier Health Sciences (2007).
2. Karakousis CP, De Young C, Driscoll DL. Soft tissue sarcomas of the hand and foot: management and survival. *Ann Surg Oncol* (1998) **5**(3):238–40. doi:10.1007/BF02303779
3. Lin PP, Guzel VB, Pisters PW, Zagars GK, Weber KL, Feig BW, et al. Surgical management of soft tissue sarcomas of the hand and foot. *Cancer* (2002) **95**(4):852–61. doi:10.1002/cncr.10750
4. Billingsley KG, Lewis JJ, Leung DH, Casper ES, Woodruff JM, Brennan MF. Multifactorial analysis of the survival of patients with distant metastasis arising from primary extremity sarcoma. *Cancer* (1999) **85**(2):389–95. doi:10.1002/(SICI)1097-0142(19990115)85:2<389::AID-CNCR17>3.3.CO;2-A
5. Steinau HU, Daigeler A, Langer S, Steinstrasser L, Hauser J, Goertz O, et al. Limb salvage in malignant tumors. *Semin Plast Surg* (2010) **24**(1):18–33. doi:10.1055/s-0030-1253240
6. Kandel R, Coakley N, Werier J, Engel J, Ghert M, Verma S, et al. Surgical margins and handling of soft-tissue sarcoma in extremities: a clinical practice guideline. *Curr Oncol* (2013) **20**(3):e247–54. doi:10.3747/co.20.1308
7. Stojadinovic A, Jaques DP, Leung DH, Healey JH, Brennan MF. Amputation for recurrent soft tissue sarcoma of the extremity: indications and outcome. *Ann Surg Oncol* (2001) **8**(6):509–18. doi:10.1007/s10434-001-0509-3
8. Stojadinovic A, Leung DH, Allen P, Lewis JJ, Jaques DP, Brennan MF. Primary adult soft tissue sarcoma: time-dependent influence of prognostic variables. *J Clin Oncol* (2002) **20**(21):4344–52. doi:10.1200/JCO.2002.07.154
9. Stojadinovic A, Leung DH, Hoos A, Jaques DP, Lewis JJ, Brennan MF. Analysis of the prognostic significance of microscopic margins in 2,084 localized primary adult soft tissue sarcomas. *Ann Surg* (2002) **235**(3):424–34. doi:10.1097/00000658-200203000-00015
10. Gronchi A, Casali PG, Mariani L, Miceli R, Fiore M, Lo Vullo S, et al. Status of surgical margins and prognosis in adult soft tissue sarcomas of the extremities: a series of patients treated at a single institution. *J Clin Oncol* (2005) **23**(1):96–104. doi:10.1200/JCO.2005.04.160
11. Steinau HU, Steinstrasser L, Hauser J, Tilkorn D, Stricker I, Daigeler A. [Soft tissue sarcoma. Resection and plastic reconstruction]. *Orthopade* (2012) **41**(2):165–75. doi:10.1007/s00132-011-1876-5
12. Lehnhardt M, Daigeler A, Homann HH, Schwaiberger V, Goertz O, Kuhnen C, et al. MFH revisited: outcome after surgical treatment of undifferentiated pleomorphic or not otherwise specified (NOS) sarcomas of the extremities – an analysis of 140 patients. *Langenbecks Arch Surg* (2009) **394**(2):313–20. doi:10.1007/s00423-008-0368-5
13. Karakousis CP. Refinements of surgical technique in soft tissue sarcomas. *J Surg Oncol* (2010) **101**(8):730–8. doi:10.1002/jso.21563
14. Kaushal A, Citrin D. The role of radiation therapy in the management of sarcomas. *Surg Clin North Am* (2008) **88**(3):629–46. doi:10.1016/j.suc.2008.03.005
15. Pisters PW, Pollock RE, Lewis VO, Yasko AW, Cormier JN, Respondek PM, et al. Long-term results of prospective trial of surgery alone with selective use of radiation for patients with T1 extremity and trunk soft tissue sarcomas. *Ann Surg* (2007) **246**(4):675–81. doi:10.1097/SLA.0b013e318155a9ae
16. Karakousis CP, Zografos GC. Radiation therapy for high grade soft tissue sarcomas of the extremities treated with limb-preserving surgery. *Eur J Surg Oncol* (2002) **28**(4):431–6. doi:10.1053/ejso.2002.1264
17. Potter BK, Hwang PF, Forsberg JA, Hampton CB, Graybill JC, Peoples GE, et al. Impact of margin status and local recurrence on soft-tissue sarcoma outcomes. *J Bone Joint Surg Am* (2013) **95**(20):e1511–8. doi:10.2106/JBJS.L.01149
18. Kasper B, Ouali M, van Glabbeke M, Blay JY, Bramwell VH, Woll PJ, et al. Prognostic factors in adolescents and young adults (AYA) with high risk soft tissue sarcoma (STS) treated by adjuvant chemotherapy: a study based on pooled European Organisation for Research and Treatment of Cancer (EORTC) clinical trials 62771 and 62931. *Eur J Cancer* (2013) **49**(2):449–56. doi:10.1016/j.ejca.2012.08.007
19. Daigeler A, Harati K, Goertz O, Hirsch T, Steinau HU, Lehnhardt M. [Prognostic factors and surgical tactics in patients with locally recurrent soft tissue sarcomas]. *Handchir Mikrochir Plast Chir* (2015) **47**(2):118–27. doi:10.1055/s-0034-1394425
20. Daigeler A, Zmarsly I, Hirsch T, Goertz O, Steinau HU, Lehnhardt M, et al. Long-term outcome after local recurrence of soft tissue sarcoma: a retrospective analysis of factors predictive of survival in 135 patients with locally recurrent soft tissue sarcoma. *Brit J Cancer* (2014) **110**(6):1456–64. doi:10.1038/bjc.2014.21
21. Lewis JJ, Leung D, Casper ES, Woodruff J, Hajdu SI, Brennan MF. Multifactorial analysis of long-term follow-up (more than 5 years) of primary extremity sarcoma. *Arch Surg* (1999) **134**(2):190–4. doi:10.1001/archsurg.134.2.190
22. Trovik CS. Scanadinavian Sarcoma Group P. Local recurrence of soft tissue sarcoma. A Scandinavian Sarcoma Group Project. *Acta Orthop Scand Suppl* (2001) **72**(300):1–31. doi:10.1080/000164701317323417
23. Deroose JP, Eggermont AM, van Geel AN, Burger JW, den Bakker MA, de Wilt JH, et al. Long-term results of tumor necrosis factor alpha- and melphalan-based isolated limb perfusion in locally advanced extremity soft tissue sarcomas. *J Clin Oncol* (2011) **29**(30):4036–44. doi:10.1200/JCO.2011.35.6618
24. Deroose JP, Grunhagen DJ, de Wilt JH, Eggermont AM, Verhoef C. Treatment modifications in tumour necrosis factor-alpha (TNF)-based isolated limb perfusion in patients with advanced extremity soft tissue sarcomas. *Eur J Cancer* (2015) **51**(3):367–73. doi:10.1016/j.ejca.2014.11.020
25. Hidalgo DA, Shaw WW. Anatomic basis of plantar flap design. *Plast Reconstr Surg* (1986) **78**(5):627–36.
26. Shaw WW, Hidalgo DA. Anatomic basis of plantar flap design: clinical applications. *Plast Reconstr Surg* (1986) **78**(5):637–49. doi:10.1097/00006534-198611000-00012
27. Gahalaut P, Pinto J, Pai GS, Kamath J, Joshua TV. A novel treatment for plantar ulcers in leprosy: local superficial flaps. *Lepr Rev* (2005) **76**(3):220–31.
28. Hidalgo DA, Shaw WW. Reconstruction of foot injuries. *Clin Plast Surg* (1986) **13**(4):663–80.
29. Spyropoulou A, Jeng SF. Microsurgical coverage reconstruction in upper and lower extremities. *Semin Plast Surg* (2010) **24**(1):34–42. doi:10.1055/s-0030-1253244
30. Chang SM, Li XH, Gu YD. Distally based perforator sural flaps for foot and ankle reconstruction. *World J Orthop* (2015) **6**(3):322–30. doi:10.5312/wjo.v6.i3.322
31. Jordan DJ, Malahias M, Hindocha S, Juma A. Flap decisions and options in soft tissue coverage of the lower limb. *Open Orthop J* (2014) **8**:423–32. doi:10.2174/1874325001408010423
32. Mileto D, Cotrufo S, Cuccia G, Delia G, Risitano G, Colonna MR, et al. The distally based sural flap for lower leg reconstruction: versatility in patients with associated morbidity. *Ann Ital Chir* (2007) **78**(4):323–7.

33. Akhtar S, Hameed A. Versatility of the sural fasciocutaneous flap in the coverage of lower third leg and hind foot defects. *J Plast Reconstr Aesthet Surg* (2006) **59**(8):839–45. doi:10.1016/j.bjps.2005.12.009
34. Kneser U, Bach AD, Polykandriotis E, Kopp J, Horch RE. Delayed reverse sural flap for staged reconstruction of the foot and lower leg. *Plast Reconstr Surg* (2005) **116**(7):1910–7. doi:10.1097/01.prs.0000189204.71906.c2
35. Ali F, Harunarashid H, Yugasmavanan K. Delayed reverse sural flap for cover of heel defect in a patient with associated vascular injury. A case report. *Indian J Surg* (2013) **75**(Suppl 1):148–9.
36. Ali MA, Chowdhury P, Ali M, Ifteker Ibne Z, Dev J. Distally-based sural island flap for soft tissue coverage of ankle and heel defects. *J Coll Physicians Surg Pak* (2010) **20**(7):475–7.
37. Mendieta MJ, Roblero C, Vega JC. Neurotized distally based sural flap for heel reconstruction. *J Reconstr Microsurg* (2013) **29**(8):501–4. doi:10.1055/s-0033-1348034
38. Tan O, Aydin OE, Demir R, Barin EZ, Cinal H, Algan S. Neurotized sural flap: an alternative in sensory reconstruction of the foot and ankle defects. *Microsurgery* (2015) **35**(3):183–9. doi:10.1002/micr.22325
39. Bibbo C. Plantar heel reconstruction with a sensate plantar medial artery musculocutaneous pedicled island flap after wide excision of melanoma. *J Foot Ankle Surg* (2012) **51**(4):504–8. doi:10.1053/j.jfas.2012.04.017
40. Kwan MK, Merican AM, Ahmad TS. Reconstruction of the heel defect with in-step island flap. A report of four cases. *Med J Malaysia* (2005) **60**(Suppl C):104–7.
41. Mourougayan V. Medial plantar artery (instep flap) flap. *Ann Plast Surg* (2006) **56**(2):160–3. doi:10.1097/01.sap.0000190830.71132.b8
42. Yang D, Yang JF, Morris SF, Tang M, Nie C. Medial plantar artery perforator flap for soft-tissue reconstruction of the heel. *Ann Plast Surg* (2011) **67**(3):294–8. doi:10.1097/SAP.0b013e3181f9b278
43. Georgescu AV. Propeller perforator flaps in distal lower leg: evolution and clinical applications. *Arch Plast Surg* (2012) **39**(2):94–105. doi:10.5999/aps.2012.39.2.94
44. Pignatti M, Ogawa R, Hallock GG, Mateev M, Georgescu AV, Balakrishnan G, et al. The "Tokyo" consensus on propeller flaps. *Plast Reconstr Surg* (2011) **127**(2):716–22. doi:10.1097/PRS.0b013e3181fed6b2
45. Dong KX, Xu YQ, Fan XY, Xu LJ, Su XX, Long H, et al. Perforator pedicled propeller flaps for soft tissue coverage of lower leg and foot defects. *Orthop Surg* (2014) **6**(1):42–6. doi:10.1111/os.12081
46. Georgescu AV, Matei IR, Capota IM. The use of propeller perforator flaps for diabetic limb salvage: a retrospective review of 25 cases. *Diabet Foot Ankle* (2012) **3**. doi:10.3402/dfa.v3i0.18978
47. Fischer S, Klinkenberg M, Behr B, Hirsch T, Kremer T, Hernekamp F, et al. Comparison of donor-site morbidity and satisfaction between anterolateral thigh and parascapular free flaps in the same patient. *J Reconstr Microsurg* (2013) **29**(8):537–44. doi:10.1055/s-0033-1351394
48. Klinkenberg M, Fischer S, Kremer T, Hernekamp F, Lehnhardt M, Daigeler A. Comparison of anterolateral thigh, lateral arm, and parascapular free flaps with regard to donor-site morbidity and aesthetic and functional outcomes. *Plast Reconstr Surg* (2013) **131**(2):293–302. doi:10.1097/PRS.0b013e31827786bc
49. Sauerbier M, Dittler S, Kreutzer C. Microsurgical chest wall reconstruction after oncologic resections. *Semin Plast Surg* (2011) **25**(1):60–9. doi:10.1055/s-0031-1275172
50. Saba SC, Shaterian A, Tokin C, Dobke MK, Wallace AM. The pedicled myocutaneous flap as a choice reconstructive technique for immediate adjuvant brachytherapy in sarcoma treatment. *Curr Oncol* (2012) **19**(6):e491–5. doi:10.3747/co.19.1141
51. Hughes TM, Thomas JM. Sarcoma metastases due to iatrogenic implantation. *Eur J Surg Oncol* (2000) **26**(1):50–2. doi:10.1053/ejso.1999.0740
52. Mehling I, Lanz U, Prommersberger KJ, Fuhrmann RA, van Schoonhoven J. [Transfer of the posterior tibialis tendon to restore an active dorsiflexion of the foot]. *Handchir Mikrochir Plast Chir* (2012) **44**(1):29–34. doi:10.1055/s-0031-1291316
53. Kremer T, Riedel K, Germann G, Heitmann C, Sauerbier M. [Tendon transfers for peroneal palsy – functional outcome]. *Handchir Mikrochir Plast Chir* (2011) **43**(2):95–101. doi:10.1055/s-0030-1269930
54. Steinau HU, Tofaute A, Huellmann K, Goertz O, Lehnhardt M, Kammler J, et al. Tendon transfers for drop foot correction: long-term results including quality of life assessment, and dynamometric and pedobarographic measurements. *Arch Orthop Trauma Surg* (2011) **131**(7):903–10. doi:10.1007/s00402-010-1231-z
55. Vigasio A, Marcoccio I, Patelli A, Mattiuzzo V, Prestini G. New tendon transfer for correction of drop-foot in common peroneal nerve palsy. *Clin Orthop Relat Res* (2008) **466**(6):1454–66. doi:10.1007/s11999-008-0249-9
56. Dellon AL, Mackinnon SE. Results of posterior tibial nerve grafting at the ankle. *J Reconstr Microsurg* (1991) 7(2):81–3. doi:10.1055/s-2007-1006764
57. Nunley JA, Gabel GT. Tibial nerve grafting for restoration of plantar sensation. *Foot Ankle* (1993) **14**(9):489–92. doi:10.1177/107110079301400901
58. Lee MC, Kim DH, Jeon YR, Rah DK, Lew DH, Choi EC, et al. Functional outcomes of multiple sural nerve grafts for facial nerve defects after tumor-ablative surgery. *Arch Plast Surg* (2015) **42**(4):461–8. doi:10.5999/aps.2015.42.4.461

5

# 3D Volumetric Modeling and Microvascular Reconstruction of Irradiated Lumbosacral Defects after Oncologic Resection

*Emilio Garcia-Tutor[1,2], Marco Romeo[1], Michael P. Chae[3,4], David J. Hunter-Smith[3,4] and Warren Matthew Rozen[3,4]**

*[1]Department of Plastic and Reconstructive Surgery, Hospital de Guadalajara, Guadalajara, Spain, [2]MD Anderson Cancer Center, Madrid, Spain, [3]Department of Surgery, School of Clinical Science at Monash Health, Faculty of Medicine, Monash University, Monash Medical Centre, Clayton, VIC, Australia, [4]Monash University Plastic and Reconstructive Surgery Unit (Peninsula Clinical School), Peninsula Health, Frankston, VIC, Australia*

**Background:** Locoregional flaps are sufficient in most sacral reconstructions. However, large sacral defects due to malignancy necessitate a different reconstructive approach, with local flaps compromised by radiation and regional flaps inadequate for broad surface areas or substantial volume obliteration. In this report, we present our experience using free muscle transfer for volumetric reconstruction, in such cases, and demonstrate three-dimensional (3D) haptic models of the sacral defect to aid preoperative planning.

**Methods:** Five consecutive patients with irradiated sacral defects secondary to oncologic resections were included, surface area ranging from 143–600 cm$^2$. Latissimus dorsi (LD)-based free flap sacral reconstruction was performed in each case, between 2005 and 2011. Where the superior gluteal artery was compromised, the subcostal artery (SA) was used as a recipient vessel. Microvascular technique, complications, and outcomes are reported. The use of volumetric analysis and 3D printing is also demonstrated, with imaging data converted to 3D images suitable for 3D printing with Osirix software (Pixmeo, Geneva, Switzerland). An office-based, desktop 3D printer was used to print 3D models of sacral defects, used to demonstrate surface area and contour and produce a volumetric print of the dead space needed for flap obliteration.

**Results:** The clinical series of LD free flap reconstructions is presented, with successful transfer in all cases, and adequate soft-tissue cover and volume obliteration achieved. The original use of the SA as a recipient vessel was successfully achieved. All wounds healed uneventfully. 3D printing is also demonstrated as a useful tool for 3D evaluation of volume and dead space.

**Conclusion:** Free flaps offer unique benefits in sacral reconstruction where local tissue is compromised by irradiation and tumor recurrence, and dead space requires accurate volumetric reconstruction. We describe for the first time the use of the SA as a recipient in free flap sacral reconstruction. 3D printing of haptic bio-models is a rapidly evolving field with a substantial role in preoperative planning.

**Keywords: volumetric analysis, preoperative imaging, planning, free flap, model**

***Edited by:***
*Iain Stuart Whitaker, Swansea University School of Medicine, UK*

***Reviewed by:***
*Fatih Zor, Gulhane Military Medical Academy, Turkey*
*Safak Uygur, Koc University Hospital, Turkey*

***Correspondence:***
*Warren Matthew Rozen*
*warrenrozen@hotmail.com*

***Specialty section:***
*This article was submitted to Reconstructive and Plastic Surgery, a section of the journal Frontiers in Surgery*

## INTRODUCTION

A vast majority of sacral wounds derived from pressure sores can be treated with either a local or regional flap, as conventionally taught (1). However, where wounds span a large area from oncological resection, have substantial volume deficits or involve areas compromised by radiotherapy, locoregional flaps are relatively contraindicated. Radiation induces hypocellularity and hypovascularity in the normal tissue surrounding the tumor compromising its vascularity and, hence, its viability as a flap option (2, 3). Furthermore, reconstruction of the irradiated lumbosacral defects is curtailed by the reduced number and caliber of the vessels at the recipient site. Moreover, the need to restore a composite defect and the proximity of the anal region potentially increases the infection risk and present significant challenges for reconstructive surgeons.

In recent times, reconstructive surgeons have benefited from the availability of three-dimensional (3D) haptic bio-models for preoperative planning and flap designing (4). These models are produced by rapid prototyping (RP) techniques that use scan data from the conventional imaging modalities, such as the computed tomography (CT) and the magnetic resonance imaging (MRI). RP has been utilized in industrial design for decades; however, it has been adopted for medical application only in the last two decades. RP has introduced a convenient method of fabricating physical 3D models that accurately represent the anatomical structures and provide a tactile, or haptic, feedback to the clinician facilitating a superior understanding of the spatial relationship between structures (5). In medicine, stereolithography and 3D printing are the most extensively studied RP techniques. In contrast to stereolithography, 3D printing is a newer technology that is more affordable, quicker, and more convenient (6). 3D-printed haptic models have demonstrated utility in numerous surgical disciplines, such as maxillofacial (6) and orthopedic surgery (7). In plastic and reconstructive surgery, they have been useful in flap designing for soft-tissue defects (8) and preoperative volumetric assessment of breast asymmetry (9).

The current paper reports our experience using a large voluminous free flap for a single-stage reconstruction of irradiated lumbosacral oncologic defects. The technique and surgical outcomes are assessed. The use of 3D haptic models of the sacral defect to aid preoperative planning and volumetric analysis is presented.

## PATIENTS AND METHODS

A case series of five consecutive patients were included, each of which were planned for microvascular reconstruction of an irradiated sacral defect, between 2005 and 2011. The series comprised one female and four males, with a mean age of 41.5 (range: 32–69). Each patient presented with a malignancy in the sacral region that was reconstructed by the senior author (EGT) following oncologic resection and irradiation. The resection was either of a primary or a recurrent tumor and all patients received radiotherapy (**Table 1**). For each case, consideration of a muscle only, myocutaneous or fasciocutaneous flap was considered,

**TABLE 1 | Patient demographics and operative details.**

| Case | Age | Sex | Pathology | Primary/ recurrence | Recipient vessels | Immediate/ delayed | Flap surface dimensions and area | Colostomy required | Complications | Follow-up (years) | Survival outcomes |
|---|---|---|---|---|---|---|---|---|---|---|---|
| 1 | 69 | Male | Squamous cell carcinoma | Recurrence | Superior gluteal artery (SGA) | Immediate | 25 cm x 10 cm = 250 $cm^2$ | Yes | Nil | 3 | Long-term survival |
| 2 | 38 | Male | Squamous cell carcinoma | Primary | Subcostal artery (SA) | Immediate | 18 cm x 20 cm = 360 $cm^2$ | Yes | Nil | 3 | Long-term survival |
| 3 | 35 | Female | Radiation-induced sarcoma | Recurrence | SGA | Immediate | 11 cm x 13 cm = 143 $cm^2$ | No | Nil | 9 | Mortality |
| 4 | 32 | Male | Ewing's sarcoma | Recurrence | SGA | Immediate | 20 cm x 10 cm = 200 $cm^2$ | No | Nil | 7 | Long-term survival |
| 5 | 54 | Male | Squamous cell carcinoma | Primary | SA | Delayed | 20 cm x 30 cm = 600 $cm^2$ | Yes | Wound dehiscence requiring local flap | 5 | Mortality |

with selection based on donor-site availability, volume filling and contour requirements. The specific flap selected in each case is described below.

## Surgical Technique

In delayed reconstructions, the volume and soft-tissue deficit was mapped preoperatively, while in immediate cases, this was able to be estimated based on resection planning. The 2D images from CT and MRI were used for initial evaluation of the planned reconstruction. Preoperative planning also involved the oncologic surgeon in surgical and reconstructive planning, in planning for estimated resection volumes. Flap choice was thus achieved, and where a skin paddle was sought, surface area able to be rapidly and accurately achieved.

The average wound surface was 359 $cm^2$ (range: 200–600 $cm^2$). In two cases, the skin surface defect was small enough for the skin island of the flap to adequately fill the surface defect. In two cases, the surface defects were larger and skin grafting was necessary. In one patient, the defect surface width was too broad and required closure with a tensor fascia lata flap. Regarding wound depth and volume, the LD flaps provided adequate tissue to fill and obliterate the cavity in all cases.

Consideration of a muscle only, myocutaneous or fasciocutaneous flap was considered, with selection based on donor-site availability, volume filling, and contour requirements as evaluated from imaging and bio-models. Ultimately, muscle only or myocutaneous latissimus dorsi (LD) flaps were selected in each case. In all cases, there was a volume requirement that exceeded the filling achievable with a fasciocutaneous flap, and the added benefits the longest pedicle possible was considered. Originally, deep inferior epigastric artery perforator flaps were also considered but were not used ultimately utilized as options.

Whenever they were available (three cases), superior gluteal artery (SGA) was the first-choice recipient vessel. In other cases where the gluteal arteries were damaged during the tumor resection or discarded due to their proximity to the tumor (two cases), subcostal artery (SA) of the eleventh rib was selected. All flap arteries and veins were anastomosed to recipient vessels in an end-to-end fashion. The location of a diverting stoma was planned based on imaging preoperatively and undertaken for wound care and patient positioning considerations.

## Creation of a 3D-Printed Haptic Bio-Model

Imaging with either CT and/or MRI of the sacral region was used for volumetric analysis (see **Figure 1**). Haptic models of sacral defects were fabricated using a 3D printer similar to a technique described previously (9). The 2D scan data from CT or MRI was uploaded on to a computer using a free, third-party software called Osirix (Pixmeo, Geneva, Switzerland). The data were 3D-reconstructed using the "surface rendering" function (see **Figure 2**) and exported into a universal 3D file format called standard tessellation language (STL). The STL file was configured suitable for 3D printing using computer software, Cubify (3D Systems, Rock Hill, SC, USA), which accompanies the 3D printer (Cube 2 printer, 3D Systems). In Cubify (3D Systems), the model was reduced in size to fit within the maximum dimension of the printer (16 cm × 16 cm × 16 cm) and also orientated prone so that the defect was "pointing up" (see **Figure 3**). Due to the mechanism of 3D printing where the thermoplastic filament was deposited in a layer-by-layer fashion, where the defect was "pointing sideways," the printer deposited a support structure to fill the "gap in height" (8). Although the support structures were easily removable, they left a rough surface that compromised the aesthetics of the model. The model was comparable to scan data for volumetric

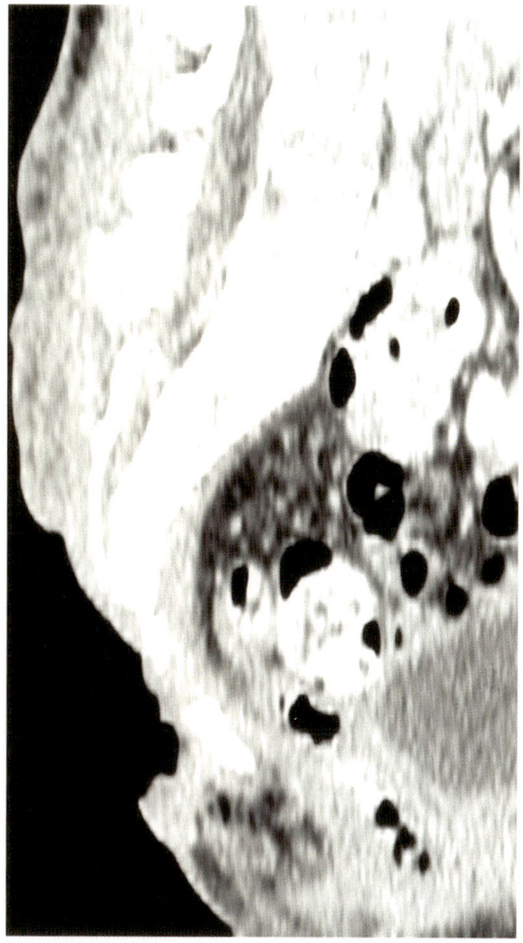

**FIGURE 1** | **Preoperative computed tomography scan, showing the three-dimensional nature of a sacral defect.**

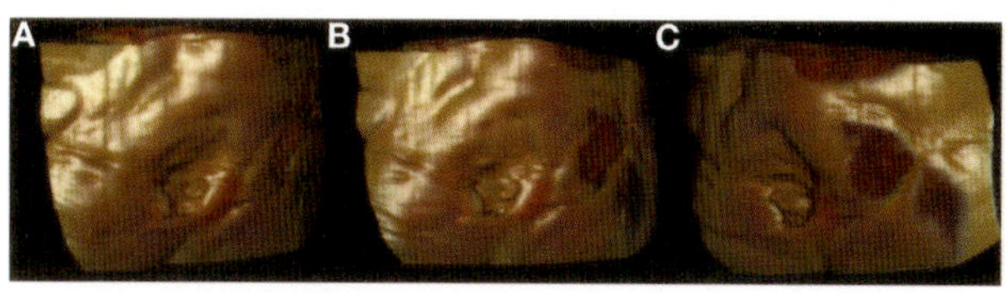


**FIGURE 2** | **Surface-rendered reconstruction images derived from a preoperative computed tomography scan, showing the three-dimensional nature of a sacral defect (A–C: three dimensional rotating views).**

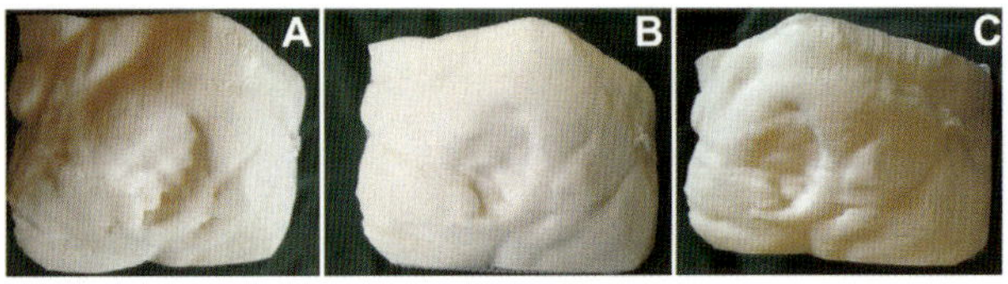


**FIGURE 3 | Three-dimensional (3D) printed model of the sacral defect shown in Figure 2, produced using a 3D printer (Cube 2 printer, 3D Systems, Rock Hill, SC, USA) (A–C: three dimensional rotating views).**

analysis, and the benefits of a 3D model with haptic feedback were assessed.

## RESULTS

The LD free flap was successfully transferred in all cases (100% survival), with adequate soft-tissue cover and volume obliteration achieved. Each microvascular reconstruction with a free flap was performed in either the immediate post-resection setting or delayed if further irradiation or chemotherapy was planned. In the delayed cases, the open resected area was managed with local dressings and VAC therapy (KCI, San Antonio, TX, USA). In three cases, colostomy was necessary and presented an added advantage of preventing fecal contamination. Operative features of the patients are summarized in **Table 1**.

All wounds healed completely except one case, in which a minimal wound dehiscence occurred in the upper aspect of the sacrum defect, which required a lumbar artery perforator rotation flap to close. In three patients who had a colostomy, the wounds healed faster, especially in the caudal aspect of the flap near thee perianal region, and required less postoperative care. There were no wound infections and obliteration of the dead space and volumetric defect in all cases.

The anastomoses to the SGA and SA were performed without any major complications that necessitated an intraoperative or a postoperative revision of the flap. Of note, the anastomoses to the SGA differed to those to the SA due to their shorter and ramified pedicle, which arose vertically between the muscle fibers. At 3 years follow-up, three patients had survived. Two patients died within a year after the reconstruction secondary to tumor recurrence. All wounds had healed, with no donor-site complications and no need for secondary surgery.

Three-dimensional printing of sacral wound defects was achievable with either CT and/or MRI for all prints undertaken. The mean printing time for the scans was 12.5 h, and approximately 40% of the printer cartridge was required for each case (see **Figure 3**). The print was able to establish the cavity itself for haptic analysis, or able to be printed in a reverse manner, to demonstrate the volumetric defect itself.

### Case Examples

#### Case 1

A 69-year-old man presented with a Marjolin's ulcer secondary to a 20-year history of pilonidal cyst. Originally, the lesion was resected from another institution and reconstructed with a bilateral V-Y advancement flap. The patient represented a year later with extensive local recurrence. Preoperative imaging was performed with both CT and MRI. 3D volumetric analysis was undertaken with this imaging, and planned resection margins were recorded, able to preoperatively map the need for a 25 cm by 10 cm surface area defect and modeling highlighting a depth ranging from 10 to 13 cm. Resection planning thus highlighted the need for sacrectomy, colectomy, and a definitive colostomy with bladder exposure within ultimate the wound (see **Figure 4**).

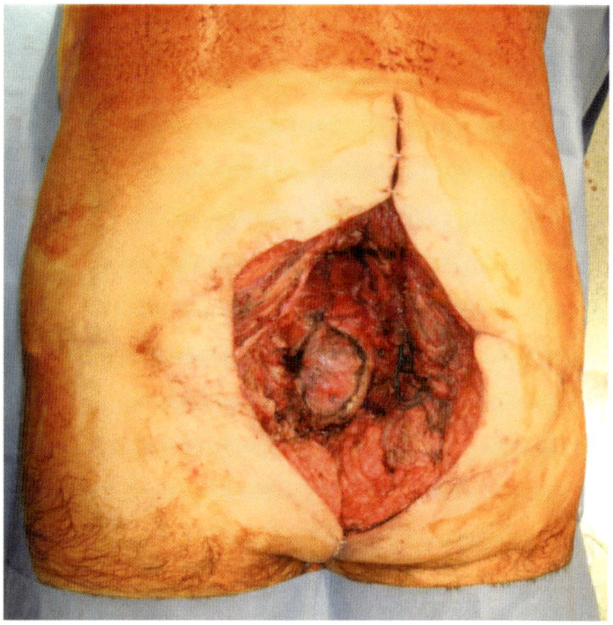

**FIGURE 4 | A 25 cm × 10 cm surface area sacral defect requiring reconstruction.**

A free LD flap with a 25 cm × 10 cm skin paddle was chosen for reconstruction (see **Figure 5**). The flap was harvested with the entirety of the muscle and skin paddle (see **Figure 6**), with arterial anastomosis performed to the SGA using an end-to-end technique and vein anastomosis performed using a Synovis microvascular coupler (Synovis Life Technologies, Birmingham, AL, USA). The flap was thus able to fill the 3D volumetric dead space and cover the defect (see **Figure 7**). There were no complications and good donor and recipient outcomes.

#### Case 2

A 38-year-old man presented with a Marjolin's ulcer following a long-standing pilonidal cyst for 15 years. The lesion had been previously resected, including the cortical portion of the sacrum, and irradiated. The general surgeons planned for an immediate reconstruction, with resection and colostomy planned.

Preoperative imaging was performed with both CT and MRI. 3D volumetric analysis was undertaken with this imaging, and planned resection margins were recorded, with an 18 cm by 20 cm surface area defect planned and modeling highlighting a depth ranging from 5 to 11 cm. This closely mirrored the ultimate

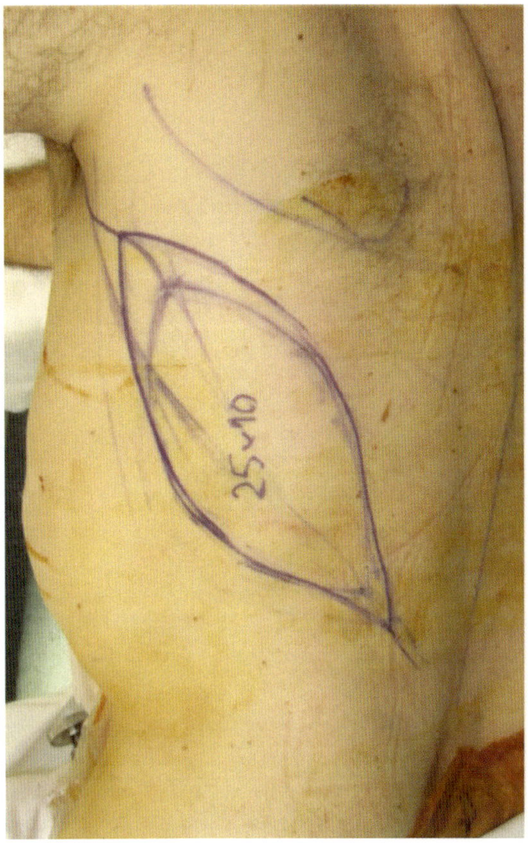


**FIGURE 5 | A free latissimus dorsi myocutaneous flap was selected for reconstruction of the defect, with donor site marked.**

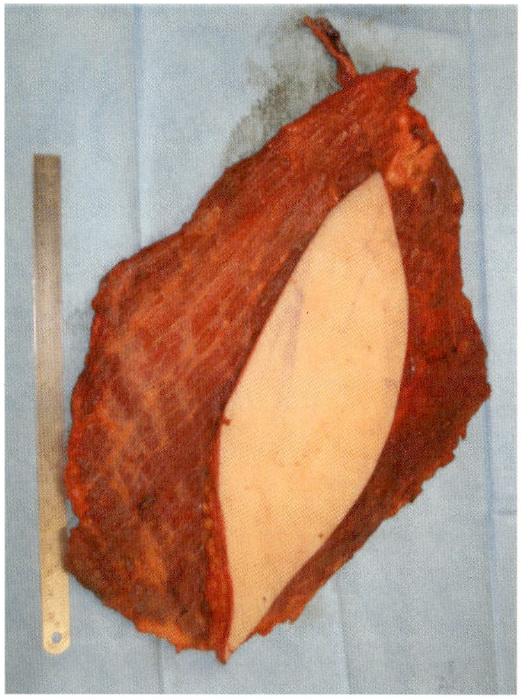

**FIGURE 6 | Free latissimus dorsi myocutaneous flap harvested, with templated skin paddle and muscle for volumetric filling.**

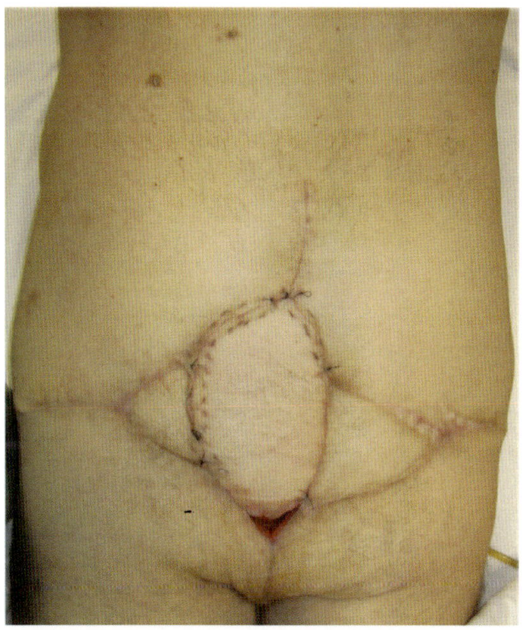

**FIGURE 7 | Flap inset into sacral defect, with adjacent remnants of previous locoregional reconstructive flaps.**

resection, where the defect comprised an 18 cm × 20 cm surface area defect, with substantial dead space volume (see **Figure 8**).

An LD muscle flap was chosen for reconstruction, and for the recipient vessel, the SA was chosen, since the SGA was too close to the resection area posing a risk of local recurrence and endangering the pedicle. The SA was exposed 15 cm cranial to the upper edge of the sacral defect, preventing the need for further operative morbidity. The vessels were anastomosed end-to-end, and despite some notable discrepancy in the caliber of donor and recipient veins, no complications eventuated. The flap suitably filled the defect (see **Figure 9**), was skin-grafted and healed uneventfully.

## DISCUSSION

According to the traditional reconstructive ladder, microsurgical free flap repairs exist at the top. Recent advancements in preoperative imaging and operative techniques demand a re-ordering of the reconstructive ladder (10, 11). With 3D templating for soft-tissue reconstruction, a decision as to where to step on the ladder is made clearer. 3D analysis and volumetric planning have been used extensively and published broadly in a range of fields: breast reconstruction, cutaneous defects, and dead space filling (4, 6, 7). The ability to interact hands-on with the haptic bio-models that accurately represent the anatomical structures has revolutionized the way reconstructive surgeons would plan preoperatively and design free flaps (8, 9). In this field of sacral reconstruction, the specific dead space and volumetric needs of

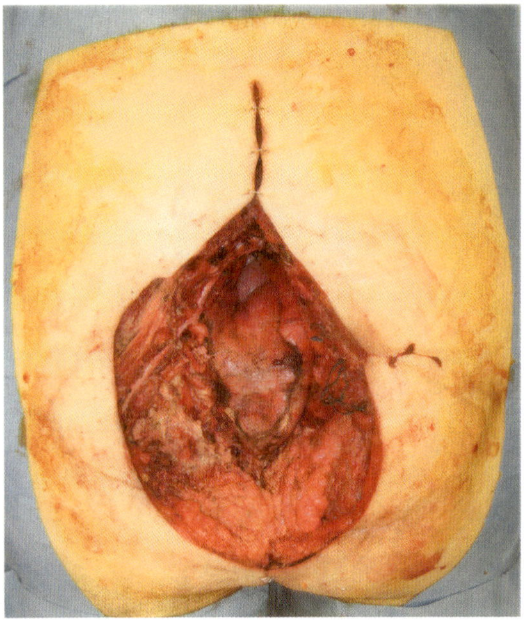

**FIGURE 8 | An 18 cm × 20 cm surface area sacral defect requiring reconstruction.**

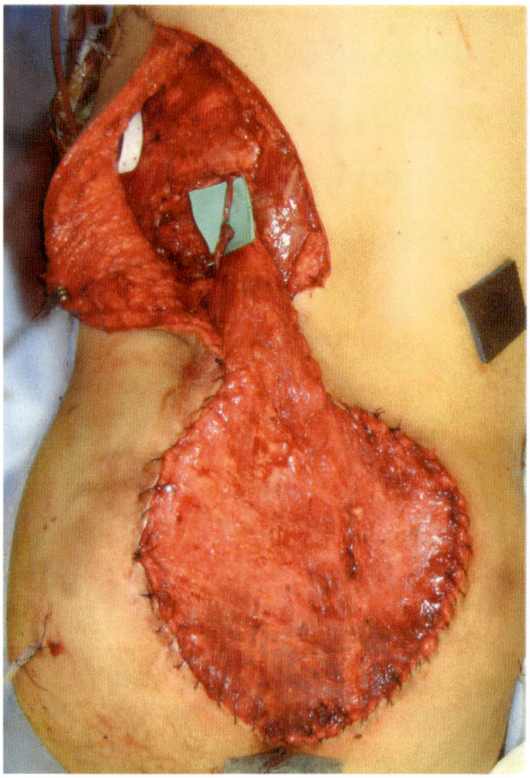

**FIGURE 9 | Free latissimus dorsi muscle only flap inset into the defect.**

a reconstructive choice makes the technology of 3D analysis and 3D printing well-suited. The optimal choice of flap, approach to harvest and technique of inset to adequately replace volume and surface tissues can be achieved successfully.

One current limitation of this technology arises from having to outsource the fabrication of the bio-models to external companies that incur significant costs and a long production time. As the 3D printers become mainstream and more affordable, clinicians are able to quickly produce anatomical models at their own desktop (4, 8, 9, 12). The model used in this study was small-size replica of a sacral defect due to the maximal dimensions afforded by a desktop, office-based 3D printer (16 cm × 16 cm × 16 cm). Although the product was sufficiently detailed for the clinicians to appreciate the shape and depth of the defect, we expect to be able to print these lesions in life-size as the prices of larger 3D printers decrease. There are a range of office-based 3D printers available, the cheapest and the smallest of which make small models (16 cm × 16 cm × 16 cm), while there are other printers, such as MakerBot Z18 (MakerBot Industries, Brooklyn, NY, USA), that can print larger models (30 cm × 30 cm × 45 cm) exceeding the size of the defects described in this paper. We currently use both of these printers in our practice, and it is up to the individual surgeon to decide which is more preferred in terms of size, cost, and level of complexity. The smaller printer options are still useful in terms of comparative scale.

The current series comprises large defects, with substantial needs in volume and surface replacement. While locoregional flaps are the standard of care in most sacral wound defects, they are not plausible in many scenarios. Numerous local flap options have been reported, including gluteal artery perforator flaps (13–16), gluteus maximus sliding flaps (17), paraspinal flaps (18), V-Y advancement flaps (19, 20), and regional anterolateral thigh flaps (21). However, they are relatively contraindicated in oncological sacral defects. Local flaps are compromised by the collateral damage to the normal surrounding tissues from radiotherapy, and margins may not be completely clear of tumor spread. Regional flaps are disfiguring and may require more than one flap where a large defect needs to be covered, increasing donor-site morbidity. As a result, where a wide, heavily irradiated tissue area needs to be covered, locoregional flaps frequently necessitate multiple procedures. In contrast, there is currently insufficient evidence regarding the use of a free-tissue transfer for reconstruction of large complex defects.

From our case series, we demonstrate that microsurgical free flaps provide an alternative that is safe and facilitates a single-stage reconstruction that, as overall, results in a reduction in operative exposure. Conventional wisdom dictates that free flaps naturally require longer operative time due to their technical complexity. However, from our experience working with two surgical teams operating simultaneously on the donor site and the recipient site, there was a minimal difference between the operative length of a local flap and a free flap. Where wound dehiscence occurred, most commonly in the transitional area between the irradiated and the non-irradiated tissues, locoregional flaps have been useful as an adjunct.

Less discussion of free flaps for sacral reconstruction exist, with interpolation flaps utilizing omentum (22), the vertical rectus abdominis myocutaneous flap (23–25), the LD flaps, the chimeric LD flaps combined with the serratus anterior, and the free fibula flap all used in this setting (26, 27). Consistent with previous authors' choice, the LD flap is reliable, easier, faster, and associated with less morbidities than many of the other options. Particularly for volumetric filling, LD flaps provide increased volume and depth by the ability to fold on themselves. Recipient vessels are of particular importance in sacral reconstruction, with superior and inferior gluteal, deep femoral and inferior epigastric arteries all considered (26, 27), often requiring intra-abdominal access or an arteriovenous loop (27). We describe an alternate option, the SA, which has consistent anatomy, few side branches and a long pedicle (up to 10 cm) (28). The use of a free flap based on the eleventh intercostal artery was first described by Badran et al. (29), and in 2006, Hamdi et al. classified the intercostal perforator flaps into dorsal, lateral or anterior depending on the portion of the SA being used (30).

## CONCLUSION

Free flaps may be a first-choice approach for sacral defects that are of substantial volume and have been irradiated. The relative lack of recipient vessels should not be a limitation, and we describe for the first time that the SA is a useful recipient in this setting. The volume of such defects can be assessed with traditional 2D imaging techniques, or with 3D-printed bio-models. Facilitated by modern preoperative planning technologies, 3D-printed haptic bio-models can map surface area and volume defects and may facilitate easier reconstruction planning.

## AUTHOR NOTES

Full authorship and ownership of the manuscript is with the authors above. The content of this article has not been submitted or published elsewhere. All the authors contributed significantly, and all the authors are in agreement with the content of the manuscript. The first and second authors' contribution included manuscript preparation and literature review, the third and fourth authors were involved in all imaging aspects and manuscript preparation.

## AUTHOR CONTRIBUTIONS

The authors of this manuscript have full ownership of the illustrations presented and permit their reproduction for the purposes of this publication. Both authors contributed equally and completely to the manuscript.

## REFERENCES


1. Phan TQ, Spilker G, Theodorou P, Gossmann A, Heiss M, Weinand C. Combined latissimus dorsi and serratus anterior flaps for pelvic reconstruction. *Microsurgery* (2011) 31(7):529–34. doi:10.1002/micr.20917
2. Stone HB, Coleman CN, Anscher MS, McBride WH. Effects of radiation on normal tissue: consequences and mechanisms. *Lancet Oncol* (2003) 4(9):529–36. doi:10.1016/S1470-2045(03)01191-4
3. Marx RE. A new concept in the treatment of osteoradionecrosis. *J Oral Maxillofac Surg* (1983) 41(6):351–7. doi:10.1016/0278-2391(83)90294-X
4. Chae MP, Hunter-Smith DJ, Rozen WM. Image-guided 3D-printing and haptic modeling in plastic surgery. In: Saba L, Rozen WM, Alonso-Burgos A, Ribuffo D, editors. *Imaging in Plastic Surgery*. London, UK: CRC Taylor and Francis Press (2014). p. 819–30.
5. Way TP, Barner KE. Automatic visual to tactile translation – part II: evaluation of the TACTile image creation system. *IEEE Trans Rehabil Eng* (1997) 5(1):95–105. doi:10.1109/86.559354
6. Cohen A, Laviv A, Berman P, Nashef R, Abu-Tair J. Mandibular reconstruction using stereolithographic 3-dimensional printing modeling technology. *Oral Surg Oral Med Oral Pathol Oral Radiol Endod* (2009) 108(5):661–6. doi:10.1016/j.tripleo.2009.05.023
7. Chen YX, Zhang K, Hao YN, Hu YC. Research status and application prospects of digital technology in orthopaedics. *Orthop Surg* (2012) 4(3):131–8. doi:10.1111/j.1757-7861.2012.00184.x
8. Chae MP, Lin F, Spychal RT, Hunter-Smith DJ, Rozen WM. 3D-printed haptic 'reverse' models for preoperative planning in soft tissue reconstruction. *Microsurgery* (2015) 35(2):148–53. doi:10.1002/micr.22293
9. Chae MP, Hunter-Smith DJ, Spychal RT, Rozen WM. 3D volumetric analysis for planning breast reconstructive surgery. *Breast Cancer Res Treat* (2014) 146(2):457–60. doi:10.1007/s10549-014-3028-1
10. Janis JE, Kwon RK, Attinger CE. The new reconstructive ladder: modifications to the traditional model. *Plast Reconstr Surg* (2011) 127(Suppl 1):205S–12S. doi:10.1097/PRS.0b013e318201271c
11. Gottlieb LJ, Krieger LM. From the reconstructive ladder to the reconstructive elevator. *Plast Reconstr Surg* (1994) 93(7):1503–4. doi:10.1097/00006534-199406000-00027
12. Gerstle TL, Ibrahim AM, Kim PS, Lee BT, Lin SJ. A plastic surgery application in evolution: three-dimensional printing. *Plast Reconstr Surg* (2014) 133(2):446–51. doi:10.1097/01.prs.0000436844.92623.d3
13. Gaster RS, Bhatt KA, Shelton AA, Lee GK. Free transverse rectus abdominis myocutaneous flap reconstruction of a massive lumbosacral defect using superior gluteal artery perforator vessels. *Microsurgery* (2012) 32(5):388–92. doi:10.1002/micr.21981
14. Lin CT, Chang SC, Chen SG, Tzeng YS. Modification of the superior gluteal artery perforator flap for reconstruction of sacral sores. *J Plast Reconstr Aesthet Surg* (2014) 67(4):526–32. doi:10.1016/j.bjps.2013.12.031
15. Chen YC, Huang EY, Lin PY. Comparison of gluteal perforator flaps and gluteal fasciocutaneous rotation flaps for reconstruction of sacral pressure sores. *J Plast Reconstr Aesthet Surg* (2014) 67(3):377–82. doi:10.1016/j.bjps.2013.12.029
16. Kuo PJ, Chew KY, Kuo YR, Lin PY. Comparison of outcomes of pressure sore reconstructions among perforator flaps, perforator-based rotation fasciocutaneous flaps, and musculocutaneous flaps. *Microsurgery* (2014) 34(7):547–53. doi:10.1002/micr.22257
17. Weitao Y, Qiqing C, Songtao G, Jiaqiang W. Use of gluteus maximus adipomuscular sliding flaps in the reconstruction of sacral defects after tumor resection. *World J Surg Oncol* (2013) 11:110. doi:10.1186/1477-7819-11-110
18. Gupta S, Chattopadhyay D, Agarwal AK, Guha G, Bhattacharya N, Chumbale PK, et al. Paraspinal transposition flap for reconstruction of sacral soft

tissue defects: a series of 53 cases from a single institute. *Asian Spine J* (2014) 8(3):309–14. doi:10.4184/asj.2014.8.3.309

19. Kesan K, Kothari P, Gupta R, Gupta A, Karkera P, Ranjan R, et al. Closure of large meningomyelocele wound defects with subcutaneous based pedicle flap with bilateral V-Y advancement: our experience and review of literature. *Eur J Pediatr Surg* (2015) 25(2):189–94. doi:10.1055/s-0034-1368796
20. Olenczak JB, Stanwix MG, Rosson GD. CASE REPORT complex wound closure of partial sacrectomy defect with human acellular dermal matrix and bilateral V to Y gluteal advancement flaps in a pediatric patient. *Eplasty* (2013) 13:e20.
21. Santanelli Di Pompeo F, Longo B, Pagnoni M, Laporta R. Sensate anterolateral thigh perforator flap for ischiatic sores reconstruction in meningomyelocele patients. *Microsurgery* (2015) 35(4):279–83. doi:10.1002/micr.22330
22. Unal C, Eren GG, Isil E, Alponat A, Sarlak A. Utility of the omentum in sacral reconstruction following total sacrectomy due to recurrent and irradiated giant cell tumour of the spine. *Indian J Plast Surg* (2012) 45(1):140–3. doi:10.4103/0970-0358.96617
23. Loessin SJ, Meland NB, Devine RM, Wolff BG, Nelson H, Zincke H. Management of sacral and perineal defects following abdominoperineal resection and radiation with transpelvic muscle flaps. *Dis Colon Rectum* (1995) 38(9):940–5. doi:10.1007/BF02049729
24. Garvey PB, Clemens MW, Rhines LD, Sacks JM. Vertical rectus abdominis musculocutaneous flow-through flap to a free fibula flap for total sacrectomy reconstruction. *Microsurgery* (2013) 33(1):32–8. doi:10.1002/micr.21990
25. Cheong YW, Sulaiman WA, Halim AS. Reconstruction of large sacral defects following tumour resection: a report of two cases. *J Orthop Surg (Hong Kong)* (2008) 16(3):351–4. doi:10.1177/230949900801600317
26. Hung SJ, Chen HC, Wei FC. Free flaps for reconstruction of the lower back and sacral area. *Microsurgery* (2000) 20(2):72–6. doi:10.1002/(SICI)1098-2752(2000)20:2<72::AID-MICR5>3.3.CO;2-T
27. Feliciano B, Paige KT, Beshlian KM. Latissimus dorsi free flaps for complex ischiosacral defects. *Am J Surg* (2007) 193(5):648–50. doi:10.1016/j.amjsurg.2006.12.027
28. Feinendegen DL, Niederhauser T, Herrmann G, Abderhalden S, Vogelin E, Banic A, et al. The subcostal artery perforator flap; an anatomical study. *J Plast Reconstr Aesthet Surg* (2008) 61(12):1496–502. doi:10.1016/j.bjps.2007.09.021
29. Badran HA, El-Helaly MS, Safe I. The lateral intercostal neurovascular free flap. *Plast Reconstr Surg* (1984) 73(1):17–26. doi:10.1097/00006534-198401000-00003
30. Hamdi M, Van Landuyt K, de Frene B, Roche N, Blondeel P, Monstrey S. The versatility of the inter-costal artery perforator (ICAP) flaps. *J Plast Reconstr Aesthet Surg* (2006) 59(6):644–52. doi:10.1016/j.bjps.2006.01.006

# 6

# Microsurgical reconstruction of extensive oncological scalp defects

*Ole Goertz[1]*, Leon von der Lohe[1], Ramón Martinez-Olivera[2], Adrien Daigeler[1], Kamran Harati[1], Tobias Hirsch[1], Marcus Lehnhardt[1] and Jonas Kolbenschlag[1]*

*[1] Department of Plastic Surgery, BG University Hospital Bergmannsheil, Ruhr-University, Bochum, Germany, [2] Neurosurgical Unit, Department of Surgery, BG University Hospital Bergmannsheil, Ruhr-University, Bochum, Germany*

Although most small to medium defects of the scalp can be covered by local flaps, large defects or complicating factors, such as a history of radiotherapy, often require a microsurgical reconstruction. Several factors need to be considered in such procedures. A sufficient preoperative planning is based on adequate imaging of the malignancy and a multi-disciplinary concept. Several flaps are available for such reconstructions, of which the latissimus dorsi and anterior-lateral thigh flaps are the most commonly used ones. In very large defects, combined flaps, such as a parascapular/latissimus dorsi flaps, can be highly useful or necessary. The most commonly used recipient vessels for microsurgical scalp reconstructions are the superficial temporal vessels, but various other feasible choices exist. If the concomitant veins are not sufficient, the jugular veins represent a safe back-up alternative but require a vessel interposition or long pedicle. Post-operative care and patient positioning can be difficult in these patients but can be facilitated by various devices. Overall, microsurgical reconstruction of large scalp defects is a feasible undertaking if the mentioned key factors are taken into account.

**Keywords: plastic surgery, reconstruction, oncology, calvarial defect, head**

***Edited by:***
*Wim Ceelen, Ghent University Hospital, Belgium*

***Reviewed by:***
*Andreas Arkudas, University Hospital of Erlangen, Germany*
*Thomas Kremer, BG Trauma Center Ludwigshafen, Germany*

****Correspondence:***
*Ole Goertz, Department of Plastic Surgery, BG University Hospital Bergmannsheil, Buerkle-de-la-Camp-Platz 1, Bochum 44789, Germany*
*ole.goertz@rub.de*

***Specialty section:***
*This article was submitted to Surgical Oncology, a section of the journal Frontiers in Surgery*

## Introduction

The scalp covers the calvarium and consists of skin, subcutaneous tissue, the galea aponeurotica, loose areolar tissue, and the pericranium. If this cover is disrupted by trauma or the resection of malignancies, the exposed bone can succumb to infection and its potentially life-threatening complications. Therefore, timely reconstruction of such defects is paramount.

For small and medium sized defects, local flaps are often sufficient. Such coverage by means of adjacent tissue gives a good color and texture match and even allows the reconstruction of the hair bearing area. However, in large defects or in patients with a history of radiation therapy, such options are often not feasible. In these cases, free tissue transfer becomes the first choice (1).

Interestingly, the microsurgical reconstruction of the scalp was one of the earliest applications of free tissue transfer. Already in 1972, McLean and Buncke covered a large scalp defect with a free omentum majus flap (2). Microsurgery and its reconstructive possibilities have evolved since then, but some general principles still remain of unchanged importance.

Therefore, the aim of this review is to illustrate several general and specific considerations in patients undergoing microsurgical reconstruction of large oncological scalp defects.

## General Considerations

A sufficient preoperative planning is essential for an extensive surgical procedure, such as the oncological resection and microsurgical reconstruction of malignancies of the scalp.

First, the surgical resectability of the tumor needs to be evaluated. Although MRI provides good visualization of the soft tissues and the tumor, CT-scans can aid in assessing the amount of involvement of the calvarium bone. In patients with an extensive history of operative interventions, such as neck dissections or radiation therapy, an angiography of the possible recipient vessels can support preoperative decision-making and facilitate the intraoperative dissection. Based on the angiography findings (as well as in their absence), one should also devise a back-up plan in case the primary vessel can not be dissected due to scarring or does not show adequate flow after dissection.

Multiple soft-tissue and bone biopsies can aid in both an exact diagnosis of the malignancy and the planning of the surgical margins. Also, an adequate staging of the disease is paramount. Such complex cases should be preoperatively discussed in an interdisciplinary board of oncologists, neurosurgeons, and plastic surgeons. Here, not only the resection and reconstruction but also the use of (neo-)adjuvant radio- or chemotherapy should be discussed. Especially noteworthy in this regard is the trend toward less aggressive resections of sarcomas. Although the wide resection is still commonly recommended in sarcoma surgery, such an approach would render most of the sarcomas of the scalp to be considered not resectable. According to the findings in sarcomas of the extremities and recurrent sarcomas, less radical resections might be sufficient for most entities, as long as clear surgical margins are achieved (3, 4).

Only by incorporating all these findings, a reasonable treatment plan can be devised. However, even the most elaborate surgical treatment plan cannot stand on its own and needs to be adjusted to the individual patient and their respective wishes. Especially in a palliative situation, invasiveness of the procedure and its potential complications need to be weighted carefully against the expected gain in quality of life. Nonetheless, even large reconstructions should not be shunned in the face of palliation, if the patient is capable and willing to undertake such a journey. In this way, defects that are painful, bleeding, and demand extensive wound care can be covered, enabling the patient to regain their independence and quality of life (5, 6).

The possibility to cover nearly any oft-tissue defect of the scalp via free tissue transfer enables a radical surgical resection. Often, this resection also has to include the calvarium bone and the dura. Such defects are commonly covered by custom-made methyl acrylate implants or titanium mesh implants and dura patch plasties. In some cases, a microvascular transplant can be used as a dermal reinforcement of such a dura plasty (7).

## Soft-Tissue Reconstruction

A variety of free flaps have been described for the microsurgical reconstruction of the scalp (2, 8–10). The choice of free flap is mainly dependent on the size of the defect and the required pedicle length. Due to its size, the latissimus dorsi has become one of the work horse flaps for scalp reconstruction (11). It can be harvested as a sole muscle flap or musculocutaneous flap with an overlying skin paddle. Although this skin paddle facilitates clinical perfusion monitoring or/and could be use for extension of coverage, it is often very bulky due to the subcutaneous fat. In high risk cases requiring intense monitoring of the flap (coagulopathies, history of radiation, e.g.) such a skin paddle might be easier to monitor than the muscle itself. In such cases, one or more perforating vessel that supply the overlying skin paddle can be dissected in the initial operation. After isolating the paddle on these perforators, the muscle surface of the flap can be skin grafted, leaving only small gaps for the vessels (12). When the need for an intense clinical monitoring has subsided, the perforator-based skin paddle can be easily removed by ligating the vessels without the need for additional surgery. The initial bulk of the latissimus declines over the course of time and together with a split thickness graft results in a reasonable esthetic outcome. The case of a patient undergoing free latissimus dorsi coverage of the scalp following oncological resection is depicted in **Figures 1–5**.

In the beginning, we designed those skin islands on multiple perforators, but such large skin islands are often hard to fix to the underlying surface and can be compromised by shearing off due to their own weight. Therefore, a smaller island with one singled

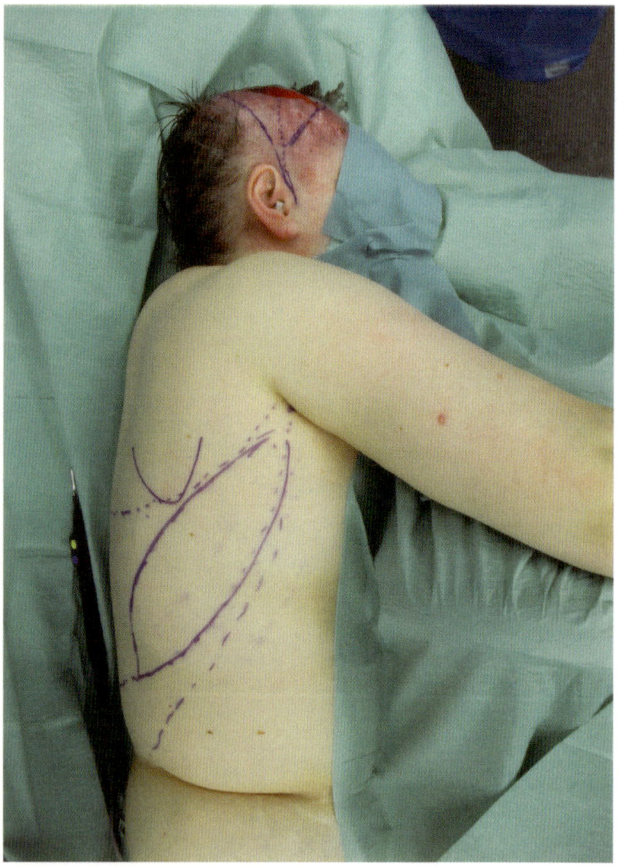

**FIGURE 1 | Intraoperative view of a patient with an oncological defect of the scalp**. The latissimus skin paddle as well as the anatomical landmarks are marked.

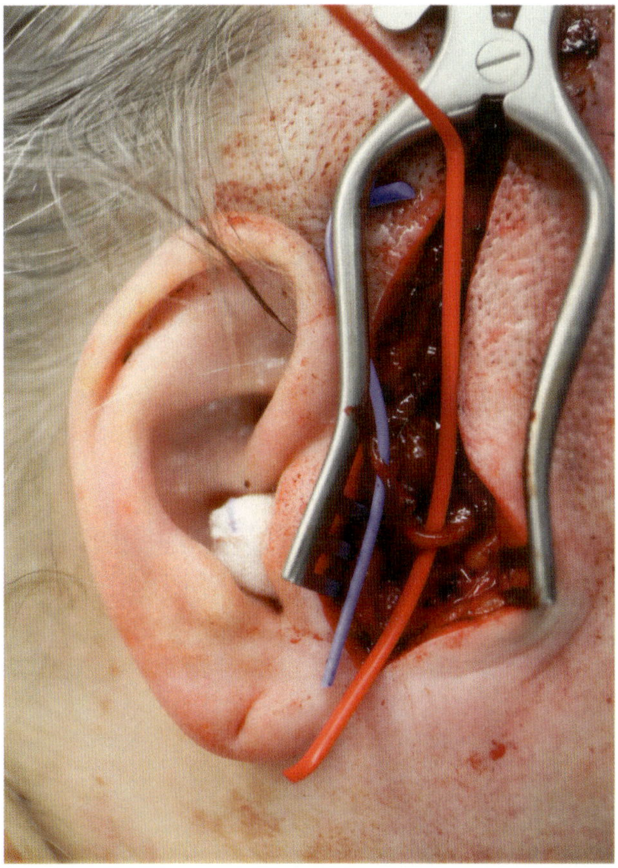

**FIGURE 2 | The dissected superficial temporal vessels that will be utilized as recipient vessels.**

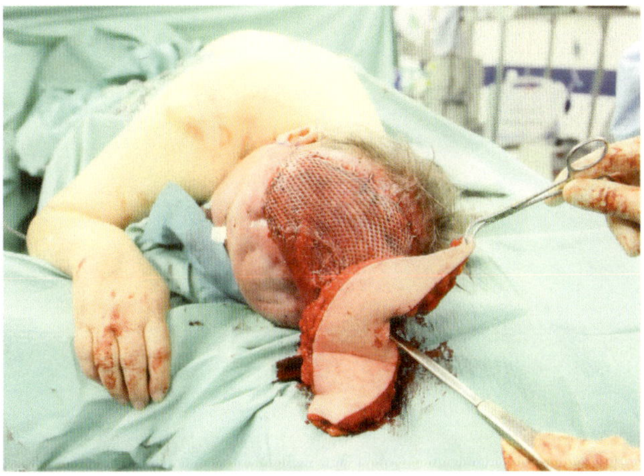

**FIGURE 3 | After fitting of the flap**. Note the skin grafted muscle surface with leaves only small gaps for the vessels.

out perforator is often more feasible, especially since the option to use such a perforator island as another flap to close secondary defects is undesirable in this constellation due to the bulk of the subcutaneous fat.

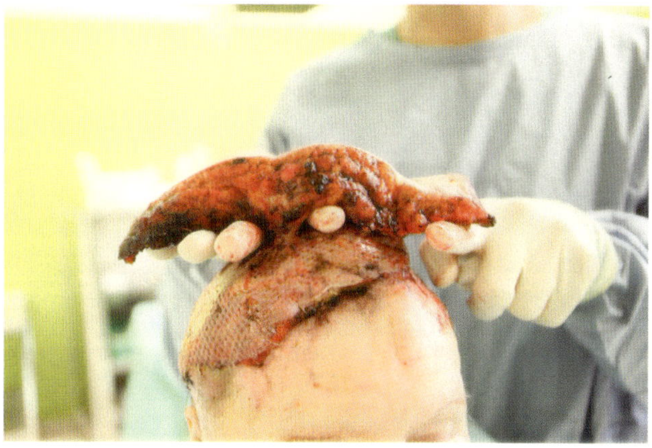

**FIGURE 4 | Skin paddle of a latissimus dorsi free flap based on three perforator vessels 1 week after surgery.**

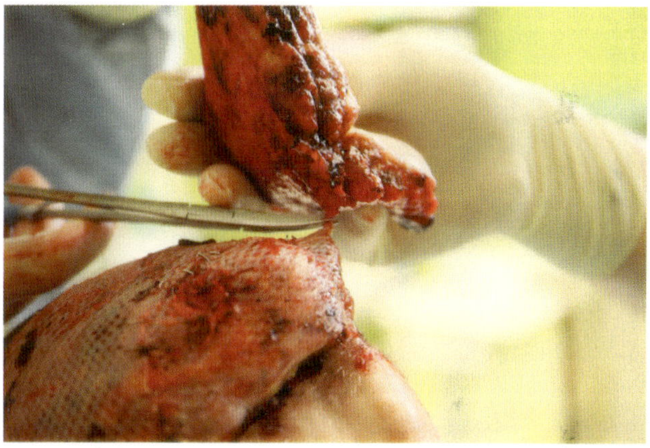

**FIGURE 5 | Removal of the skin paddle after ligation and severing of the perforating vessels.**

Based on the same vascular tree, the (para-) scapular flap can be raised as a fascio-cutaneous flap that carries little bulk and sufficient pedicle length (13). Due to their common vascular tree, both the (para-)scapular and the latissimus flap can be harvested together, thus allowing for even larger defects to be covered. A disadvantage of harvesting the common vascular tree is the extensive diameter of the venular confluence and its mismatch with the tiny vein of the superficial temporal vessels. To achieve a smooth passage at the anastomosis, we utilize a chamfering technique that is discussed later. We prefer to place the parascapular flap with its good skin quality over the occipital bone and the latissimus muscle over the mid part of the calvarium. This way, the more resilient skin of the parascapular flap allows for a better cover when resting the head. **Figures 6–9** depict the case of a patient undergoing total scalp resection for an angiosarcoma and the microsurgical reconstruction with a chimeric Latissimus/Parascapular flap.

Another commonly used free flap is the anterior-lateral thigh flap (ALT). The mean achievable flap size is smaller than in the

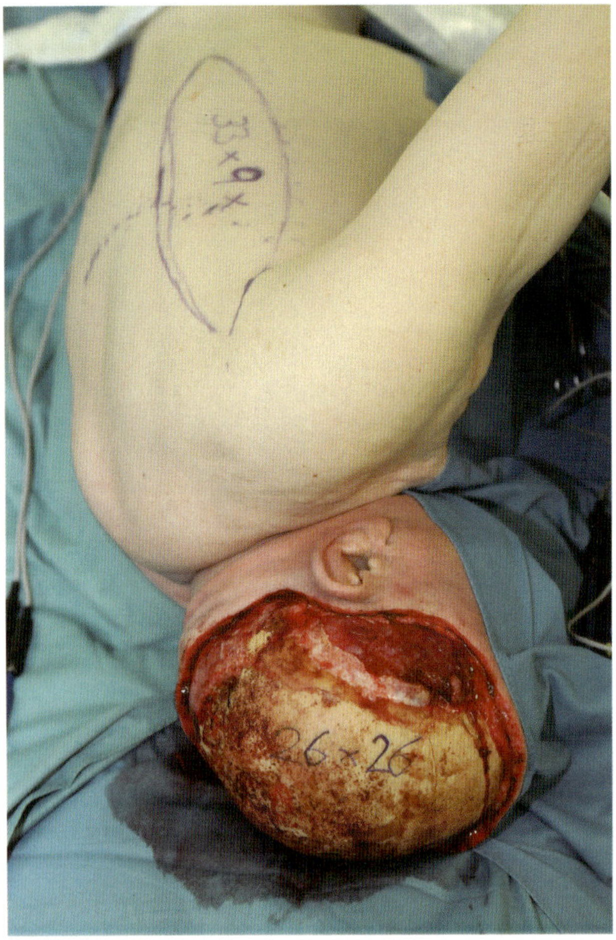

**FIGURE 6 | Intraoperative view after total full thickness scalp resection due to an angiosarcoma.** Note the 26 cm × 26 cm sized defect and the planned parascapular flap with a size of 33 cm × 9 cm.

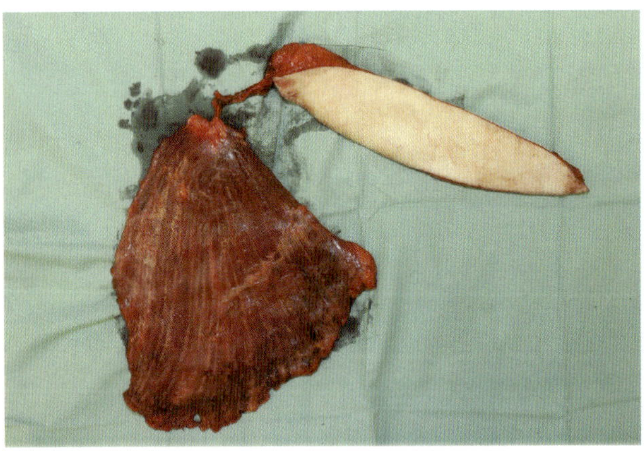

**FIGURE 7 | The combined latissimus/parascapular flap after its elevation on the common vascular pedicle.**

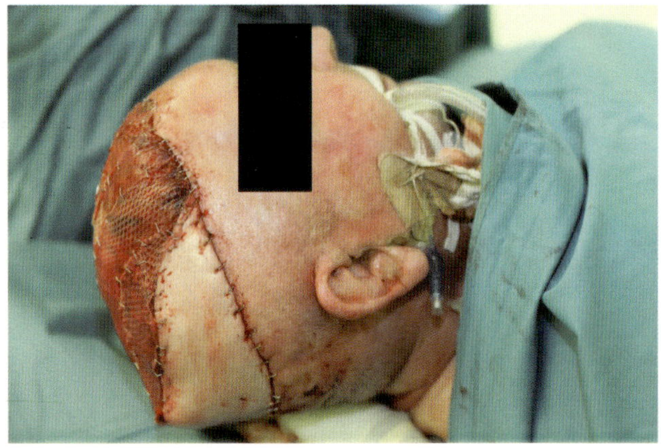

**FIGURE 8 | Intraopearative view after fitting of the flaps.** Note the more resilient skin cover of the parascapular flap over the occiput on which the head rests.

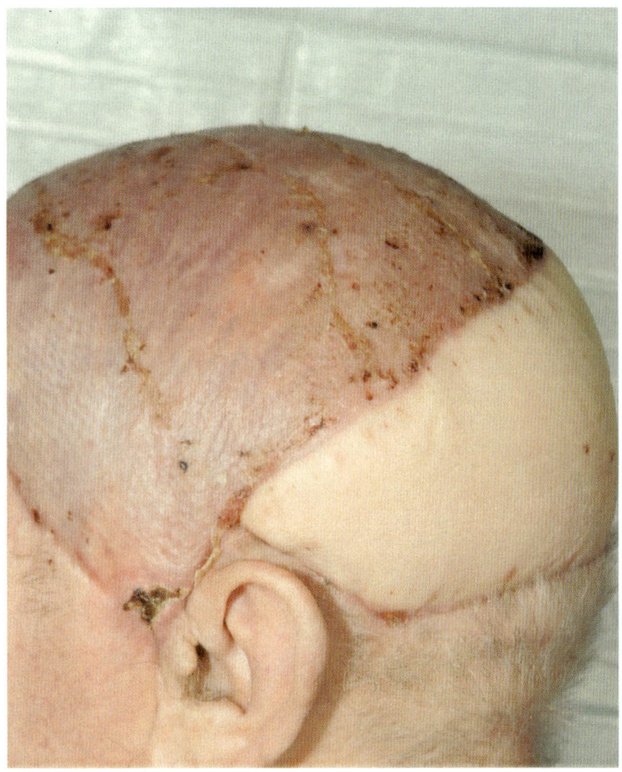

**FIGURE 9 | Follow up after 4 weeks.**

latissimus; however, it carries less initial bulk in slender patients. In cases where obliteration of dead space is required, the flap can be raised as a musculocutaneous flap that incorporates the vastus lateralis muscle. One of the main advantages of the ALT flap over the latissimus and the (para-)scapular flap is the possibility to harvest it in a supine position. However, in extensive scalp defects, the patient is often positioned in either a prone or lateral position to allow access to the entire defect thus negating this advantage.

A good alternative for medium to large defects is the gracilis muscle free flap. It can be expanded and also flattened by intramuscular dissection, allowing for a stable coverage without too much bulk (14). Also, similar to the latissimus flap, the appearance of the grafted muscle surface is often superior to the patch-like appearance of fascio-cutaneous flaps.

Other potential flap choices include the ulnar and radial forearm flaps. Both deliver little bulk and often require a less complex dissection than perforator flaps. However, the donor site including the loss of a major artery can be problematic. Therefore, these flaps are not the first choice in our hands.

## Specific Considerations

One of the main things to be considered in microsurgical reconstructions is the recipient vessels. Although there are several potential vessels available in the head and neck, the choice of the optimal vessel depends on various factors. Depending on the localization of the defect, the recipient vessels should be easily reachable with the anticipated pedicle length, thus eliminating the need for vein grafts. In patients with extensive previous operations, such as neck dissections or history of radiotherapy, the integrity of the vessels might be compromised or its dissection can be hindered by scars. Therefore, preoperative evaluation of their patency is recommended in such cases. Often, hand-held Doppler assessment is sufficient. However, in selected cases, an angiography can aid in the preoperative planning. As mentioned above, sometimes the primary "go-to" vessel can not be dissected due to scarring or shows insufficient flow. Therefore, a back-up plan needs to be devised beforehand.

Due to its easy access in the preauricular space and reliable course, the superficial temporal artery is one of the most commonly used recipient vessels in microsurgical scalp reconstruction (10, 15). However, there can be a serious discrepancy of the caliber between the flap and the recipient vessels, especially in chimeric flaps. To reach an appropriate size of recipient vessels, one can either extend the dissection proximally, which in turn can bring the need for the interposition of vein grafts. Although such grafts carry an intrinsic risk, a proximal anastomosis often has less tendency for spasms and can deliver a higher blood flow to perfuse even very large flaps. Also, in our experience, the superficial temporal artery reacts quite sensitive to manipulation and its flow can easily become compromised due to vasoconstriction. However, by dissection of the artery to the level of the ear lobe the flow becomes sufficient in most cases.

Another option is to perform an end-to-end anastomosis after preparing both vessels in the way depicted in **Figure 10**. By chamfering the larger lumen of the flap vessel, a cone-like configuration can be achieved. This cone can then be adapted to the size of the recipient vessels by the numbers of sutures placed. In this way, the lumen can be tailored to the required size in a safe and reliable way. Such a procedure does also carry some intrinsic risk for thrombosis, therefore careful consideration of the recipient vessels need to be taken.

Other options of recipient vessels include the superior thyroid and the facial artery. In cases where the concomitant veins are not sufficient, the internal and external jugular veins represent a reliable alternative (10, 16).

Due to the tendency to rest the head on the occipital bone, post-operative positioning of patients with total scalp reconstruction can be problematic. To avoid pressure on the flap, the patient can be positioned in a sitting position with some support of the cervical spine. If post-operative ventilation is required, the patient can be brought into a prone position to allow for an absolute pressure free environment for the flap. To facilitate this, special beds for the prone positioning of patients as seen in burn units can be used. However, both in sitting and prone positions, the risk for pressure sores is increased and therefore requires meticulous assessment of the soft tissues over high pressure areas.

**Figures 11–15** depict the case of a patient with a neglected carcinoma of the skull and a reduced compliance due to a mental handicap. Even despite complete resection of the malignancy, the

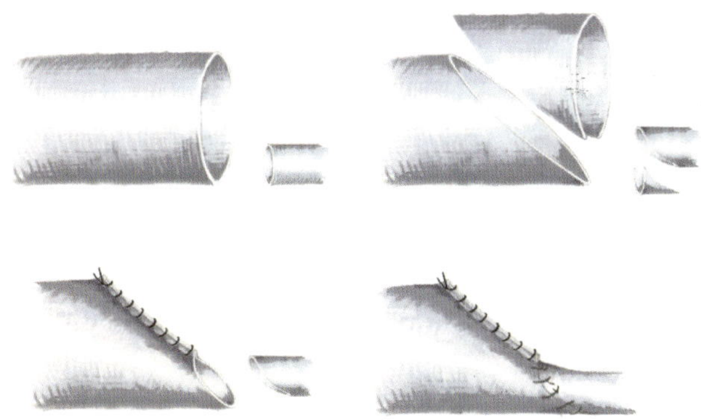

**FIGURE 10 | Schematic drawing of the technique employed in cases of large caliber differences between recipient and flap vessels by chamfering the lumen.**

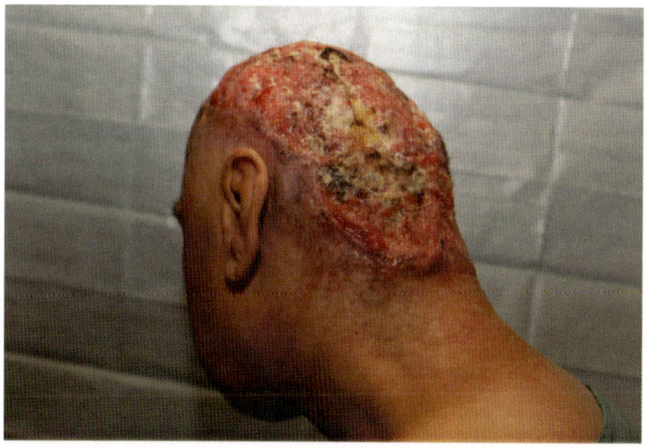

**FIGURE 11 | A case of extensive squamous cell carcinoma of the scalp with infiltration of the calvarium.**

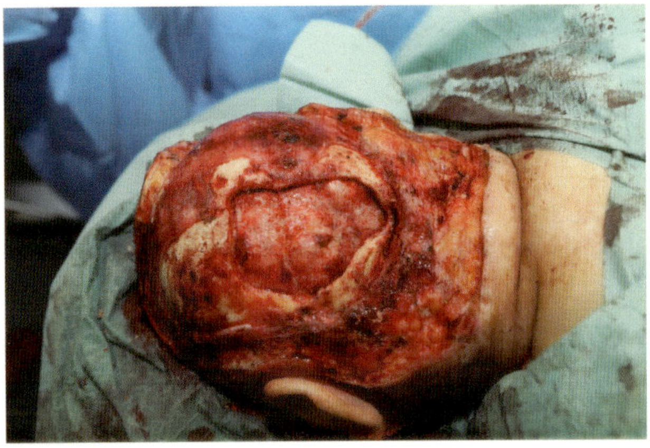

**FIGURE 12 | Intraoperative view after resection of the scalp and the infiltrated calvarium.**

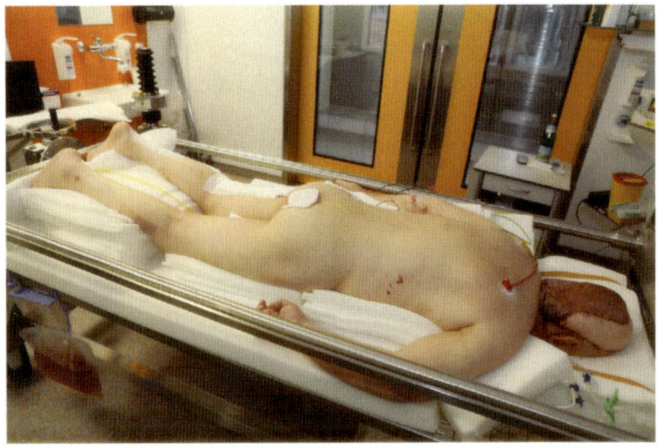

**FIGURE 14 | The patient was initially positioned in a prone position.** Note the extensive padding to reduce the incidence of pressure sores and the apparatus on the end of the bed that facilitates rotating the bed.

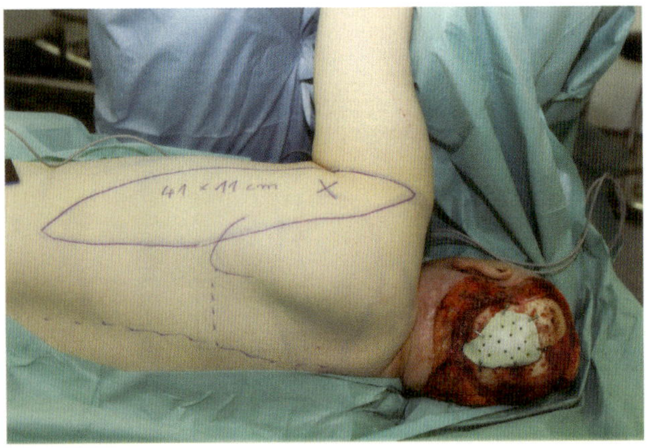


**FIGURE 13 | The calvarial defect was closed with a custom-made methyl acrylate implant.** Note the anatomical landmarks and the outline of the planned skin paddle of the parascapular flap.

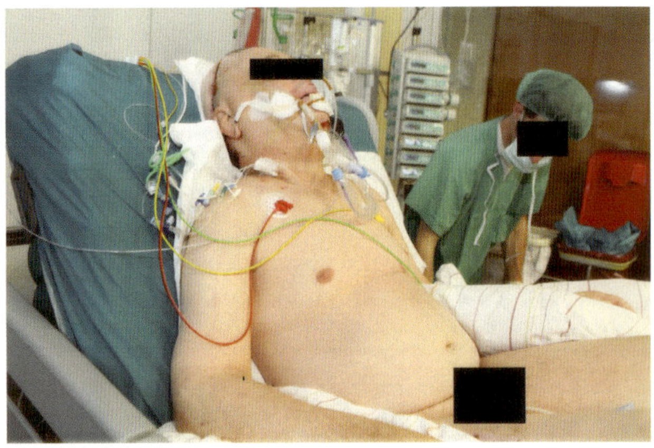

**FIGURE 15 | The same patient in a sitting position to prepare for extubation.**

patient deceased 12 months after surgery due to metastatic disease. However, the painful daily dressing changes were discontinued, improving the quality of life of the patient. Therefore, such complex reconstructions can also be feasible in a palliative setting. In such cases, the invasiveness of the procedure needs to be weighted very carefully against the expected gains in quality of life.

Also, the site of the anastomosis itself needs to be protected from any pressure. If the anastomosis is in the area of the lateral face and neck, a modified cervical spine collar with sufficient space over the area of the anastomosis can aid in protecting it.

## Conclusion

The ability to reconstruct even total scalp defects via free tissue transfer enables the radical surgical resection of malignancies.

A variety of free flaps are available for this task, most prominently the latissimus dorsi and the ALT flap. In very large defects, the latissimus dorsi and a parascapular flap can be elevated on their common vascular tree and used as a chimeric flap. Although the reconstruction itself as well as the perioperative management can be challenging, the overall outcomes with regards to the reconstruction is good.

## References


1. Desai SC, Sand JP, Sharon JD, Branham G, Nussenbaum B. Scalp reconstruction: an algorithmic approach and systematic review. *JAMA Facial Plast Surg* (2015) **17**(1):56–66. doi:10.1001/jamafacial.2014.889
2. McLean DH, Buncke HJ Jr. Autotransplant of omentum to a large scalp defect, with microsurgical revascularization. *Plast Reconstr Surg* (1972) **49**(3):268–74. doi:10.1097/00006534-197203000-00005
3. Daigeler A, Zmarsly I, Hirsch T, Goertz O, Steinau HU, Lehnhardt M, et al. Long-term outcome after local recurrence of soft tissue sarcoma: a retrospective analysis of factors predictive of survival in 135 patients with locally recurrent soft tissue sarcoma. *Br J Cancer* (2014) **110**(6):1456–64. doi:10.1038/bjc.2014.21
4. Steinau HU, Steinstrasser L, Langer S, Stricker I, Goertz O. [Surgical margins in soft tissue sarcoma of the extremities]. *Pathologe* (2011) **32**(1):57–64. doi:10.1007/s00292-010-1394-y

5. Daigeler A, Harati K, Kapalschinski N, Goertz O, Hirsch T, Lehnhardt M, et al. Plastic surgery for the oncological patient. *Front Surg* (2014) **1**:42. doi:10.3389/fsurg.2014.00042
6. Kippenhan T, Hirche C, Lehnhardt M, Daigeler A. [Palliative plastic surgery in multidisciplinary therapeutic concepts]. *Zentralbl Chir* (2015) **140**(2):228–34. doi:10.1055/s-0032-1328184
7. Lessard L, Tahiri Y. Complex scalp, skull, and dural defect reconstruction using a turnover "tournedos" myocutaneous free flap. *J Craniofac Surg* (2013) **24**(1):62–5. doi:10.1097/SCS.0b013e318272db28
8. Chao AH, Yu P, Skoracki RJ, Demonte F, Hanasono MM. Microsurgical reconstruction of composite scalp and calvarial defects in patients with cancer: a 10-year experience. *Head Neck* (2012) **34**(12):1759–64. doi:10.1002/hed.21999
9. Lee B, Bickel K, Levin S. Microsurgical reconstruction of extensive scalp defects. *J Reconstr Microsurg* (1999) **15**(4):255–62. doi:10.1055/s-2007-1000099
10. Takamatsu A, Harashina T, Inoue T. Selection of appropriate recipient vessels in difficult, microsurgical head and neck reconstruction. *J Reconstr Microsurg* (1996) **12**(8):499–507. doi:10.1055/s-2007-1006622
11. Lin SJ, Hanasono MM, Skoracki RJ. Scalp and calvarial reconstruction. *Semin Plast Surg* (2008) **22**(4):281–93. doi:10.1055/s-0028-1095887
12. Beier JP, Horch RE, Dragu A, Arkudas A, Kneser U. Perforator-based monitoring skin islands in free muscle flaps: teaching old dogs new tricks. *Plast Reconstr Surg* (2012) **129**(3):586e–7e. doi:10.1097/PRS.0b013e3182419c54
13. Sachs C, Lehnhardt M, Daigeler A, Goertz O. [Free fasciocutaneous parascapular flap: Coverage of extensive skin and soft tissue defects]. [Article in German] *Unfallchirurg* (2015). doi:10.1007/s00113-014-2686-0.
14. Huemer GM, Dunst KM, Maurer H, Ninkovic M. Area enlargement of the gracilis muscle flap through microscopically aided intramuscular dissection: ideas and innovations. *Microsurgery* (2004) **24**(5):369–73. doi:10.1002/micr.20050
15. Medved F, Manoli T, Medesan R, Janghorban Esfahani B, Stahl S, Schaller HE, et al. In vivo analysis of the vascular pattern of the superficial temporal artery based on digital subtraction angiography. *Microsurgery* (2014) **35**(5):380–6. doi:10.1002/micr.22348
16. van Driel AA, Mureau MA, Goldstein DP, Gilbert RW, Irish JC, Gullane PJ, et al. Aesthetic and oncologic outcome after microsurgical reconstruction of complex scalp and forehead defects after malignant tumor resection: an algorithm for treatment. *Plast Reconstr Surg* (2010) **126**(2):460–70. doi:10.1097/PRS.0b013e3181de2260

# 7

# A Systematic Review of the Role of Robotics in Plastic and Reconstructive Surgery—From Inception to the Future

*Thomas D. Dobbs[1,2]*, Olivia Cundy[3], Harsh Samarendra[3], Khurram Khan[4] and Iain Stuart Whitaker[1,2]*

[1] Reconstructive Surgery and Regenerative Medicine Research Group (ReconRegen), Institute of Life Science, Swansea University Medical School, Swansea, United Kingdom, [2] The Welsh Centre for Burns and Plastic Surgery, Morriston Hospital, Swansea, United Kingdom, [3] Oxford University Medical School, Oxford, United Kingdom, [4] Department of Plastic Surgery, Birmingham Children's Hospital, Birmingham, United Kingdom

**Background:** The use of robots in surgery has become commonplace in many specialties. In this systematic review, we report on the current uses of robotics in plastic and reconstructive surgery and looks to future roles for robotics in this arena.

**Methods:** A systematic literature search of Medline, EMBASE, and Scopus was performed using appropriate search terms in order to identify all applications of robot-assistance in plastic and reconstructive surgery. All articles were reviewed by two authors and a qualitative synthesis performed of those articles that met the inclusion criteria. The systematic review and results were conducted and reported in accordance with the Preferred Reporting Items for Systematic Reviews and Meta Analysis (PRISMA) guidelines.

**Results:** A total of 7,904 articles were identified for title and abstract review. Sixty-eight studies met the inclusion criteria. Robotic assistance in plastic and reconstructive surgery is still in its infancy, with areas such as trans-oral robotic surgery and microvascular procedures the dominant areas of interest currently. A number of benefits have been shown over conventional open surgery, such as improved access and greater dexterity; however, these must be balanced against disadvantages such as the lack of haptic feedback and cost implications.

**Conclusion:** The feasibility of robotic plastic surgery has been demonstrated in several specific indications. As technology, knowledge, and skills in this area improve, these techniques have the potential to contribute positively to patient and provider experience and outcomes.

**Edited by:**
*Vincenzo Neri, University of Foggia, Italy*

**Reviewed by:**
*David J. Hunter-Smith, Monash University Plastic and Reconstructive Surgery Group, Australia*
*Oren Lapid, Academic Medical Center (AMC), Netherlands*
*Jeffrey B. Friedrich, University of Washington Tacoma, United States*

***Correspondence:**
*Thomas D. Dobbs*
*tomdobbs@doctors.org.uk*

**Specialty section:**
*This article was submitted to Reconstructive and Plastic Surgery, a section of the journal Frontiers in Surgery*

**Keywords: robotic surgery, plastic surgery, microsurgery, head and neck, technology, innovation**

## INTRODUCTION

The use of robotics in surgery has captured the imagination of many. It is a growth area across the breadth of surgical specialties, with many procedures becoming routinely classed as "robot-assisted." The rapid increase in surgical research involving robotic assistance can be witnessed by the rising number of articles published in consecutive years related to the subject (**Figure 1**).

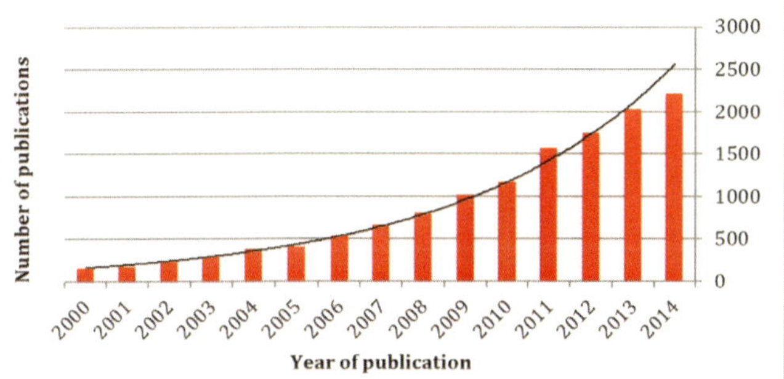


**FIGURE 1** | A 15-year literature review of the number of publications relating to robotic surgery demonstrating a highly significant exponential increase. Each column represents the number of papers published in that year, rising from 168 in 2000 to over 2,000 in the year 2014 (Source; Pubmed, searched using the terms "robot" and "surgery" from January 2000 to December 2014).

Since the first reported use of the daVinci® Surgical Robotic System (Intuitive Surgical, Sunnyvale, CA, USA) in a robotic-assisted laparoscopic cholecystectomy (1), Intuitive Surgical has become the leading force in surgical robotics. The daVinci® robot has been widely implemented in many surgical specialties, from cardiac surgery (2, 3) to gynecology (4, 5). In the USA, 80% of radical prostatectomies are now being performed robotically (6). With updates to the daVinci® robot including a fourth instrument arm, its application is broadening to other specialties such as colorectal surgery (7). The dominance of the daVinci® system is, however, beginning to be challenged with new competitors entering the market.

Plastic and reconstructive surgery is an innovative specialty, often at the forefront of technical innovation within surgery. It is also a specialty that works collaboratively with many other surgical disciplines and, therefore, those practicing it will likely come across advances in robotic surgery in these other specialties. It is, therefore, important for plastic surgeons to embrace this new surgical platform, explore potential uses for it, and learn from those who have already incorporated robotics into their surgical armamentarium.

This systematic review aimed to identify all current reported uses of robotic assistance in plastic and reconstructive surgery, from cadaveric to clinical examples. We have provided and up-to-date list of all areas of interest to the plastic and reconstructive surgeon, evaluating the relevant advantages and disadvantages of the use of robotics in these areas.

## METHODS

A database search was performed to identify all articles describing the use of robotic assistance in plastic and reconstructive surgery. The search strategy was constructed in line with the Preferred Reporting Items for Systematic Reviews and Meta Analysis (PRISMA) guidelines (8) and the Cochrane handbook (9). Key words and Medical Subject Heading terms were combined using Boolean logic and refined with the help of an information specialist (see **Figure 2** for an example of the full search strategy). Medline (1946-present), EMBASE (1980-present), and Scopus electronic databases were all searched using the developed search strategy up to May 2017.

All studies identified were downloaded into EndNote V8 for Mac (Clarivate Analytics) and duplicates removed. De-duplicated results were then uploaded to Covidence (www.covidence.org) for screening. Titles and abstracts were reviewed by two independent reviewers (OC and HS) against the inclusion and exclusion criteria and discrepancies resolved through discussion with a third, independent reviewer (TD). Studies were considered eligible for qualitative synthesis if they met the following inclusion criteria:

- the study was published in English
- the study design was one of the following: case reports, case cohorts, case–control and randomized controlled studies. Both prospective and retrospectively designed studies were included.
- the study reports the use of a robotic surgical system for a potential plastic surgery-related operation, with both preclinical and clinical applications included.

Full-text articles of those included studies were subsequently reviewed independently for final inclusion. References were checked for further, un-identified articles, and these were added in if appropriate.

A data extraction sheet was developed to extract the following data from studies: Author, date of publication, location of study, study design, number of operations performed, operations/techniques, outcomes measured. This was piloted on a random sample of papers and subsequently refined. All data were extracted and tabulated using Microsoft Word and Excel (Redmond, Washington, DC, USA).

## RESULTS

**Figure 3** illustrates the PRISMA flow diagram demonstrating the process of article retrieval and screening. A total of 7,904 articles were identified after de-duplication for screening. Of these 213 made it to full-text review. A total of 68 studies met the inclusion criteria and were eligible for inclusion in this systematic review. Included papers were divided into groups based on operative type or body location and a qualitative synthesis of the outcomes reported performed.

### Microsurgery

A total of 13 studies were identified discussing the use of robotics for a microsurgery application (**Table 1**). Eleven of these were preclinical studies in synthetic, animal, and cadaveric models (10–20) while two were clinical studies (21, 22). Katz et al. performed the first daVinci® system assisted anastomosis in a porcine model in 2005 (10), closely followed by work in canine tarsal and femoral vessels (13). In these studies, they concluded significant advantages such as the elimination of tremor at a microsurgical level, but that the lack of purpose-built microsurgical instruments was an important limitation. Further animal and human cadaveric work cemented the idea that robotically assisted microvascular surgery is both feasible and in some instances

1 Robotics/ (17637)
2 robot*.ti,ab. (29433)
3 davinci.ti,ab. (271)
4 "da vinci".ti,ab. (2389)
5 "remote operation*".ti,ab. (72)
6 1 or 2 or 3 or 4 or 5 (33732)
7 Surgery, Plastic/ (25253)
8 exp Reconstructive Surgical Procedures/ (173916)
9 Microsurgery/ (24806)
10 exp Surgical Flaps/ (54700)
11 Facial Nerve/ or Peripheral Nerves/ or Brachial Plexus Neuropathies/ (33304)
12 Cleft Lip/ or Cleft Palate/ (21272)
13 exp Lymphatic Vessels/ or Lymphedema/ (16357)
14 exp Upper Extremity/ (151103)
15 exp Lower Extremity/ (153770)
16 11 or 12 or 13 or 14 or 15 (352969)
17 6 and 16 (1977)
18 "plastic surgery".ti,ab. (12358)
19 "cosmetic surgery".ti,ab. (1694)
20 "aesthetic surgery".ti,ab. (1036)
21 "esthetic surgery".ti,ab. (181)
22 microsurg*.ti,ab. (22364)
23 "flap surgery".ti,ab. (1591)
24 "surgical flap*".ti,ab. (245)
25 "reconstructive surg*".ti,ab. (12984)
26 "free flap surg*".ti,ab. (296)
27 ("trans-oral" adj3 surg*).ti,ab. (42)
28 (transoral adj3 surg*).ti,ab. (968)
29 (nerve adj3 surg*).ti,ab. (4525)
30 (cleft adj3 surg*).ti,ab. (1442)
31 (lymph* adj3 surg*).ti,ab. (5207)
32 (tendon adj3 surg*).ti,ab. (1411)
33 7 or 8 or 9 or 10 or 18 or 19 or 20 or 21 or 22 or 23 or 24 or 25 or 26 or 27 or 28 or 29 or 30 or 31 or 32 (275760)

**FIGURE 2** | Example search strategy performed in Medline. Searches conducted on 9.5.2017.

potentially beneficial, such as when working at depth and for surgeon comfort (20).

Two clinical examples were identified, with one cohort study by Boyd et al. including 22-patients where the robot was used for harvesting the internal mammary vessels in free breast reconstruction (21). Van der Hulst et al. used the robot to perform the anastomosis, commenting on the increased time taken for this over traditional methods, as would be expected early on in the learning curve (22). As in preclinical studies, the benefits of using the daVinci® robot for performing the microvascular anastomosis include elimination of tremor and motion scaling.

## Muscle Flap Harvest

Traditionally muscle free-flaps are raised through a large incision overlying the muscle belly and are, therefore, a perfect example of where the robot can have marked benefit as minimally invasive harvesting can significantly reduce the size of externally visible scarring. Laparoscopic harvesting has been attempted, but with

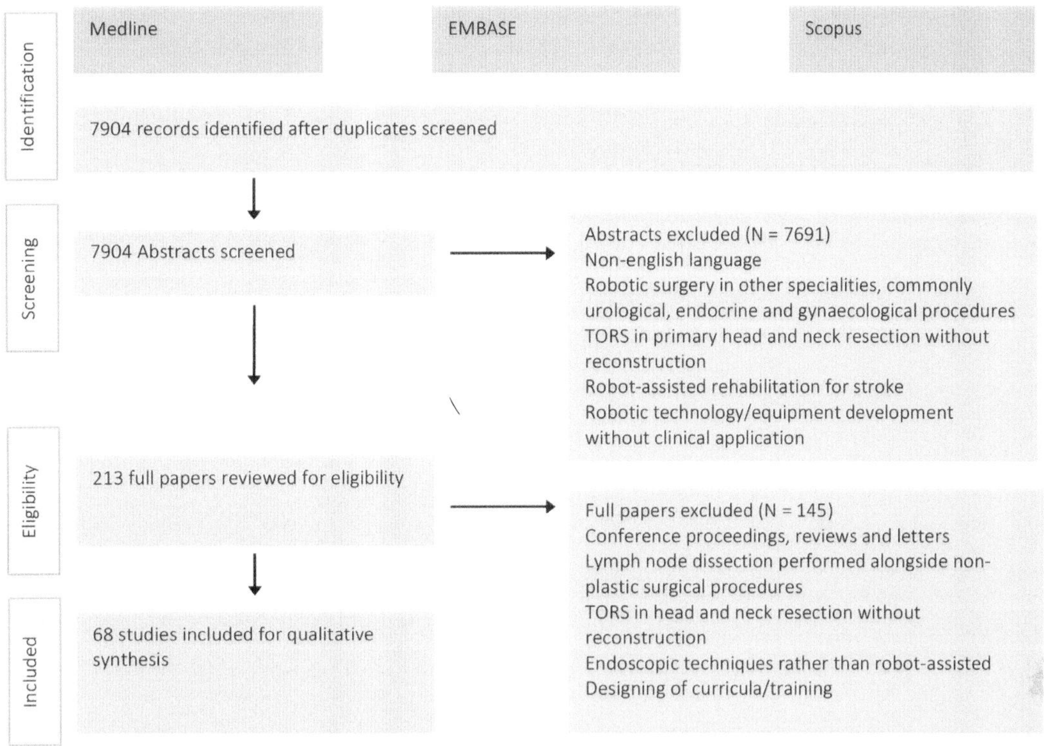


**FIGURE 3** | PRISMA flow diagram demonstrating the number of retrieved articles, those screened and final number included in the systematic review after full-text review.

poor uptake due to difficulties with visualization of the operative field and the inherent limitations of laparoscopic instruments (23, 24). Three human cadaveric studies (25–27) and five clinical reports (28–32) were identified describing the use of the robot for muscle flap harvest (**Table 2**). In those clinical studies, it is clear that the robot improves visualization, reduces the scar burden and resulted in reduced postoperative pain and hospital stay.

The traditional approach to rectus muscle harvest is with a large abdominal skin incision. Not only is this cosmetically unappealing but also, in combination with division of the anterior abdominal wall fascia, can result in incisional hernia formation. As robot-assisted colorectal surgery becomes increasingly routine, with the advantages of minimal scarring, reduced conversion to open procedure, reduced time to intestinal motility, and reduced postoperative sexual dysfunction reported (33), it would seem a retrograde step to then introduce a large abdominal wound when harvesting the rectus abdominis muscle for perineal reconstruction. In a case series by Singh et al. the robot was used in tandem with a robotically performed abdominoperineal resection for adenocarcinoma to raise the rectus abdominis flap for reconstruction (32). This produced satisfactory closure of the defect without the risk of a ventral hernia. In these combined procedures the risks associated with entering the abdominal cavity are already present from the colorectal resection and, therefore, one of the major disadvantages of robotically assisted rectus abdominis muscle harvest is not a risk purely implicated through the use of this novel muscle harvest technique.

## Nerve Surgery

A total of eight preclinical studies and five clinical studies were identified, with the majority investigating the role of robotics in brachial plexus work (**Table 3**) (34–46). Epineural nerve repair using robotic assistance has been shown to be technically feasible in animal models, with the benefits of reduced physiological tremor and improved vision of the surgical field noted (35). Nerve harvest has also been demonstrated to be feasible in cadaveric and animal models (35, 37).

In those clinical studies identified, robotic assistance was successfully used to repair a brachial plexus (45), repair the sympathetic chain to treat Horner's syndrome (42), perform a thoracic sympathectomy for palmar hyperhidrosis (43), repair a peripheral nerve following tumor excision (46), and undertake an Oberlin procedure (44).

## Upper Limb

**Table 4** illustrates those articles relating to procedures in the upper limb, with three preclinical (47–49) and one clinical study identified (50). As with a number of other areas of the body the use of the robot has so far only been for proof of concept and there has yet to be any concrete studies demonstrating a benefit.

## Trans-Oral Robotic Surgery (TORS)

Trans-oral robotic surgery has allowed head and neck surgeons to treat benign and malignant conditions of the oral

**TABLE 1** | Preclinical and clinical studies relating to the use of robotics in microvascular procedures.

| Reference | Year | Study design | Operations performed | Outcomes reported |
|---|---|---|---|---|
| **Preclinical studies** | | | | |
| Katz et al. (10) | 2005 | Animal model | Arterial and venous anastomoses and free-flap transplantation *(N = 1 pig)* | All anastomoses grossly patent, confirmed by audible Doppler signals, visibly adequate perfusion of tissues, and arterial bleeding seen after incision distal to the anastomoses 4 h after the procedure |
| Knight et al. (11) | 2005 | Animal model<br>Case controlled | Arterial end-to-end anastomoses (*N* = 31 vs *N* = 30 controls) | A remarkable degree of tremor filtration, but significantly slower operative time. All anastomoses were patent and non-leaking |
| Karamanoukian et al. (12) | 2006 | Animal tissue samples | Slit arteriotomy and end-to-end arterial anastomoses in procine hearts | The Zeus robotic system is a viable tool for microsurgical vascular reconstruction. It allows for precise movement, lack of hand tremor, enhanced microvascularisation and improved ergonomics, compared to conventional human assistance. The major advantage is the ability of the robot to scale down the surgeon's movements to a microscopic level |
| Katz et al. (13) | 2006 | Animal cadavers | Microvascular anastomoses of tarsal and superficial femoral vessels (*N* = 2 dog cadavers) | All anastomoses were successful and patent postoperatively |
| Taleb et al. (14) | 2008 | Animal cadaver | Microvascular anastomoses in rat tail transplantation (*N* = 2) | Immediate and delayed (1 h postoperation) patency of the arterial anastomoses |
| Ramdhian et al. (15) | 2011 | Animal tissue samples | Earthworm segment anastomoses (*N* = 15) | The high quality 3D vision allowed by the robotic system was excellent and compensated for loss of tactile feedback. The robotic system eliminated physiological tremor. Motion scaling by the robot improved precision of the surgical gesture |
| Lee et al. (16) | 2012 | Live animal models | Femoral artery end-to-end anastomoses (*N* = 20) | Generation of learning curves for robot-assisted microvascular anastomosis. Important aspects of learning identified included starting level, learning plateau and learning rate |
| Robert et al. (17) | 2013 | Human cadaver | Radial/ulnar artery dissection and microvascular anastomoses (*N* = 2 cadavers, 4 anastomoses) | Successful anastomoses<br>The assembling and disassembling of the vascular clamp were time consuming<br>In both cases (radial and ulnar arteries), the 10/0 needle was bent and a second suture had to be used |
| Alrasheed et al. (18) | 2014 | Synthetic vessel models | Microvascular anastomoses (*N* = 50) | Successful validation of microsurgical assessment tool and characterization of learning curve<br>Proficiency gained by operators over 5 learning sessions |
| Selber and Alrasheed (19) | 2014 | Synthetic models | Microvascular anastomoses (*N* = 5 per surgeon) | Definition of a learning curve in microsurgery and the development of a structured assessment of robotic microsurgical skills |
| Willems et al. (20) | 2016 | Synthetic microvessel models<br>Case controlled | Microvascular anastomoses (*N* = 80, vs 80 control) | Manual surgery was superior to robotically assisted microsurgery in technically easy exposures. In difficult exposures (greater depth and lower sidewall angles), however, robotically assisted microsurgery had a shorter surgery time and a higher comfort rating. Objective Structured Assessment of Technical Skills scores were similar to those assessing traditional microsurgery |
| **Clinical studies** | | | | |
| Boyd et al. (21) | 2006 | Case cohort, retrospective | Robotic vessel harvest of internal mammary vessels for use in free-flap breast reconstructive procedures (11 muscle-sparing transverse rectus abdominis musculocutaneous (TRAM) flaps, six superior gluteal artery (SGA) flaps, four superficial inferior epigastric artery flaps, and one superior gluteal arterial perforator flap) (*N* = 22 free-flaps, in 20 patients) | Pedicle was harvested with robot-assisted technique<br>Microvascular anastomosis via standard technique<br>An average pedicle length of 6.7 cm is long enough to allow anastomosis without vein graft |
| Van der Hulst et al. (22) | 2006 | Case report | Breast reconstruction with muscle-sparing free TRAM-flap, using robotic arterial anastomosis (*N* = 1) | The time to perform this anastomosis was about 40 min and significantly longer than the standard technique (around 15 min) |

*The number of procedures carried out in each study is documented and represented as N number.*

**TABLE 2** | Preclinical and clinical studies relating to the use of robotics in muscle flap harvest.

| Reference | Year | Study design | Operations performed | Outcomes reported |
|---|---|---|---|---|
| **Preclinical studies** | | | | |
| Selber (25) | 2011 | Human cadaver | Latissimus dorsi muscle harvest (*N* = 10 in 8 cadavers) | Successful harvest of all muscles |
| Patel and Pedersen (26) | 2012 | Human cadaver | Rectus abdominis muscle dissection and harvest (*N* = 2) | No postoperative complications or surgical-site morbidity |
| Selber et al. (27) | 2012 | Human cadaver | Latissimus dorsi muscle harvest and transfer (*N* = 8) | Successful harvest and transfer of all flaps that left no visible incisions, with no major complications |
| **Clinical studies** | | | | |
| Patel et al. (28) | 2012 | Case report | Pedicled myocutaneous latissimus dorsi flap for shoulder reconstruction after sarcoma resection (*N* = 1) | No objective outcomes reported-flap successfully raised robotically<br>One of the limitations is the time/learning curve |
| Lazzaro et al. (29) | 2013 | Case report | Intercostal muscle flap after lobectomy (done in conjunction with VATS) (*N* = 1) | Success of surgery—no conversion to open procedures and both patients returned home 5 days postop |
| Ibrahim et al. (30) | 2014 | Case series | Rectus abdominus muscle flap harvest (*N* not reported) | Less tissue violation, compared to open technique, resulting in reduced postoperative pain, shorter duration of hospital stay, and more rapid functional recovery |
| Chung et al. (31) | 2015 | Case series | Transaxillary gasless robot-assisted latissimus dorsi muscle harvest (3 delayed reconstructions, 4 immediate after nipple sparing mastectomy, 5 corrections of deformity in Poland syndrome) (*N* = 12) | Operating time, general satisfaction, cosmetic satisfaction, scar, and symmetry satisfaction were all outcomes measured *via* survey given to all patients with follow-up longer than months<br>Robotic time decreases with experience |
| Singh et al. (32) | 2015 | Case series and retrospective review | Extralevator abdominoperineal excision with robotic rectus abdominis flap harvest, for reconstruction after resection of distal rectal adenocarcinoma (*N* = 3) | An incisionless robotic flap harvest with preservation of the anterior rectus sheath obviates the risk of ventral hernia while providing robust tissue closure of the radiated abdominoperineal excision wound |

*The number of procedures carried out in each study is documented and represented as N number.*

cavity and oropharynx avoiding more traditional jaw and lip split approaches, facilitated by the improved access and visualization afforded by the robotic instruments (51, 52). If there is no communication between the oral cavity or oropharynx and neck dissection then the defect could be left to heal by secondary intention; however, in more complex or advanced stages of disease, reconstruction using local flaps or free tissue transfer is required (53). If a jaw split has not been performed, access for satisfactory reconstruction can be almost impossible and thus developing reconstructive techniques using the robot in order to capitalize on the minimized morbidity associated with a TORS resection is of paramount importance.

Trans-oral robotic surgery has become the biggest area for robotic-assisted plastic surgery procedures, with 2 preclinical (54, 55) and 21 clinical studies identified (56–76) (**Table 5**). Local reconstructive options include the use of the Facial Artery Musculomucosal flap, commonly used in reconstruction of the floor of the mouth and soft palate. Bonawitz and Duvvuri have described using the robot for raising and in-setting the flap with good results (64, 65). Others demonstrated that the use of the robot to perform a musculomucosal advancement flap pharyngoplasty gives good results, both in terms of orocutaneous fistula risk and functional outcomes (60, 61).

In larger or more complex composite defects there is often the requirement for free-flap reconstruction, with specific indications including exposure of the carotid artery, large base-of-tongue defects and defects of the soft palate and tonsillar fossa which cannot be closed with local flap options. The commonest reported free-flap used following TORS resection is the radial forearm flap; however, others such as the anterolateral thigh flap are also described. In the majority of cases the robot was used for flap inset, with authors reporting good access and visualization that allowed a water-tight inset to be achieved and no flap complications despite the lack of a traditional jaw spilled. The robot was also used in a number of studies to perform the vascular anastomosis (58, 62, 63, 69).

## Trans-Oral Robotic Cleft Surgery (TORCS)

Trans-oral robotic cleft surgery is still in its infancy with only three articles identified (77–79) (**Table 6**); however, it builds upon the same benefit profile achieved by TORS that has been outlined previously for access to the oral cavity and oropharynx in cleft lip and palate patients.

## Other Indications

**Table 7** demonstrates four other studies identified in the systematic review, which do not fit into the categories above (80–83). Of these indications, it is likely that only lymph node based procedures are likely to progress in the future, with some benefits such as the ability to perform supermicro-surgery an obvious advantage in lymph node transfer.

**TABLE 3** | Preclinical and clinical studies relating to the use of robotics in nerve surgery.

| Reference | Year | Study design | Operations performed | Outcomes reported |
|---|---|---|---|---|
| **Preclinical studies** | | | | |
| Latif et al. (34) | 2008 | Animal model | Intercostal nerve grafting for reversal of thoracic sympathectomy (*N* = 1) | Successful anastomosis with no apparent complications |
| Nectoux et al. (35) | 2009 | Animal and human tissue samples | Extrafascicular neurolysis, donor nerve dissection and subsequent repair of peripheral nerve (*N* not reported) | The robot removed physiological tremor<br>There was some technical difficulty with the choice and manipulation of the three-dimensional stereoscopic vision enabled a better view and safe and accurate repair of peripheral nerve lesions |
| Mantovani et al. (36) | 2011 | Human cadaver | Supraclavicular brachial plexus exploration and nerve graft anastomosis and reconstruction (*N* = 2) | The robot allowed microsurgery to be performed in a very small space with telemanipulation and minimally invasive techniques |
| Garcia et al. (37) | 2012 | Human cadaver | Sural nerve graft and neurotisation using the accessory nerve (*N* = 3) | The goals of the operation were achieved without conversion to open surgery. There were no complications |
| de Melo et al. (38) | 2013 | Human cadaver | Microsurgical nerve transfer of the branches of the axillary nerve onto the nerve of the long head of the triceps brachii (*N* = 1) | Dissection and transfer achieved successfully |
| Facca et al. (39) | 2014 | Human cadaver | Sural nerge graft between C5 root or spinal nerve, and the musculocutaneous nerve (*N* = 8) | Endoscopic treatment of supraclavicular nerve palsy is feasible, however, both sural nerve grafts and C5-6 avulsions were converted to open |
| Porto de Melo et al. (40) | 2014 | Animal model | Phrenic nerve harvest and application in brachial plexus surgery (*N* = 1) | Successful nerve harvest |
| Miyamoto et al. (41) | 2016 | Animal model | Intercostal nerve harvest for brachial plexus reconstruction (*N* = 3) | Physiological tremor was eliminated and there were no major complications |
| **Clinical studies** | | | | |
| Latif et al. (42) | 2011 | Case study | Intercostal nerve graft harvesting and grafting into sympathetic chain using tension free nerve anastomoses (*N* = 1) | Successful operation, patient discharged one day postoperatively and no sign of Horner's syndrome on short term follow-up |
| Coveliers et al. (43) | 2013 | Case cohort, retrospective | Selective postganglionic thoracic sympathectomy for patients with palmar or axillary hyperhidrosis (*N* = 110 operations in 55 patients) | Of the 55 patients, 53 (96%) had sustained relief of their hyperhidrosis at a median follow-up of 24 months (range, 3 to 36 months), and compensatory sweating was seen in four patients (7.2%) |
| Naito et al. (44) | 2012 | Case cohort | The Oberlin procedure of nerve transfer for restoration of elbow flexion (*N* = 4) | At 12 months' mean follow-up, all patients had recovered to useful elbow flexion, with no sensory/motor deficit in the ulnar nerve territory |
| Berner (45) (book chapter) | 2013 | Case series | Repair of brachial plexus injury (*N* = 12) | Considering the microsurgical gesture, all nerve repairs were achieved under excellent conditions<br>Need to convert to open surgery in nine cases |
| Tigan et al. (46) | 2014 | Case cohort | Nerve grafting after excision of benign peripheral nerve tumors (*N* = 7) | In postoperative surveys, neuropathic pain halved from 6/10 to 3/10 postop, with no worsening of sensory deficits |

*The number of procedures carried out in each study is documented and represented as N number.*

## DISCUSSION

In the 30 years since the first robot was used in a surgical procedure the arena of robotic surgery has changed at a breathtaking pace, with the use of the daVinci® robot now common place in some specialties. This revolution has taken longer to impact on the plastic surgery community. It is, therefore, somewhat ironic that it was a plastic surgeon who was at the forefront of robotic and tele-surgery at its inception (84). However, this systematic review has shown that significant developments have been made in the last few years.

The benefits of robotic surgery have been well documented, albeit with no large scale studies, and include reduced blood loss, reduced postoperative pain, faster recovery, and improved cosmesis (85). In relation to plastic and reconstructive surgery the elimination of tremor, greater degree of freedom of the instrument and motion scaling all have the potential to improve the accuracy and reproducibility of microsurgery. The evidence suggests that while the initial learning curve is steep, proficiency in microsurgical skills using the robot can be gained in a short number of sessions (18).

Of the areas identified in this systematic review there are some that are further down the development road than others and some, where the advantages of robotic assistance are greater. For example, with the recent uptake of free-perforator flaps in the field of reconstructive surgery we are beginning to approach the limits of human dexterity at which point the robot may prove to

**TABLE 4** | Preclinical and clinical studies relating to the use of robotics in upper limb procedures.

| Reference | Year | Study design | Operations performed | Outcomes reported |
|---|---|---|---|---|
| **Preclinical studies** | | | | |
| Taleb et al. (47) | 2009 | Animal cadaver | Humeral cross-section, amputation, and replantation of the left forelimb. Stages done with surgical robot were soft tissue repair and vessel patency tests during limb replantation (not any microvascular procedures) ($N$ = 1) | Patency tests were all positive. Venous bleeding demonstrated vascular success of replantation<br>The robot removed physiological tremor and allowed for a smaller operating field |
| Huart et al. (48) | 2012 | Human cadaver | Kite flap hand surgery ($N$ = 1) | Operating time was longer with the robot, but kite flap transfer was successful |
| Maire et al. (49) | 2012 | Human cadaver | Removal of left hallux medial hemipulp (with sensory nerve, collateral artery and dorsal vein) and transfer to left thumb radial hemipulp ($N$ = 1) | Successful free hallux hemipulp transfer, however, operating time was increased by non-microsurgical moments which could be improved by instrumentation improvement |
| **Clinical studies** | | | | |
| Facca and Liverneaux (50) | 2010 | Case report | Robotic anastomosis of vein grafts for hypothenar hammer syndrome ($N$ = 1) | No postoperative problems of note<br>Successful cure of vasomotor disorder |

*The number of procedures carried out in each study is documented and represented as N number.*

**TABLE 5** | Preclinical and clinical studies relating to the use of robotics in trans-oral robotic surgery (TORS) for a plastic surgery application.

| Reference | Year | Study design | Operations performed | Outcomes reported |
|---|---|---|---|---|
| **Preclinical studies** | | | | |
| Selber et al. (54) | 2010 | Coffee cup models, pig cadavers, human cadavers | TORS free radial forearm flap reconstruction of oropharyngeal defect ($N$ = 2)<br>Robotic microvascular anastomosis | Successful reconstruction of the oropharynx by trans-oral robotic flap inset and microvascular anastomosis |
| Smartt et al. (55) | 2013 | Human cadaver | Superiorly based posterior pharyngeal flap transfer ($N$ = 3) | Successful transfer of posterior pharyngeal flaps, with mean surgical time of 113 min. Technically, the learning curve for using the robot telemanipulator was steep<br>There was no damage to adjacent structures |
| **Clinical studies** | | | | |
| Desai et al. (56) | 2008 | Case cohort, retrospective analysis | Mucosal flap and pyriform sinus flap reconstructions ($N$ = 7) | No intra- or postoperative complications, one patient required tracheostomy |
| Mukhija et al. (57) | 2009 | Case series | Radial forearm fasciocutaneous free-flap harvest and reconstruction of oral cavity ($N$ = 2) | Successful positioning of the flap, shorter operating time compared to conventional techniques, shorter hospital stay compared to mandibulotomy approach |
| Selber (58) | 2010 | Case series | Free-flap reconstruction of oropharynx (radial forearm free-flap, anterolateral thigh flap, facial artery, myomucosal flap), primary closure after tumor resection, and microvascular anastomosis ($N$ = 5) | Better access and improved precision within the oropharynx, compared to conventional tecnhiques<br>Successful microvascular anastomosis |
| Garfein et al. (59) | 2011 | Case report | Radial forearm flap for reconstruction of the tounge base, vallecula and pre-epiglotic space, due to soft tissue and hyoid radionecrosis ($N$ = 1) | The patient passed a swallow evaluation after 1 week, and started an oral diet 8 days after the operation<br>There was good function showed by video oesophagram 6 week postoperatively |
| Genden et al. (60) | 2011 | Prospective non-randomized case–control study | Free-flap reconstruction of oropharynx—sternocleidomastoid free-flap, mucosal mulscular flaps and pharyngoplasty ($N$ = 30) | Equivalent rates of loco-regional and distant control of malignancy and better short-term eating ability, compared to conventional techniques<br>No major long term sequelae |
| Genden et al. (61) | 2011 | Prospective non-randomized case–control study | Musculomucosal advancement flap pharyngoplasty ($N$ = 30)<br>Radial forearm free-flap reconstruction | Postoperatively, patients regained excellent function, with near-normal scores on the Functional Oral Intake Scale and Performance Status Scale for Head and Neck Cancer Patients at 1 year after surgery |
| Bonawitz and Duvvuri (62) | 2012 | Case cohort, retrospective | Free-flap oropharyngeal reconstruction, with microvascular anastomoses in the tongue base and soft palate ($N$ not reported) | No major complications and no flap loss |

(Continued)

**TABLE 5** | Continued

| Reference | Year | Study design | Operations performed | Outcomes reported |
|---|---|---|---|---|
| Longfield et al. (63) | 2012 | Case series | Robotic reconstruction after resection squamous cell carcinoma of the oropharynx using local and distant free-flaps, with microvascular anastomoses (*N* not reported) | Patients can be safely reconstructed (locally or with free tissue transfer) robotically after TORS |
| Bonawitz and Duvvuri (64) | 2013 | Case series | Local random transposition flaps from buccal mucosa, the hard palate or the pharyngeal wall (*N* not reported)<br>Facial artery musculomucosal (FAMM) flap for larger defects of the soft palate | No major complications |
| Bonawitz and Duvvuri (65) | 2013 | Case cohort, retrospective | FAMM flap reconstruction after removal of malignant tumors of the soft palate ($N = 5$) | No major complications, no flap loss |
| Duvvuri et al. (66) | 2013 | Case cohort, retrospective | Oropharyngeal reconstruction with FAMM free-flaps, ALT free-flaps, radial forearm flaps and uvular flaps ($N = 12$) | No major complications, some minor flap dehiscence, two revision procedures needed (one fistula, one bulky flap) |
| Hans et al. (67) | 2013 | Case series | Radial forearm free-flap reconstruction after resection of hypopharyngeal carcinoma ($N = 2$) | A complication of a neck hematoma requiring draining under general anesthesia, no fistulae |
| Park et al. (68) | 2013 | Case series, prospective study | Radial forearm muscle free-flap reconstruction of oropharynx ($N = 7$) | No surgery-related complications of infections, viable and functioning free-flaps in all patients, one hundred percent of patients happy with postoperative appearance and could tolerate an oral diet |
| Song et al. (69) | 2013 | Case series | Robotic ablation surgery, free-flap reconstruction (radial forearm free-flaps, anterolateral thigh flap), and microvascular anastomosis ($N = 5$) | Flap insetting and microanastomoses were achieved using a specially manufactured robotic instrument<br>No complications |
| De Almeida et al. (70) | 2014 | Case cohort, retrospective | Velopharyngoplasty reconstructinos with local flaps alone, regional and free-flaps, and secondary healing ($N = 92$) | Good swallowing outcomes, no carotid artery ruptures |
| Byeon et al. (71) | 2015 | Case series | Reconstruction and lymph node dissection for head and neck malignancy ($N = 37$) | Good cosmetic outcomes and no major complications |
| Perrenot et al. (72) | 2014 | Case series | Infra-hyoid myocutaneous flap reconstructions ($N = 8$) | Good esthetic results<br>One case required re-operating due to hemostasis<br>No other complications<br>Seven out of eight patients tolerated oral feeding postoperatively |
| Lai et al. (73) | 2015 | Case cohort | Free radial forearm fasciocutaneous flap reconstruction after resection of oropharyngeal cancer ($N = 5$) | All reconstructive surgeries were successful, with no flap failure or take-backs, no wound infections and no fistulae |
| Meccariello et al. (74) | 2016 | Case report | Resection and reconstruction, with temporalis muscle flap, of squamous cell carcinoma of the lateral oropharyngeal wall extending into the soft palate ($N = 1$) | Restoration of a competent velopharyngeal sphincter, with water-tight seal between pharynx and neck<br>Timely healing and enhanced postoperative functional results |
| Gorphe et al. (75) | 2017 | Non-randomized phase II muti-center prospective trial | FAMM and free ALT flap reconstructions of the oropharynx ($N = 9$) | Robotic surgery proved feasible, and further technological progress in developing robotic systems specifically for trans-oral surgery will be of benefit to patients |
| Biron et al. (76) | 2017 | Case–control series | Radial forearm free-flap reconstruction after excision of oropharyngeal squamous cell carcinoma ($N = 18$) | Significantly shorter admission duration and fewer postoperative complications |

*The number of procedures carried out in each study is documented and represented as N number.*

be advantageous. However, to fully exploit this there needs to be focused development in the field of robotic instrument design, expanding the portfolio of micro-instruments. It is our opinion that the potential for robotic head and neck reconstruction is huge and is one of the areas that will most definitely see growth due to the obvious benefits it offers. This will be especially true as the indications for TORS resection continue to widen, resulting in larger and more complex defects. The current limitation to more widespread utilization is instrument design in order to perform microvascular anastomoses and easier inset and it is

**TABLE 6** | Preclinical and clinical studies relating to the use of robotics in trans-oral robotic cleft surgery.

| Reference | Year | Study design | Operations performed | Outcomes reported |
|---|---|---|---|---|
| **Preclinical studies** | | | | |
| Khan et al. (77) | 2016 | Airway manikin and human cadaver | The Hynes pharyngoplasty ($N$ = 1) | With each variation, a subjective assessment (rated as poor, fair, good or excellent) was made for vision and access to either the posterior pharynx or palate, and it was validated by two of the authors for each set-up |
| Podolsky et al. (78) | 2017 | Cleft palate simulator test bed | The von Langenbeck cleft palate repair procedure ($N$ = 1) | Excellent close up visualization of the anatomy, the ability to articulate the wrist intra-orally (not possible with standard instruments), tremor reduction, better ambidexterity and more precise dissection and tissue manipulation, compared to conventional open techniques |
| **Clinical studies** | | | | |
| Nadjmi (79) | 2015 | Controlled cohort study | The robot was used to dissection and repair the palatine muscles in 10 patients with a cleft of the palate ($N$ = 10, 30 controls) | Increased dexterity and operative view using the robot<br>Overall operative time was longer using the robot compared to the control group in which the traditional method was used |

*The number of procedures carried out in each study is documented and represented as N number.*

**TABLE 7** | Preclinical and clinical studies relating to the use of robotics in other, miscellaneous areas of plastic and reconstructive surgery.

| Reference | Year | Study design | Operations performed | Outcomes reported |
|---|---|---|---|---|
| **Microvascular surgery** | | | | |
| Dombre et al. (80) | 2003 | Live animal model | Skin graft ($N$ not reported) | Robotically harvested skin samples were of the same quality as manually harvested ones |
| Taghizadeh et al. (81) | 2014 | Human cadaver | "Necklift" platysmaplasty—a short incision facelift with concomitant robot-assisted neck lift ($N$ = 6) | Successful necklift procedures, with certain areas for improvement in surgical methodology suggested when using robotic systems (hard to interpret) |
| Shi et al. (82) | 2017 | Live animal model | Mandibular bone drilling osteotomy ($N$ = 1) | The robotically assisted drilling demonstrated more accurate drill positioning, increased stability and accuracy, and relieved surgeon fatigue so as to reduce facial trauma |
| **Clinical studies** | | | | |
| Ciudad et al. (83) | 2016 | Case-report | Tight gastroepiploic lymph node flap (RGE-LNF) for the treatment of lymphedema of the extremities ($N$ = 1)<br>Microvascular procedures performed with standard technique | Successful flap harvest, but no postoperative surgical outcomes reported |

*The number of procedures carried out in each study is documented and represented as N number.*

this area that research should focus. This may also be the case with TORCS. As with cancer resection, there are many circumstances where adequate access to the pharynx and palate in the pediatric cleft patient can pose a significant challenge. The space in which to operate, as well as access for instrumentation, can be severely restricted, especially in cases with abnormal anatomy, poor jaw opening, or anomalies of the nasopharyngeal space. Adequate illumination and visualization can also be difficult. Early work has shown that performing posterior pharyngeal wall surgery using the daVinci® robot is feasible, with benefits such as an improved view, easier dissection, reduced secondary surgical insult and preferential ergonomics for the operating surgeon (77). Its use may also open up avenues of new surgical interventions to areas of the oropharynx that were previously inaccessible.

There is currently less convincing evidence for the use of robotics in areas such as nerve and upper limb surgery. In brachial plexus reconstruction nerve harvest is often required and, therefore, reduced donor site morbidity through robotic harvest, such as with trans-thoracic harvest of intercostal and phrenic nerves, is an area that has the potential for future advancement. It will be important, however, to also demonstrate its safety and cost-effectiveness in order to justify the marginal reductions in scarring when compared to more traditional harvest sites. To date all of the preclinical and clinical studies investigating robotic nerve surgery have demonstrated that it is technically feasible. However, it is still mostly at a proof of concept level and while does have benefits in terms of reduced tremor, it is most likely to be of benefit in difficult to assess areas or when the robot is already being used to perform other parts of the procedure. Finally, at present the indications for the use of robotics in hand surgery are probably more limited than other areas discussed, especially as access is not normally a problem in hand surgery. However, the benefits as discussed for microsurgical anastomosis may prove to be useful in specific indications such as traumatic replantation or congenital reconstruction.

Robotic surgery's main disadvantage remains the high cost of purchasing and maintaining the equipment. This will undoubtedly improve with time as a greater number of procedures are performed using the robot and the unit cost per operation reduces. A recent comparison of the cost of TORS compared to radiotherapy demonstrated that TORS is currently more expensive; however, this is likely to reduce through the creation of high-volume centers performing TORS (86). It has also been shown that in a center where the learning curve had already been overcome, robotic surgery was cheaper than equivalent open surgery for the surgical treatment of endometrial cancer (87).

Lack of haptic feedback is also often cited as another disadvantage of robotic surgery, with studies demonstrating that operators of augmented robotic surgical systems prefer those with haptic feedback (88). However, other studies such as by Hagen and colleagues who looked at 52 individuals and their perception of haptic feedback while performing robotic surgery demonstrated that visual cues are able to give the perception of haptic feedback, even when true haptic feedback is not present (89). Despite this evidence there is still a tremendous amount of working looking at ways to incorporate haptic feedback into robotic systems, summarized in a review by Okamura (90).

Finally, robotic surgery often results in longer operative times, although this improves with proficiency and in some cases is now comparable to traditional techniques.

The future of robotics in plastic surgery is clearly exciting. Over the last 5 years the range of procedures using the daVinci® robot being attempted by the plastic surgery community has increased significantly and, as technology continues to improve, this will gain further momentum. Of the 68 studies included in this review, only three used a robotic system other than the daVinci®. This dominance is beginning to be challenged and while equipment additions such as a micro-forcep is currently available for the daVinci® robot and external companies have developed micro-doppler probes and hydrojet dissectors (91) it will be the development of further microsurgical instruments that will allow greater use of the robot in the field of plastic and reconstructive surgery. The combination of motion scaling and tremor-free instrument manipulation with new instrument design will also allow new avenues in microsurgery that have to date been too technically demanding to be explored. Furthermore, the introduction of a new single port addition to the daVinci® system will allow greater access in trans-oral surgery, improving instrument maneuverability within the tight confines of the intra-oral cavity.

## CONCLUSION

The potential value of robotic plastic surgery has already been investigated in several specific indications. It is still early days for the field and only time will tell if the use of robotics in plastic surgery is truly of benefit. As the technology, knowledge, and skills in this area improve, it is likely that in specific indications the use of robotic surgery will further contribute positively to patient and provider experience and outcomes. It is, therefore, imperative that the plastic surgery community embraces this new technology platform, but in doing so conducts well-designed, patient-focused research to ensure that it is only being used when there is true benefit to our patients.

## AUTHOR CONTRIBUTIONS

TD, KK, and IW developed the idea for this paper. TD, OC, and HS developed the search strategy and performed the systematic review and data extraction. TD, KK, IW, OC, and HS wrote the manuscript and all authors edited and agreed the final version.

## FUNDING

This work has received no specific funding. TD is funded by the Welsh Clinical Academic Training Fellowship.

## REFERENCES

1. Ballantyne GH. Robotic surgery, telerobotic surgery, telepresence, and telementoring. Review of early clinical results. *Surg Endosc* (2002) 16(10):1389–402. doi:10.1007/s00464-001-8283-7
2. Kappert U, Cichon R, Schneider J, Gulielmos V, Tugtekin SM, Matschke K, et al. Robotic coronary artery surgery – the evolution of a new minimally invasive approach in coronary artery surgery. *Thorac Cardiovasc Surg* (2000) 48(4):193–7. doi:10.1055/s-2000-6904
3. Ishikawa N, Watanabe G, Iino K, Tomita S, Yamaguchi S, Higashidani K, et al. Robotic internal thoracic artery harvesting. *Surg Today* (2007) 37(11):944–6. doi:10.1007/s00595-007-3542-4
4. Cadière GB, Himpens J, Germay O, Izizaw R, Degueldre M, Vandromme J, et al. Feasibility of robotic laparoscopic surgery: 146 cases. *World J Surg* (2001) 25(11):1467–77. doi:10.1007/s00268-001-0132-2
5. Bush SH, Apte SM. Robotic-assisted surgery in gynecological oncology. *Cancer Control* (2015) 22(3):307–13. doi:10.1177/107327481502200308
6. Barbash GI, Glied SA. New technology and health care costs – the case of robot-assisted surgery. *N Engl J Med* (2010) 363(8):701–4. doi:10.1056/NEJMp1006602
7. Pappou EP, Weiser MR. Robotic colonic resection. *J Surg Oncol* (2015) 112(3):315–20. doi:10.1002/jso.23953
8. Moher D, Liberati A, Tetzlaff J, Altman DG. Preferred reporting items for systematic reviews and meta-analyses: the PRISMA statement. *Ann Intern Med* (2009) 151(4):264–9. doi:10.1016/j.jclinepi.2009.06.005
9. Higgins JPT, Green S, editors. Cochrane handbook for systematic reviews of interventions version 5.1.0 [updated March 2011]. *The Cochrane Collaboration*. (2011).
10. Katz RD, Rosson GD, Taylor JA, Singh NK. Robotics in microsurgery: use of a surgical robot to perform a free flap in a pig. *Microsurgery* (2005) 25:566–9. doi:10.1002/micr.20160
11. Knight CG, Lorincz A, Cao A, Gidell K, Klein MD, Langenburg SE. Computer-assisted, robot-enhanced open microsurgery in an animal model. *J Laparoendosc Adv Surg Tech A* (2005) 15(2):182–5. doi:10.1089/lap.2005.15.182
12. Karamanoukian RL, Finley DS, Evans GR, Karamanoukian HL. Feasibility of robotic-assisted microvascular anastomoses in plastic surgery. *J Reconstr Microsurg* (2006) 22(06):429–32. doi:10.1055/s-2006-947697
13. Katz RD, Taylor JA, Rosson GD, Brown PR, Singh NK. Robotics in plastic and reconstructive surgery: use of a telemanipulator slave robot to perform microvascular anastomoses. *J Reconstr Microsurg* (2006) 22:53–7. doi:10.1055/s-2006-931908
14. Taleb C, Nectoux E, Liverneaux PA. Telemicrosurgery: a feasibility study in a rat model. *Chir Main* (2008) 27(2–3):104–8. doi:10.1016/j.main.2008.04.001

15. Ramdhian RM, Bednar M, Mantovani GR, Facca SA, Liverneaux PA. Microsurgery and telemicrosurgery training: a comparative study. *J Reconstr Microsurg* (2011) 27(09):537–42. doi:10.1055/s-0031-1285985
16. Lee JY, Mattar T, Parisi TJ, Carlsen BT, Bishop AT, Shin AY. Learning curve of robotic-assisted microvascular anastomosis in the rat. *J Reconstr Microsurg* (2012) 28(07):451–6. doi:10.1055/s-0031-1289166
17. Robert E, Facca S, Atik T, Bodin F, Bruant-Rodier C, Liverneaux P. Vascular microanastomosis through an endoscopic approach: feasibility study on two cadaver forearms. *Chir Main* (2013) 32(3):136–40. doi:10.1016/j.main.2013.01.002
18. Alrasheed T, Liu J, Hanasono MM, Butler CE, Selber JC. Robotic microsurgery: validating an assessment tool and plotting the learning curve. *Plast Reconstr Surg* (2014) 134:794–803. doi:10.1097/PRS.0000000000000550
19. Selber JC, Alrasheed T. Robotic microsurgical training and evaluation. *Semin Plast Surg* (2014) 28(1):005–010. doi:10.1055/s-0034-1368161
20. Willems JI, Shin AM, Shin DM, Bishop AT, Shin AY. A comparison of robotically assisted microsurgery versus manual microsurgery in challenging situations. *Plast Reconstr Surg* (2016) 137(4):1317–24. doi:10.1097/PRS.0000000000002030
21. Boyd B, Umansky J, Samson M, Boyd D, Stahl K. Robotic harvest of internal mammary vessels in breast reconstruction. *J Reconstr Microsurg* (2006) 22(4):261–6. doi:10.1055/s-2006-939931
22. van der Hulst R, Sawor J, Bouvy N. Microvascular anastomosis: is there a role for robotic surgery? *J Plast Reconstr Aesthetic Surg* (2007) 60(1):101–2. doi:10.1016/j.bjps.2006.05.011
23. Greensmith A, Januszkiewicz J, Poole G. Rectus abdominis muscle free flap by laparoscopic sheath-sparing technique. *Plast Reconstr Surg* (2000) 105(4):1438–41. doi:10.1097/00006534-200004040-00026
24. Aijaz T, Singhal D, Tan SA, Iqbal A. A novel method of minimally invasive rectus abdominis muscle flap harvest: laparoscopic surgeons take note. *J Minim Access Surg* (2017) 13(2):146–7. doi:10.4103/0972-9941.186688
25. Selber JC. Robotic latissimus dorsi muscle harvest. *Plast Reconstr Surg* (2011) 128(2):88.e–90.e. doi:10.1097/PRS.0b013e31821ef25d
26. Patel NV, Pedersen JC. Robotic harvest of the rectus abdominis muscle: a preclinical investigation and case report. *J Reconstr Microsurg* (2012) 28:477–80. doi:10.1055/s-0031-1287674
27. Selber JC, Baumann DP, Holsinger CF. Robotic harvest of the latissimus dorsi muscle: laboratory and clinical experience. *J Reconstr Microsurg* (2012) 28:457–64. doi:10.1055/s-0032-1315789
28. Patel NP, Van Meeteren J, Pedersen J. A new dimension: robotic reconstruction in plastic surgery. *J Robot Surg* (2012) 6(1):77–80. doi:10.1007/s11701-011-0300-9
29. Lazzaro RS, Guerges M, Kadosh B, Gulkarov I. Robotic harvest of intercostal muscle flap. *J Thorac Cardiovasc Surg* (2013) 146(2):486–7. doi:10.1016/j.jtcvs.2013.03.037
30. Ibrahim AE, Sarhane KA, Pederson JC, Selber JC. Robotic harvest of the rectus abdominis muscle: principles and clinical applications. *Semin Plast Surg* (2014) 28(1):26–31. doi:10.1055/s-0034-1368164
31. Chung JH, You HJ, Kim HS, Lee BI, Park SH, Yoon ES. A novel technique for robot assisted latissimus dorsi flap harvest. *J Plast Reconstr Aesthet Surg* (2015) 68:966–72. doi:10.1016/j.bjps.2015.03.021
32. Singh P, Teng E, Cannon LM, Bello BL, Song DH, Umanskiy K. Dynamic article: tandem robotic technique of extralevator abdominoperineal excision and rectus abdominis muscle harvest for immediate closure of the pelvic floor defect. *Dis Colon Rectum* (2015) 58(9):885–91. doi:10.1097/DCR.0000000000000419
33. Lee SH, Lim S, Kim JH, Lee KY. Robotic versus conventional laparoscopic surgery for rectal cancer: systematic review and meta-analysis. *Ann Surg Treat Res* (2015) 89:190–201. doi:10.4174/astr.2015.89.4.190
34. Latif MJ, Afthinos JN, Connery CP, Perin N, Bhora FY, Chwajol M, et al. Robotic intercostal nerve graft for reversal of thoracic sympathectomy: a large animal feasibility model. *Int J Med Robot* (2008) 4(3):258–62. doi:10.1002/rcs.205
35. Nectoux E, Taleb C, Liverneaux P. Nerve repair in telemicrosurgery: an experimental study. *J Reconstr Microsurg* (2009) 25:261–5. doi:10.1055/s-0028-1104562
36. Mantovani G, Liverneaux P, Garcia JC Jr, Berner SH, Bednar MS, Mohr CJ. Endoscopic exploration and repair of brachial plexus with telerobotic manipulation: a cadaver trial. *J Neurosurg* (2011) 115(3):659–64. doi:10.3171/2011.3.JNS10931
37. Garcia JC Jr, Lebailly F, Mantovani G, Mendonca LA, Garcia J, Liverneaux P. Telerobotic manipulation of the brachial plexus. *J Reconstr Microsurg* (2012) 28:491–4. doi:10.1055/s-0032-1313761
38. de Melo PP, Garcia JC, de Souza Montero EF, Atik T, Robert EG, Facca S, et al. Feasibility of an endoscopic approach to the axillary nerve and the nerve to the long head of the triceps brachii with the help of the Da Vinci Robot. *Chir Main* (2013) 32(4):206–9. doi:10.1016/j.main.2013.05.003
39. Facca S, Hendriks S, Mantovani G, Selber JC, Liverneaux P. Robot- assisted surgery of the shoulder girdle and brachial plexus. *Semin Plast Surg* (2014) 28:39–44. doi:10.1055/s-0034-1368167
40. Porto de Melo P, Miyamoto H, Serradori T, Ruggiero Mantovani G, Selber J, Facca S, et al. Robotic phrenic nerve harvest: a feasibility study in a pig model. *Chir Main* (2014) 33:356–60. doi:10.1016/j.main.2014.07.006
41. Miyamoto H, Serradori T, Mikami Y, Selber J, Santelmo N, Facca S, et al. Robotic intercostal nerve harvest: a feasibility study in a pig model. *J Neurosurg* (2016) 124(1):264–8. doi:10.3171/2015.1.JNS14603
42. Latif MJ, Park K, Razi SS, Bhora F, Todd G, Perin N, et al. Robotic microsurgical nerve grafting for sympathectomy reversal: technique and feasibility for first human case. *Int J Med Robot Comput Assist Surg* (2011) 7:27.
43. Coveliers H, Meyer M, Gharagozloo F, Wisselink W, Rauwerda JM, Tempesta B, et al. Robotic selective postganglionic thoracic sympathectomy for the treatment of hyperhidrosis. *Ann Thorac Surg* (2013) 95(1):269–74. doi:10.1016/j.athoracsur.2012.08.013
44. Naito K, Facca S, Lequint T, Liverneaux PA. The Oberlin procedure for restoration of elbow flexion with the da Vinci robot: four cases. *Plast Reconstr Surg* (2012) 129(3):707–11. doi:10.1097/PRS.0b013e318241287f
45. Berner S. Nerve repair. In: Liverneaux P, Berner S, Bednar M, Parekattil S, Mantovani Ruggiero G, Selber J, editors. *Telemicrosurgery*. Paris: Springer (2013) p. 119–22.
46. Tigan L, Miyamoto H, Hendriks S, Facca S, Liverneaux P. Interest of telemicrosurgery in peripheral nerve tumors: about a series of seven cases. *Chir Main* (2014) 33(1):13–6. doi:10.1016/j.main.2013.10.177
47. Taleb C, Nectoux E, Liverneaux P. Limb replantation with two robots: a feasibility study in a pig model. *Microsurgery* (2009) 29(3):232–5. doi:10.1002/micr.20602
48. Huart A, Facca S, Lebailly F, Garcia JC, Liverneaux PA. Are pedicled flaps feasible in robotic surgery? Report of an anatomical study of the kite flap in conventional surgery versus robotic surgery. *Surg Innov* (2012) 19(1):89–92. doi:10.1177/1553350611415869
49. Maire N, Naito K, Lequint T, Facca S, Berner S, Liverneaux P. Robot-assisted free toe pulp transfer: feasibility study. *J Reconstr Microsurg* (2012) 28:481–4. doi:10.1055/s-0032-1313760
50. Facca S, Liverneaux P. Robotic assisted microsurgery in hypothenar hammer syndrome: a case report. *Comput Aided Surg* (2010) 15(4–6):110–4. doi:10.3109/10929088.2010.507942
51. Hockstein NG, Nolan JP, O'Malley BW, Woo YJ. Robotic microlaryngeal surgery: a technical feasibility study using the daVinci surgical robot and an airway mannequin. *Laryngoscope* (2005) 115:780–5. doi:10.1097/01.MLG.0000159202.04941.67
52. Weinstein GS, O'Malley BW, Desai SC, Quon H. Transoral robotic surgery: does the ends justify the means? *Curr Opin Otolaryngol Head Neck Surg* (2009) 17:126–31. doi:10.1097/MOO.0b013e32832924f5
53. Weinstein GS, O'Malley BW, Snyder W, Sherman E, Quon H. Transoral robotic surgery: radical tonsillectomy. *Arch Otolaryngol Head Neck Surg* (2007) 133:1220–6. doi:10.1001/archotol.133.12.1220
54. Selber JC, Robb G, Serletti JM, Weinstein G, Weber R, Holsinger FC. Transoral robotic free flap reconstruction of oropharyngeal defects: a preclinical investigation. *Plast Reconstr Surg* (2010) 125(3):896–900. doi:10.1097/01.prs.0000371802.58729.30
55. Smartt JM Jr, Gerety P, Serletti JM, Taylor JA. Application of a robotic telemanipulator to perform posterior pharyngeal flap surgery: a feasibility study. *Plast Reconstr Surg* (2013) 131(4):841–5. doi:10.1097/PRS.0b013e318282761b
56. Desai SC, Sung CK, Jang DW, Genden EM. Transoral robotic surgery using a carbon dioxide flexible laser for tumors of the upper aerodigestive tract. *Laryngoscope* (2008) 118(12):2187–9. doi:10.1097/MLG.0b013e31818379e4

57. Mukhija VK, Sung CK, Desai SC, Wanna G, Genden EM. Transoral robotic assisted free flap reconstruction. *Otolaryngol Head Neck Surg* (2009) 140(1):124–5. doi:10.1016/j.otohns.2008.09.024
58. Selber JC. Transoral robotic reconstruction of oropharyngeal defects: a case series. *Plast Reconstr Surg* (2010) 126:1978–87. doi:10.1097/PRS.0b013e3181f448e3
59. Garfein ES, Greaney PJ, Easterlin B, Schiff B, Smith RV. Transoral robotic reconstructive surgery reconstruction of a tongue base defect with a radial forearm flap. *Plast Reconstr Surg* (2011) 127:2352–4. doi:10.1097/PRS.0b013e318213a0e4
60. Genden EM, Kotz T, Tong CC, Smith C, Sikora AG, Teng MS, et al. Transoral robotic resection and reconstruction for head and neck cancer. *Laryngoscope* (2011) 121(8):1668–74. doi:10.1002/lary.21845
61. Genden EM, Park R, Smith C, Kotz T. The role of reconstruction for transoral robotic pharyngectomy and concomitant neck dissection. *Arch Otolaryngol Head Neck Surg* (2011) 137:151–6. doi:10.1001/archoto.2010.250
62. Bonawitz SC, Duvvuri U. Robot-assisted oropharyngeal reconstruction with free tissue transfer. *J Reconstr Microsurg* (2012) 28:485–90. doi:10.1055/s-0032-1313758
63. Longfield EA, Holsinger FC, Selber JC. Reconstruction after robotic head and neck surgery: when and why. *J Reconstr Microsurg* (2012) 28(7):445–50. doi:10.1055/s-0032-1306376
64. Bonawitz SC, Duvvuri U. Robotic-assisted oropharyngeal reconstruction with local flaps. *Oper Tech Otolaryngol* (2013) 24:115–9. doi:10.1016/j.otot.2013.04.001
65. Bonawitz SC, Duvvuri U. Robotic-assisted FAMM flap for soft palate reconstruction. *Laryngoscope* (2013) 123:870–4. doi:10.1002/lary.23578
66. Duvvuri U, Bonawitz SC, Kim S. Robotic-assisted oropharyngeal reconstruction. *J Robot Surg* (2013) 7:9–14. doi:10.1007/s11701-011-0326-z
67. Hans S, Jouffroy T, Veivers D, Hoffman C, Girod A, Badoual C, et al. Transoral robotic-assisted free flap reconstruction after radiation therapy in hypopharyngeal carcinoma: report of two cases. *Eur Arch Otorhinolaryngol* (2013) 270(8):2359–64. doi:10.1007/s00405-013-2566-1
68. Park YM, Lee WJ, Yun IS, Lee DW, Lew DH, Lee JM, et al. Free flap reconstruction after robot-assisted neck dissection via a modified face-lift or retroauricular approach. *Ann Surg Oncol* (2013) 20(3):891–8. doi:10.1245/s10434-012-2731-6
69. Song HG, Yun IS, Lee WJ, Lew DH, Rah DK. Robot-assisted free flap in head and neck reconstruction. *Arch Plast Surg* (2013) 40:353–8. doi:10.5999/aps.2013.40.4.353
70. de Almeida JR, Park RC, Villanueva NL, Miles BA, Teng MS, Genden EM. Reconstructive algorithm and classification system for transoral oropharyngeal defects. *Head Neck* (2014) 36(7):934–41. doi:10.1002/hed.23353
71. Byeon HK, Holsinger FC, Kim DH, Kim JW, Park JH, Koh YW, et al. Feasibility of robot-assisted neck dissection followed by transoral robotic surgery. *Br J Oral Maxillofac Surg* (2015) 53:68–73. doi:10.1016/j.bjoms.2014.09.024
72. Perrenot C, Berengère P, Mastronicola R, Gangloff P, Dolivet G. Infrahyoid myocutaneous flap for reconstruction after robotic transoral surgery for oropharyngeal tumors. *Plast Reconstr Surg* (2014) 133(2):236.e–7.e. doi:10.1097/01.prs.0000437236.07930.fd
73. Lai CS, Chen IC, Liu SA, Lu CT, Yen JH, Song DY. Robot-assisted free flap reconstruction of oropharyngeal cancer—a preliminary report. *Ann Plast Surg* (2015) 74:S105–8. doi:10.1097/SAP.0000000000000464
74. Meccariello G, Montevecchi F, Deganello A, D'Agostino G, Bellini C, Zeccardo E, et al. The temporalis muscle flap for reconstruction of soft palate and lateral oropharyngeal wall after transoral robotic surgery. *Auris Nasus Larynx* (2016). doi:10.1016/j.anl.2016.11.011
75. Gorphe P, Von Tan J, El Bedoui S, Hartl DM, Auperin A, Qassemyar Q, et al. Early assessment of feasibility and technical specificities of transoral robotic surgery using the da Vinci Xi. *J Robotic Surg* (2017). doi:10.1007/s11701-017-0679-z
76. Biron VL, O'Connell DA, Barber B, Clark JM, Andrews C, Jeffery CC, et al. Transoral robotic surgery with radial forearm free flap reconstruction: case control analysis. *J Otolaryngol Head Neck Surg* (2017) 46(1):20. doi:10.1186/s40463-017-0196-0
77. Khan K, Dobbs T, Swan MC, Weinstein GS, Goodacre TEE. Trans-oral robotic cleft surgery (TORCS) for palate and posterior pharyngeal wall reconstruction: a feasibility study. *J Plast Reconstr Aesthet Surg* (2016) 69(1):97–100. doi:10.1016/j.bjps.2015.08.020
78. Podolsky DJ, Fisher DM, Riff KWW, Looi T, Drake JM, Forrest CR. Infant robotic cleft palate surgery: a feasibility assessment using a realistic cleft palate simulator. *Plast Reconstr Surg* (2017) 139(2):455.e–65.e. doi:10.1097/PRS.0000000000003010
79. Nadjmi N. Transoral robotic cleft palate surgery. *Cleft Palate Craniofac J* (2015) 53(3):326–31. doi:10.1597/14-077
80. Dombre E, Duchemin G, Poignet P. Dermarob: a safe robot for reconstructive surgery. *IEEE Trans Robot Autom* (2003) 19:876–84. doi:10.1109/TRA.2003.817067
81. Taghizadeh F, Reiley C, Mohr C, Paul M. Evaluation of robotic- assisted platysmaplasty procedures in a cadaveric model using the da Vinci Surgical System. *J Robot Surg* (2014) 8(1):63–71. doi:10.1007/s11701-013-0431-2
82. Shi Y, Lin L, Zhou C, Zhu M, Xie L, Chai G. A study of an assisting robot for mandible plastic surgery based on augmented reality. *Minim Invasive Ther Allied Technol* (2017) 26(1):23–30. doi:10.1080/13645706.2016.1216864
83. Ciudad P, Date S, Lee MH, Lo Torto F, Nicoli F, Araki J, et al. Robotic harvest of a right gastroepiploic lymph node flap. *Arch Plast Surg* (2016) 43(2):210–2. doi:10.5999/aps.2016.43.2.210
84. Bowersox JC. Telepresence surgery. *Br J Surg* (1996) 83(4):433–4. doi:10.1002/bjs.1800830402
85. Ponnusamy K, Mohr C, Curet MJ. Clinical outcomes with robotic surgery. *Curr Probl Surg* (2011) 48(9):577–656. doi:10.1067/j.cpsurg.2011.05.002
86. Rudmik L, An W, Livingstone D, Matthews W, Seikaly H, Scrimger R, et al. Making a case for high-volume robotic surgery centers: a cost-effectiveness analysis of transoral robotic surgery. *J Surg Oncol* (2015) 112(2):155–63. doi:10.1002/jso.23974
87. Ind TEJ, Marshall C, Hacking M, Harris M, Bishop L, Barton D, et al. Introducing robotic surgery into an endometrial cancer service–a prospective evaluation of clinical and economic outcomes in a UK institution. *Int J Med Robot Comp* (2016) 12(1):137–44. doi:10.1002/rcs.1651
88. Koehn JK, Kuchenbecker KJ. Surgeons and non-surgeons prefer haptic feedback of instrument vibrations during robotic surgery. *Surg Endosc* (2015) 29(10):2970–83. doi:10.1007/s00464-014-4030-8
89. Hagen ME, Meehan JJ, Inan I, Morel P. Visual clues act as a substitute for haptic feedback in robotic surgery. *Surg Endosc* (2008) 22(6):1505–8. doi:10.1007/s00464-007-9683-0
90. Okamura AM. Haptic feedback in robot-assisted minimally invasive surgery. *Curr Opin Urol* (2009) 19(1):102–7. doi:10.1097/MOU.0b013e32831a478c
91. Brahmbhatt JV, Gudeloglu A, Liverneaux P, Parekattil SJ. Robotic microsurgery optimization. *Arch Plast Surg* (2014) 41(3):225–30. doi:10.5999/aps.2014.41.3.225

# 8

# Endoscopic-Assisted Linea Alba Reconstruction plus Mesh Augmentation for Treatment of Umbilical and/or Epigastric Hernias and Rectus Abdominis Diastasis – Early Results

*Ferdinand Köckerling[1]*, Marinos Damianos Botsinis[1], Christine Rohde[1] and Wolfgang Reinpold[2]*

*[1] Department of Surgery, Centre for Minimally Invasive Surgery, Vivantes Hospital Berlin, Academic Teaching Hospital of Charité Medical School, Berlin, Germany, [2] Department of Surgery, Wilhelmsburger Hospital Groß Sand, Academic Teaching Hospital of University Hamburg, Hamburg, Germany*

***Edited by:***
*Hakan Kulacoglu,*
*Rize University, Turkey*

***Reviewed by:***
*Premkumar Balachandran,*
*Apollo Hospitals Chennai, India*
*Volkan Genç,*
*Ankara University, Turkey*

****Correspondence:***
*Ferdinand Köckerling*
*ferdinand.koeckerling@vivantes.de*

***Specialty section:***
*This article was submitted to Visceral Surgery,*
*a section of the journal*
*Frontiers in Surgery*

**Introduction:** Symptomatic umbilical and/or epigastric hernias are often seen concomitantly with rectus abdominis diastasis (RAD), and suture repair of such defects has a high recurrence rate. In the literature, there are reports of both endoscopic and open techniques for repair of symptomatic umbilical and/or epigastric hernias in association with RAD. This paper now reports on the early results of a hybrid technique used for reconstruction of the linea alba and mesh augmentation [endoscopic-assisted linea alba reconstruction plus mesh augmentation (ELAR plus)].

**Materials and methods:** Between 15 June 2015 and 31 January 2016, 40 patients with symptomatic umbilical and/or epigastric hernia and concomitant RAD underwent reconstruction of the linea alba using a hybrid technique involving a small umbilical incision and the use of video-endoscopic equipment. The patients comprised 29 men and 11 women with a mean age of 53.6 years and mean BMI of 32.6. The mean operating time was 120 min. The mesh had a mean longitudinal extension of 18.6 cm and transverse extension of 9.1 cm.

**Results:** Thirty-day follow-up results are available for all patients. Thirty-seven out of 40 patients (92.5%) experienced no postoperative complication. Two cases of discrete impaired umbilical wound healing and one seroma were successfully managed with conservative treatment. On 30-day follow-up, 3 out of 40 patients (7.5%) complained of intermittent pain on exertion, and 2 out of 40 patients (5%) still took painkillers when required.

**Conclusion:** ELAR plus is a novel minimally invasive procedure for repair of symptomatic umbilical and/or epigastric hernias with concomitant RAD. Reconstruction of the linea alba *via* a minimally invasive access route is able to restore the normal anatomy of the abdominal wall.

**Keywords: rectus abdominis diastasis, umbilical hernia, epigastric hernia, linea alba reconstruction, video-endoscopic technique**

## INTRODUCTION

Rectus abdominis diastasis (RAD) describes a condition in which the two rectus abdominis muscles are separated by an abnormally wide distance (1). Any separation of more than 2 cm is considered to be abnormal (1). RAD is usually quite apparent on physical examination (1). When a patient with RAD raises his or her head and begins to sit up, the increase in intra-abdominal pressure as the two rectus muscles contract can result in a diffuse fusiform bulge (1). The linea alba can become thinned due to stretching, which can be caused by elevated intra-abdominal pressure, such as in pregnancy and obesity (1). Patients with RAD typically have one of two profiles: middle-aged and older men with central obesity, or small, fit women who have carried a large fetus or twins to term (1).

It has been demonstrated that RAD produces deterioration in the functions of the abdominal wall with associated muscular imbalance and chronic back pain (2).

Rectus abdominis diastasis is often seen in association with primary abdominal wall hernia (umbilical and/or epigastric hernia) (3). For example, Köhler et al. (3) diagnosed RAD in 45% of patients with small (<2 cm) umbilical and epigastric hernias. The 31.2% of those patients with small umbilical and epigastric hernias, with concomitant RAD, who underwent suture repair had a significantly higher recurrence rate after mean follow-up of 31 months compared with non-RAD patients (3). The authors concluded that even small umbilical and epigastric hernias frequently occur concomitantly with RAD. The results support the theory that midline hernias, regardless of size, with concomitant rectus diastasis require mesh repair due to unacceptably higher recurrence rates (3).

At present, there is no consensus among the international surgical community on the surgical treatment of RAD as regards indications or surgical techniques (2). If RAD is symptomatic or is associated with midline hernias (umbilical and/or epigastric), corrective surgery of all pathologies at the same time could represent the most recommended approach (2).

There are many methods with which RAD can be repaired (1). These differ by approach (open versus laparoscopic), numbers of layers of sutures, the position of suture placement, suture material used, and whether or not mesh is used (4).

Laparoscopic plication of the linea alba is recommended as a mesh-free approach for treatment of RAD (5). Plication of the linea alba can be combined with mesh augmentation in the IPOM technique for enhanced stabilization of the abdominal wall (6).

Alternatively, following umbilical incision an endoscopic procedure can be performed in a space created between the subcutaneous tissue and the anterior layer of the rectus sheath (2), while repositioning or resecting the contents of an umbilical or epigastric hernia. Next, *via* the defects caused by rectus diastasis, meshes are introduced into the preperitoneal space where they are fixed. This is followed by endoscopic plication of the anterior layers of the rectus sheath (2).

The sublay technique (7) and resection of the rectus diastasis and thinned linea alba followed by placement of sutures are open surgical procedures cited in the literature for repair of RAD with concomitant primary ventral hernia.

A third hybrid technique was pioneered by Reinpold (8) where the sublay technique is implemented *via* a minimal skin incision; this is known as the "mini-incision less open sublay" (MILOS).

Rectus abdominis diastasis is also often corrected in the course of abdominoplasty (9–20).

The traditional method of correcting RAD during abdominoplasty is by plicating one intact anterior rectus sheath against the opposite member (9, 12–19). This method usually creates significant tension as the anterior rectus fascia is advanced over the encased rectus muscles toward the midline. This technique may produce significant postoperative pain (12). To avoid these problems, Ramirez (12) has applied to his abdominoplasties a technique he has called "rectus abdominis myofascial release" (12). The first step is to incise the anterior rectus sheath at the junction of the inner one-third with the middle third of the rectus muscle width (12). These incisions meet at the level of the xiphoid process superiorly and the subumbilical area inferiorly (12). The rectus myofascial release allows the centrifugal forces of the rectus muscles to push the muscles toward the midline, facilitating closure with decreased tension (12).

The open rectus abdominis myofascial release method described by Ramirez (12) for RAD repair during abdominoplasty has been used by several working groups with good results for treatment of incisional hernias with reconstruction of the linea alba and mesh augmentation in open technique (21–26).

Below is now described the technique of endoscopic-assisted linea alba reconstruction plus mesh augmentation (ELAR plus) for treatment of RAD with concomitant primary ventral hernia, in addition to the early results. Like the MILOS technique described by Reinpold (8), this is a hybrid technique implemented *via* a small incision.

## MATERIALS AND METHODS

### Operative Technique

On raising their head and beginning to sit up from a supine position during clinical examination, all patients operated on in this technique exhibited marked bulging extending from the xiphoid process to the subumbilical area (**Figure 1**) Furthermore, all patients had a symptomatic umbilical hernia or epigastric hernia or both (**Figure 2**). Evidence of these findings was demonstrated on ultrasound, computed tomography (CT), and magnetic resonance imaging (MRI) (**Figure 2**).

In addition to repairing the symptomatic umbilical hernia and/or epigastric hernia with lasting closure of the hernia defect, surgery is also aimed at elimination of the actual cause, i.e., RAD. This is best done by reconstruction of a new linea alba from autologous tissue, followed by restoration of the rectus muscles to their normal anatomic position directly at the linea alba. Mesh augmentation is used to further stabilize the reconstructed abdominal wall. In order to be able to conduct this operation *via* a relatively small access route, a hybrid technique involving video-endoscopic equipment is used.

The skin incision is made on the left side, encircling the umbilicus like a half-loop and extending 2–3 cm upwards (**Figure 3**). This is followed by stepwise diathermy dissection of the subcutaneous tissue, with detachment of the subcutaneous tissue from anterior rectus sheath on the left and right as well as below the umbilicus. Next, the umbilical hernia sac is opened, the hernia contents repositioned or resected and the umbilicus detached from the abdominal wall fascia. This is followed by further dissection beneath the abdominal skin/subcutaneous tissue and both anterior rectus sheaths using the video-endoscopic equipment. The operation can now be continued beneath the unopened abdominal skin as far as the xiphoid process by bilateral dissection of the anterior layers of the rectus sheaths. In those cases with an epigastric hernia, the hernia sac containing preperitoneal fatty tissue or parts of the greater omentum are detached from the subcutaneous fatty tissue and either repositioned or resected.

Next, both rectus sheaths are incised around 2–3 cm from the medial margin along their entire length from the xiphoid process to the subumbilical area and opened (**Figure 4**). That can be done with a scissors or the diathermy knife. After that, a new linea alba is reconstructed by suturing together the two medial parts of the right and left anterior rectus sheaths. Suturing is performed with non-absorbable suture material, assuring a stable new linea alba, with the rectus muscles restored to their normal anatomic position adjacent to the reconstructed linea alba (**Figure 5**). This suturing technique with reconstruction of the linea alba eliminates the RAD and closes the umbilical hernia and/or epigastric hernia defects. Using a continuous suturing technique, a mesh (TiMesh strong) for augmentation is then sutured to the incision margin of the right and left anterior rectus sheaths as replacement for the medial part of both anterior rectus sheaths (**Figure 6**). That completes reconstruction of the normal anatomy of the abdominal wall in this region. As a final step, a Redon drain is inserted between the mesh and subcutaneous tissue; the subcutaneous tissue is closed with single button sutures, finishing with an intracutaneous skin suture (**Figure 3**).

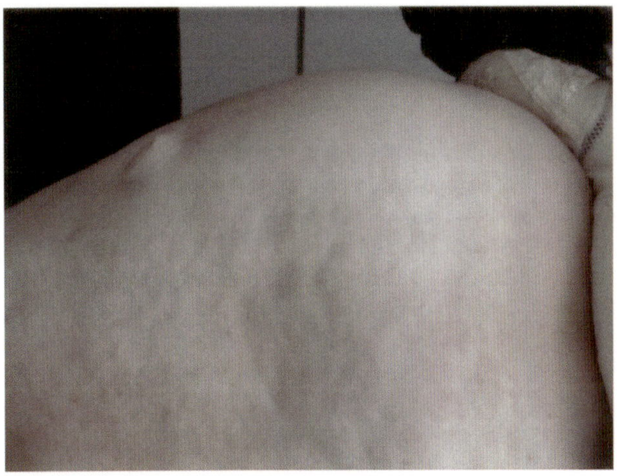

**FIGURE 1** | Clinical findings of a patient with rectus abdominis diastasis, and umbilical and epigastric hernia when beginning to sit up.

## RESULTS

### 30-Day Postoperative Outcome

Between June 15, 2015 and January 31, 2016, 40 patients with RAD and symptomatic umbilical hernia and/or epigastric hernia

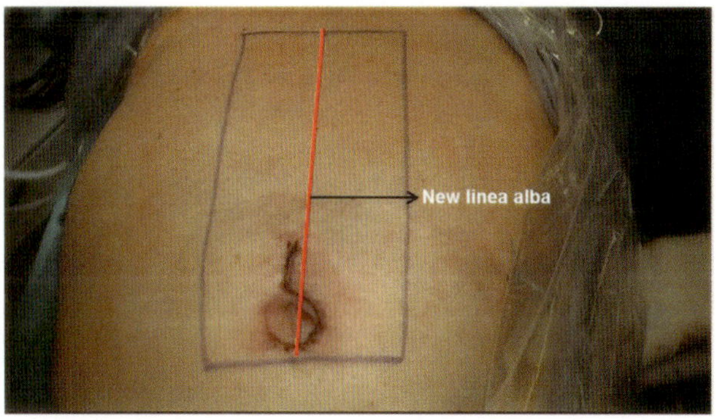


**FIGURE 3** | Extent of incision and relation of mesh placement to linea alba reconstruction.

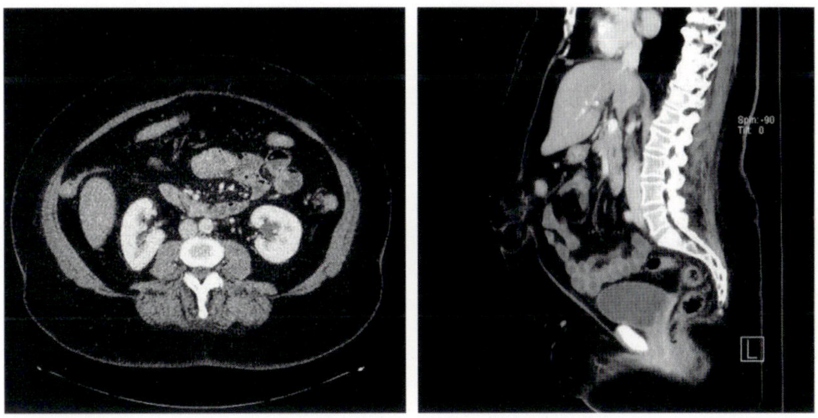

**FIGURE 2** | CT scan of the patient with rectus abdominis diastasis, and umbilical and epigastric hernia.

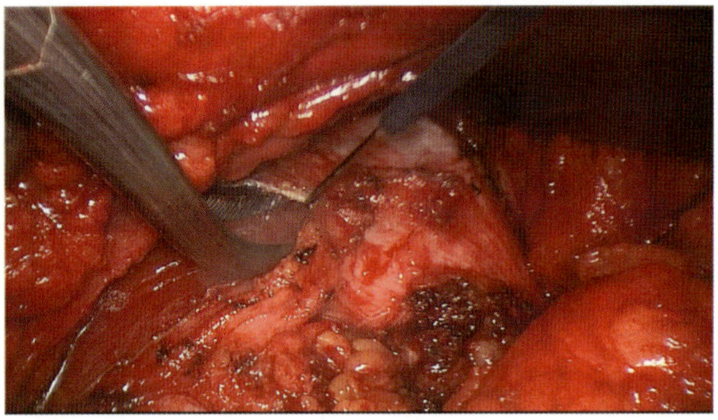

**FIGURE 4 | Incision of right rectus sheath following dissection of the latter.**

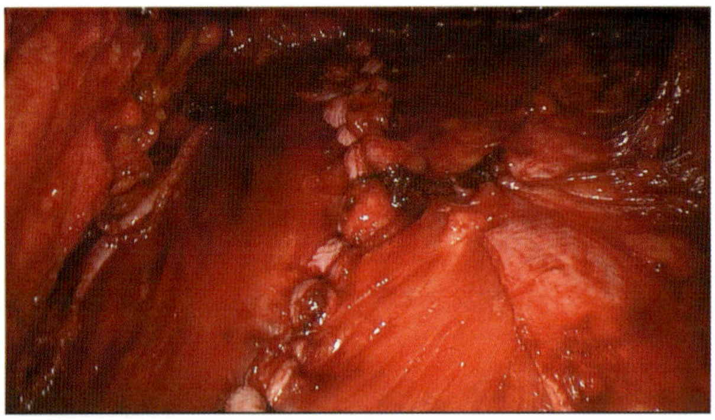

**FIGURE 5 | New linea alba after suturing together the medial portions of the two rectus sheaths at the midline.** Both rectus abdominis muscles are repositioned beside the reconstructed linea alba.

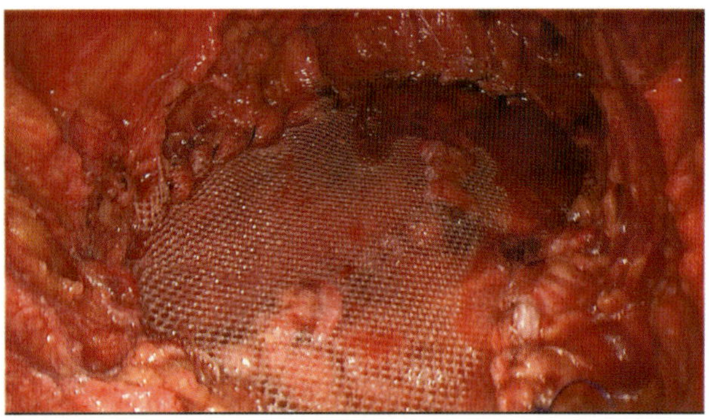

**FIGURE 6 | Replacement of the medial segments of the rectus sheaths used to reconstruct the linea with a middle-weight, large-pore polypropylene mesh (TiMesh strong).**

underwent surgery. All patients were operated on by the senior author (Ferdinand Köckerling), who since January 1, 2000 had gained experience of implementing this reconstruction technique *via* a larger skin incision (25).

**TABLE 1 | Patient characteristics, mean operating time, and mean mesh size.**

| | | |
|---|---|---|
| Sex | 29 men/11 women | |
| Age | Mean: 53.6 years | 25–76 years |
| BMI | Mean: 32.6 | 23–50 |
| ASA | Mean: 1.9 | 1–3 |
| OR duration | Mean: 120 min | 67–179 |
| Mesh length (TiMesh strong) | Mean: 18.6 cm | 15–22 |
| Mesh width (TiMesh strong) | Mean: 9.1 cm | 5–13 |

**TABLE 2 | Postoperative complication rate at the end of in-hospital treatment.**

| | | |
|---|---|---|
| None | $n = 38/40$ | 95% |
| Umbilical necrosis | $n = 1/40$ | 2.5% |
| Seroma | $n = 1/40$ | 2.5% |

**TABLE 3 | Results of 30-day follow-up visit.**

| | | |
|---|---|---|
| Discrete impaired umbilical wound healing | $n = 2/40$ | 5.0% |
| Intermittent pain on exertion | $n = 3/40$ | 7.5% |
| Painkillers still used when required | $n = 2/40$ | 5.0% |

All patients were informed about the details of the procedure and gave their consent. The patients comprised 29 men and 11 women (**Table 1**). The mean age was 53.6 years. Patients had a mean BMI of 32.6. The mean ASA score was 1.9, and mean operating time was 120 min. The mean mesh (TiMesh strong) longitudinal length extension was 18.6 cm and transverse extension was 9.1 cm. Thirty-seven out of 40 patients did not have any postoperative complications (**Table 2**). One female patient had discrete partial umbilical necrosis, which dried out, healed, and was removed without redo surgery. It was possible to preserve the umbilicus and the wound healed without any sequelae. Besides, there was one case of postoperative seroma which did not require any further treatment. On 30-day follow-up, there was also one male patient with discrete impaired umbilical wound healing that also healed without further sequelae. Three out of 40 patients still complained about intermittent pain on exertion. Two out of 40 patients took painkillers when required (**Table 3**).

## DISCUSSION

At present, there is no consensus among international hernia experts on the best surgical technique for repair of umbilical and epigastric hernias with concomitant RAD (2). Both open, e.g., sublay technique, and laparoscopic procedures are used (4). The open techniques requiring a larger incision are associated with more complications, such as impaired wound healing and wound infections, while the laparoscopic procedures are less efficient at eliminating rectus diastasis. Reinpold, Hamburg, has pioneered a third option with his MILOS technique (8), where using a hybrid technique, the sublay operation is performed *via* a very small incision (8). Inspired by his technique and experiences, we now set about modifying the technique we had practiced for more than 15 years for repair of ventral and incisional hernias. Details of this technique have been published in the literature under various names by Rehn (21), Chevrel (22), Abrahamson et al. (23), Flament et al (24), Schug-Pass et al. (25), and Joshi et al. (26). What these techniques have in common is that they all use a part of the anterior rectus sheath to reconstruct the new linea alba and thus close the hernia defects. Since implementation of this procedure involves a video-endoscopic technique, it constitutes a hybrid technique that is composed of an open and endoscopic approach. Accordingly, we have used the term "endoscopic-assisted linea alba reconstruction" to denote this technique. Since not all the techniques reported to date have used a mesh for augmentation (12, 23), we have expanded the term to include additionally "plus mesh augmentation." The new technique which is performed *via* a markedly smaller access route can be standardized in a similar way to a procedure based on a larger incision. In none of the 40 operations conducted so far with this hybrid technique has it been necessary to switch to a larger incision, i.e., to the conventional procedure. The early postoperative 30-day follow-up results show a very low complication rate. No patient needed redo surgery because of postoperative complications. Only in two cases was discrete impaired umbilical wound healing observed, and these cases were successfully managed with conservative treatment while preserving the umbilicus. One case of discrete seroma was also easily managed. Only very few patients still experienced pain on exertion or required painkillers 4 weeks later. In all patients, both the umbilical and/or epigastric hernia and RAD were successfully eliminated and, accordingly, all patients were satisfied with the cosmetic results. Based on the longer term follow-up findings, the durability of these results will, of course, need to be demonstrated in the future. This is a clear limitation of this study. Our own experiences of carrying out this technique *via* a larger access route indicate that this surgical procedure which uses stable autologous tissue and is further underpinned by mesh augmentation produces good results with low recurrence rates (25). Likewise, in a recent publication, Joshi et al. (26) reported about a zero incidence of recurrence at a minimum of 12-month follow-up in 30 cases studied. As such, the basic principle enshrined in this technique holds out promising prospects for a good long-term outcome. The mini-incision procedure reduces the rate of wound complications, has fewer postoperative drawbacks for patients, and allows earlier resumption of everyday and working activities.

With the MILOS technique pioneered by Reinpold (8) and the ELAR plus procedure presented in this paper, there are now two new minimally invasive techniques available for treatment of ventral hernias and RAD. These are also suitable for repair of incisional hernias, since both the MILOS and ELAR plus surgical procedures can be used. Both techniques aim to reduce the drawbacks associated with the conventional open and endoscopic procedures used to repair ventral and incisional hernias. As such, they represent an alternative technique to the methods used to date. Already at this stage, there is reason to believe that the MILOS and ELAR plus techniques will in the future play a role in the "tailored approach" concept for treatment of ventral and incisional hernias.

## AUTHOR CONTRIBUTIONS

FK, MB, and CR have treated the patients in their Hospital. The development of the study design and the follow-up of the patients have been also done by FK, MB, and CR. WR has first described abdominal wall hernia surgery *via* small incisions. FK, MB, CR, and WR are responsible for the content of the manuscript.

## REFERENCES


1. Brooks DC. Rectus abdominis diastasis. *UpToDate*. (2015). Available from: www.uptodate.com
2. Luque JB, Luque AB, Valdivia J, Suarez Gráu JM, Gomez Menchero J, Garcia Moreno J, et al. Totally endoscopic surgery on diastasis recti associated with midline hernias. The advantages of a minimally invasive approach. Prospective cohort study. *Hernia* (2015) **19**:493–501. doi:10.1007/s10029-014-1300-2
3. Köhler G, Luketina RR, Emmanuel K. Sutured repair of primary small umbilical and epigastric hernias: concomitant rectus diastasis is a significant risk factor for recurrence. *World J Surg* (2015) **39**:121–6. doi:10.1007/s00268-014-2765-y
4. Hickey F, Finch JG, Khanna A. A systematic review on the outcomes of correction of diastasis of the recti. *Hernia* (2011) **15**:607–14. doi:10.100/s10029-011-0839-4
5. Siddiky AH, Kapadia CR. Laparoscopic plication of the linea alba as a repair for diastasis recti – a mesh free approach. *JSCR* (2010) **5**:3.
6. Palanivelu C, Rangarajan M, Jategaonkar PA, Amar V, Gokul KS, Srikanth B. Laparoscopic repair of diastasis recti using the 'Venetian blinds' technique of plication with prosthetic reinforcement: a retrospective study. *Hernia* (2009) **13**:287–92. doi:10.1007/s10029-008-0464-z
7. Emanuelsson P, Gunnarsson U, Strigård K, Stark B. Early complications, pain, and quality of life after reconstructive surgery for abdominal rectus muscle diastasis: a 3-month follow-up. *J Plast Reconstr Aesthet Surg* (2014) **67**:1082–8. doi:10.1016/j.bjps.2014.04.015
8. Reinpold W. Neue Techniken in der Narben- und Bauchwandhernienchirurgie. *Chirurgische Allgemeine* (2013) **14**:331–7.
9. Al-Quattan MM. Abdominoplasty in multiparous women with severe musculoaponeurotic laxity. *Br J Plast Surg* (1997) **50**:450–5. doi:10.1016/S0007-1226(97)90333-7
10. Lockwood T. Rectus muscle diastasis in males: primary indication for endoscopically assisted abdominoplasty. *Plast Reconstr Surg* (1998) **101**:1685–91. doi:10.1097/00006534-199805000-00042
11. Nahas FX, Ishida J, Gemperli R, Ferreira MC. Abdominal wall closure after selective aponeurotic incision and undermining. *Ann Plast Surg* (1998) **41**:606–17. doi:10.1097/00000637-199812000-00005
12. Ramirez OM. Abdominoplasty and abdominal wall rehabilitation: a comprehensive approach. *Plast Reconstr Surg* (2000) **105**:425–35. doi:10.1097/00006534-200001000-00069
13. van Uchelen JH, Kon M, Werker PMN. The long-term durability of plication of the anterior rectus sheath assessed by ultrasonography. *Plast Reconstr Surg* (2001) **107**:1578–84. doi:10.1097/00006534-200105000-00046
14. Yousif NJ, Lifchez SD, Nguyen HH. Transverse rectus sheath plication in abdominoplasty. *Plast Reconstr Surg* (2004) **114**:778–84. doi:10.1097/01.PRS.0000131023.09405.A8

15. Nahas FX, Masako Feirreira L, Muszkat Augusto S, Ghelfond C. Long-term follow-up of correction of rectus diastasis. *Plast Reconstr Surg* (2005) **115**:1736–41. doi:10.1097/01.PRS.0000161675.55337.F1
16. Rosen A, Hartman T. Repair of the midline fascial defect in abdominoplasty with long-acting barbed and smooth absorbable sutures. *Aesthet Surg J* (2011) **31**(6):668–73. doi:10.1177/1090820X11415242
17. Tadiparthi S, Shokrollahi K, Doyle GS, Fahmy FS. Rectus sheath plication in abdominoplasty: assessment of its longevity and a review of the literature. *J Plast Reconstr Aesthet Surg* (2012) **65**:328–32. doi:10.1016/j.bjps.2011.09.024
18. Mestak O, Kullac R, Mestak J, Nosek A, Krajcova A, Sukop A. Evaluation of the long-term stability of sheath plication using absorbable sutures in 51 patients with diastasis of the recti muscles: an ultrasonographic study. *Plast Reconstr Surg* (2012) **130**:714e. doi:10.1097/PRS.0b013e318267d806
19. Huguier V, Faure JL, Doucet C, Giot JP, Dagregorio G. Couplage coelioscopie-abdominoplastie dans dix cas d'important diastasis des grands droits. *Ann Chir Plast Esthét* (2012) **57**:350–5. doi:10.1016/j.anplas.2011.08.011
20. Kulhanek J, Mestak O. Treatment of umbilical hernia and recti muscles diastasis without a periumbilical incision. *Hernia* (2013) **17**:527–30. doi:10.1007/s10029-013-1047-1
21. Rehn E. Surgery in hernias of the lower abdominal wall. 7th ed. In: Fischer AW, Gohrbrandt E, Sauerbruch F, editors. *Chirurgische Operationslehre Band V*. Leipzig: J.A. Barth Verlag (1957). p. 92–3.
22. Chevrel JP. Traitement des grandes éventrations medians par plastie en paletot et prothèse. *Nouv Presse Méd* (1979) **8**:695–6.
23. Abrahamson J. The shoelace repair. In: Bendavid R, Abrahamson J, Arregui ME, Flament JB, Phillips EH, editors. *Abdominal Wall Hernias – Principles and Management*. New York, Berlin, Heidelberg: Springer-Verlag (2001). p. 483–6.
24. Flament JB, Palot JP, Burde A, Delattre JF, Avisse C. Treatment of major incisional hernias. In: Bendavid R, Abrahamson J, Arregui ME, Flament JB, Phillips EH, editors. *Abdominal Wall Hernias – Principles and Management*. New York, Berlin, Heidelberg: Springer-Verlag (2001). p. 508–16.
25. Schug-Paß C, Trommer Y, Tamme C, Lippert H, Köckerling F. Dynamic patchplasty – a tension-free reconstruction of incisional hernias Langenbecks. *Arch Surg* (2006) **391**:403–8. doi:10.1007/s00423-006-0053-5
26. Joshi MA, Singh MB, Gadhire MA. Study of the outcome of modified shoelace repair for mid incisional hernia. *Hernia* (2015) **19**:503–8. doi:10.1007/s10029-014-1234-8

9

# The Use of Keystone Flaps in Periarticular Wound Closure: A Case Series

*Thomas H. Jovic*[1,2]*, *Zita M. Jessop*[1,2], *Robert Slade*[1], *Thomas Dobbs*[1,2] *and Iain S. Whitaker*[1,2]

[1] *Welsh Centre for Burns and Plastic Surgery, Morriston Hospital, Swansea, United Kingdom,* [2] *Reconstructive Surgery and Regenerative Medicine Research Group, Institute of Life Sciences, Swansea, United Kingdom*

The Keystone perforator island flap (Keystone flap), is a Type A fasciocutaneous advancement flap, consisting of two V to Y advancement flaps. Skin cancer excision around joints presents a number of reconstructive challenges. Owing to the mobile nature of joints, the optimal periarticular reconstructive option should possess the ability to provide adequate tissue coverage and withstand regional changes in tensile pressures. We report a single-surgeon series of five cases of periarticular keystone flap between 2014 and 2017. Data were collected from operation notes, clinical photography, histopathology, and outpatient clinic records. The indication for keystone flap was skin cancer in all cases ($n$ = 5). The largest defect size post-excision in was 75 mm × 40 mm × 15 mm. All keystone flaps demonstrate a color and cosmetic appearance comparable to adjacent tissue. There were no major postoperative complications including flap failure or impaired range of joint movement in the follow up period. Superficial wound infection occurred postoperatively in one case. This is the first case series to discuss the use of keystone flaps in periarticular wound closure. Locoregional fasciocutaneous wound coverage offered by keystone flaps may alleviate the risks of graft failure, contour defects, and donor site morbidity associated with alternative reconstructive options, with good functional and cosmetic outcomes. We advocate their use as a robust reconstructive option in periarticular areas.

***Edited by:***
*Jan A. Plock,*
*University of Zurich, Switzerland*

***Reviewed by:***
*Radu Olariu,*
*University Hospital Bern, Switzerland*
*David J. Hunter-Smith,*
*Monash University Plastic and Reconstructive Surgery Group, Australia*

****Correspondence:***
*Thomas H. Jovic*
*thjovic@doctors.org.uk*

***Specialty section:***
*This article was submitted to Reconstructive and Plastic Surgery, a section of the journal Frontiers in Surgery*

**Keywords: periarticular, wound closure, skin cancer, fasciocutaneous flaps, keystone flaps**

## INTRODUCTION

We report a single-surgeon series of five cases of periarticular keystone flap between 2014 and 2017 (**Table 1**). Data were collected from operation notes, clinical photography, histopathology, and outpatient clinic records. All patients provided written informed consent for their images and data to be used for research and publication.

The indication for keystone flap was skin cancer in all cases ($n$ = 5), consisting of two basal cell carcinomas (BCC) and three melanoma scar excisions. All cases were performed as day case operations. In all cases, melanomas were initially excised with 2 mm margins to determine Breslow thickness, and the subsequent scar revised with appropriate margins prior to reconstruction. BCC were excised with 4–5 mm margins as per British Association of Dermatology guidelines (1) and demonstrated adequately clear excision margins histologically (**Table 1**).

**TABLE 1** | Summary of lesion type, size, post-excision defect size, keystone flap subtype, and postoperative complications for included cases.

| Case | Age (gender) | Lesion | Lesion size (mm) | Area | Associated joint(s) | Defect size (mm) | | | Histology | Keystone flap | Follow-up period (months) |
|---|---|---|---|---|---|---|---|---|---|---|---|
| | | | | | | Length | Width | Depth | | | |
| 1 | 63 (M) | Nodular BCC | 18 × 18 | Left shoulder | Glenohumeral | 70 | 35 | 5 | Clear with 3 mm margins | Type 2a | 4 |
| 2 | 79 (F) | Melanoma scar | 32 × 22 | Left popliteal fossa | Knee | 55 | 40 | 12 | No residual melanoma | Type 3 | 18 |
| 3 | 71 (F) | Melanoma scar | 45 × 1 | Left forearm | Elbow | 75 | 40 | 17 | No residual melanoma | Type 3 | 10 |
| 4 | 58 (F) | Melanoma scar | 9 × 8 | Left medial malleolus | Ankle | 27 | 12 | 2 | No residual melanoma | Type 1 | 3 |
| 5 | 65 (M) | Nodular BCC | 27 × 20 | Left shoulder | Glenohumeral | 35 | 56 | 11 | Nearest margin 3.9 mm | Type 1 | 3 |

The defect size post-excision ranged from 75 mm × 40 mm × 17 mm to 27 mm × 12 mm × 2 mm with a mean size of 52 mm × 37 mm × 9 mm (**Table 1**). Two keystone flaps were Type 1, two Type 3 flaps (popliteal and antecubital fossa), and a Type 2a flap adjacent to the glenohumeral joint (**Table 1**).

All keystone flaps demonstrated a color and cosmetic appearance comparable to adjacent tissue, with minimal scar formation at the periphery (**Figure 1**). Impaired range of joint movement was neither reported subjectively nor detectable on clinical examination, plus no issues regarding contracture or problematic scarring have been identified in this series to date during the follow-up period. One patient was readmitted 7 days postoperatively with erythema and swelling underlying the keystone flap (Case 5) consistent with a superficial wound infection. Blood tests at the time of readmission demonstrated a normal white cell count and mildly elevated C-reactive protein. Methicillin-sensitive *Staphylococcus aureus* was identified from wound swabs to be the causative organism. The infection was successfully treated with 7 days of clarithromycin, with no adverse impact on the subsequent healing process. All patients have reported high levels of satisfaction with the appearance of their reconstruction.

## BACKGROUND

The Keystone perforator island flap (Keystone flap), is a local, Type A fasciocutaneous advancement flap, consisting of two V to Y advancement flaps (2). Originally described by Behan et al. (2), its use as a locoregional reconstructive tool offers an attractive alternative to skin grafting and free tissue transfer, reducing complications associated with donor site harvest, blood supply, and cosmetic donor–recipient mismatches (3).

Blood supply to the flap is based on random vascular perforators, with a dual supply from both the subcutaneous vascular plexus and perforating vessels in the fascial and muscular layers (4).

Since their introduction, keystone flaps have been subdivided into four subtypes (**Table 1**) and used for head and neck (5–8) and lower limb reconstruction (9–11), to resurface irradiated tissue or burn excisions (12, 13) and in mobile areas such as the lumbosacral spine (14, 15).

Periarticular wound closure is a unique reconstructive challenge due to multi-vector tensional forces (16). Adjacent tissue is continually subjected to stretch, compression and torsion and the reconstructive solution should possess the ability to withstand changes in tensile forces. It is widely known that periarticular skin grafts are subjected to movement and shearing forces, disrupting the formation of early fibrin bonds and leading to increased failure rates (16–18) and contracture (19, 20). In our experience, the use of locoregional flaps to reconstruct periarticular defects left from skin cancer excisions are superior to skin grafts, and we illustrate this through the use of the keystone flap in five patients.

## DISCUSSION

To our knowledge, this is the first case series to discuss the use of keystone flaps in periarticular wound closure. Our experience highlights a number of advantages and important learning points to consider during patient selection.

In our study of five patients, the cosmetic outcomes were well-received and patient satisfaction was high. This parallels studies using keystone flaps in esthetically sensitive areas such as nasal and facial reconstruction (5–7, 21–23). Despite their cosmetic appeal in matching the appearance of adjacent skin (3) a notable scar burden may still be associated with the use of these flaps, especially when under high tension, although this ameliorates with time (**Figure 1**).

Periarticular wound closure can prove challenging. Moreover, the large antecubital and popliteal fossa defects (**Table 2**) presented a range of reconstructive challenges beyond the issues of multi-vector tensile forces, such as exposed neurovascular structures needing robust soft tissue protective cover. The burden of skin cancers in mobile areas, such as the lower leg is high, especially in females (24), and to achieve clear surgical margins often creates large defects. Despite this, there is a sparsity of literature that concerns itself with the most appropriate means of periarticular wound closure. Although keystone flaps have been used previously for generic lower limb reconstruction (6, 25) they have not been used widely in the popliteal fossa or periarticular areas to our knowledge. Alternatives to fasciocutaneous flaps such as the keystone include reconstruction with skin grafts, though these do not parallel the robust tissue coverage of local flaps and may exhibit high failure rates (16), particularly in mobile areas where graft adherence may be compromised. In addition, contour defects, pigmentation mismatch (26), and secondary contractures (19) may also restrict cosmetic and functional outcomes, particularly when extrapolated to periarticular defects. Alternative flaps for lower limb wound closure may include reverse flow flaps and local

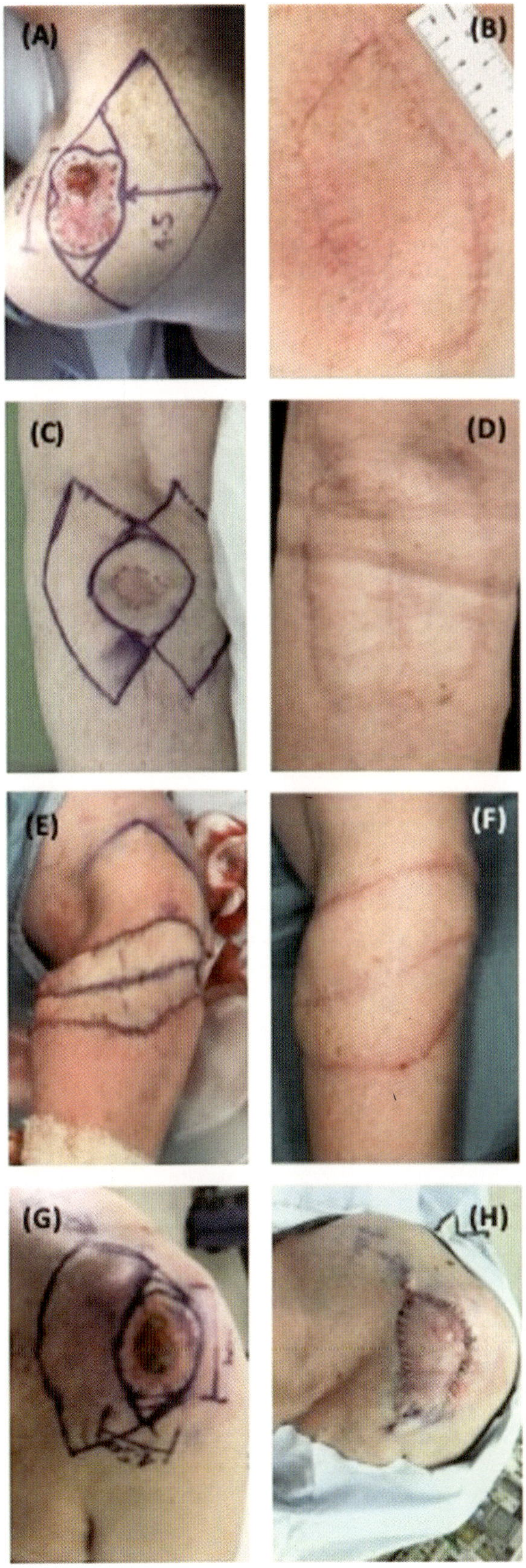


**FIGURE 1** | Continued

**FIGURE 1** | Continued
Preoperative, intra-operative and postoperative periarticular keystone flaps. **(A)** Patient 1, pre-operative; **(B)** patient 1, 2 months postoperative; **(C)** patient 2, pre-operative; **(D)** patient 2, 2 months postoperative; **(E)** patient 3, intra-operative; **(F)** patient 3, 1 month postoperative; **(G)** patient 5, pre-operative; **(H)** patient 5, intra-operative.

**TABLE 2** | Subtypes of Keystone Flap and their surgical applications [Modified from Behan et al 2003 (1); Pelissier et al 2007 (3)].

| Keystone flap subtype | Principles and surgical applications |
|---|---|
| Type I | Primary defect less than 2 cm width<br>Lateral deep fascia remains intact |
| Type IIa | Defects greater than 2 cm<br>Division of deep fascia required to facilitate tissue mobilization |
| Type IIb | Useful in large defect coverage<br>Concomitant use of split-skin graft, reduces tension on flap margins |
| Type III | Large primary defect (5–10 cm)<br>Two keystone flaps on each border of the defect |
| Type IV | Rotational keystone flap, useful in joint contracture or open fractures<br>Flap is raised with up to 50% sub-facial undermining |

transposition flaps (27). Reverse flow flaps may compromise the arterial inflow to the foot (27), and although comparable wound coverage may be achieved through transposition, defects of large size or low tissue laxity may require concomitant skin grafting to close the donor site. Similarly, pedicled fasciocutaneous flaps, such as the radial forearm flap (28) have been documented in upper limb periarticular wound closure. However, this often requires a skin graft to close the donor site, and division of the arterial inflow to the hand at the expense of wound closure (29).

It has been reported that keystone flaps around the elbow, knee, and ankle joints should be used cautiously due to reduced skin laxity and a risk of dehiscence (30), and previous studies have reported wound dehiscence following full flexion at the lumbosacral area (25). In our series, we did not immobilize the joints in plaster casts, but advise bulky dressings and enforced rest until wound checks were performed 2 weeks postoperatively. We present several examples of successful keystone flap reconstruction around the joints of the upper and lower limbs with no major complications and throughout the postoperative follow-up, both patient and clinicians were satisfied with the quality of the functional and cosmetic results.

## CONCLUDING REMARKS

Keystone flaps provide an effective means of periarticular wound closure in an area of high mobility and low skin laxity. Locoregional fasciocutaneous wound coverage offered by keystone flaps provide a good cosmetic match, robust soft tissue coverage and avoid contour defects and contracture at a cost of minimal donor site morbidity. On the basis of our experience, we advocate the increased use of the keystone flap to close periarticular defects following skin cancer excision.

## AUTHOR CONTRIBUTIONS

All authors (TJ, ZJ, RS, TD, and IW) have made substantial contributions to the conception or design of the work; or the acquisition, analysis, or interpretation of data for the work. All authors have been involved in drafting the work or revising it critically for important intellectual content and approve the final version to be published. All authors agree to be accountable for all aspects of the work in ensuring that questions related to the accuracy or integrity of any part of the work are appropriately investigated and resolved.

## FUNDING

ISW would like to acknowledge the support of the Royal College of Surgeons Pump Priming Award 2017-2018. ZJ would like to acknowledge the support of the Medical Research Council. TJ would like to acknowledge the funding of the Royal College of Surgeons Research Fellowship. TJ, TD and ZJ would like to acknowledge the support of the Welsh Clinical Academic Track.

## REFERENCES

1. Telfer NR, Colver GB, Morton CA; British Association of Dermatologists. Guidelines for the management of basal cell carcinoma. *Br J Dermatol* (2008) 159(1):35–48. doi:10.1111/j.1365-2133.2008.08666.x
2. Behan FC. The keystone design perforator island flap in reconstructive surgery. *ANZ J Surg* (2003) 73(3):112–20. doi:10.1046/j.1445-2197.2003.02638.x
3. Behan FC, Findlay MW, Lo CH. *The Keystone Perforator Island Flap Concept*. Churchill Livingstone, Elsevier (2012). 227 p. Available from: https://www.elsevier.com/books/the-keystone-perforator-island-flap-concept/behan/978-0-7295-3971-5
4. Pelissier P, Santoul M, Pinsolle V, Casoli V, Behan F. The keystone design perforator island flap. Part I: anatomic study. *J Plast Reconstr Aesthet Surg* (2007) 60(8):883–7. doi:10.1016/j.bjps.2007.01.072
5. Behan FC, Rozen WM, Wilson J, Kapila S, Sizeland A, Findlay MW. The cervico-submental keystone island flap for locoregional head and neck reconstruction. *J Plast Reconstr Aesthet Surg* (2013) 66(1):23–8. doi:10.1016/j.bjps.2012.08.027
6. Behan FC, Lo CH, Sizeland A, Pham T, Findlay M. Keystone island flap reconstruction of parotid defects. *Plast Reconstr Surg* (2012) 130(1):36e–41e. doi:10.1097/PRS.0b013e3182547f55
7. Loh IW, Rozen WM, Behan FC, Crock J. Eyelid reconstruction: expanding the applications of the keystone perforator island flap concept. *ANZ J Surg* (2012) 82(10):763–4. doi:10.1111/j.1445-2197.2012.06222.x
8. Sun Y. Keystone flap for large posterior neck defect. *Indian J Surg* (2016) 78(4):321–2. doi:10.1007/s12262-015-1406-5
9. Behan FC, Lo CH, Findlay M. Anatomical basis for the keystone island flap in the upper thigh. *Plast Reconstr Surg* (2010) 125(1):421–3. doi:10.1097/PRS.0b013e3181c2a66f
10. Hu M, Bordeaux JS. The keystone flap for lower extremity defects. *Dermatol Surg* (2012) 38(3):490–3. doi:10.1111/j.1524-4725.2011.02236.x
11. Martinez J-C, Cook JL, Otley C. The keystone fasciocutaneous flap in the reconstruction of lower extremity wounds. *Dermatol Surg* (2012) 38(3):484–9. doi:10.1111/j.1524-4725.2011.02239.x
12. Al-Busaidi AA, Semalesan N, Al-Busaidi SS. Keystone design sliding skin flap for the management of small full thickness burns. *Sultan Qaboos Univ Med J* (2011) 11(3):412–4.
13. Behan F, Sizeland A, Porcedu S, Somia N, Wilson J. Keystone island flap: an alternative reconstructive option to free flaps in irradiated tissue. *ANZ J Surg* (2006) 76(5):407–13. doi:10.1111/j.1445-2197.2006.03708.x
14. Gutman MJ, Goldschlager T, Fahardieh RD, Ying D, Xenos C, Danks RA. Keystone design perforator island flap for closure of myelomeningocele. *Childs Nerv Syst* (2011) 27(9):1459–63. doi:10.1007/s00381-011-1448-3
15. Park H-S, Morrison E, Lo C, Leong J. An application of keystone perforator island flap for closure of lumbosacral myelomeningocele defects. *Ann Plast Surg* (2016) 77(3):332–6. doi:10.1097/SAP.0000000000000600
16. Stankiewicz M, Coyer F, Webster J, Osborne S. Incidence and predictors of lower limb split-skin graft failure and primary closure dehiscence in day-case surgical patients. *Dermatol Surg* (2015) 41(7):775–83. doi:10.1097/DSS.0000000000000391
17. Farhadieh RD, Bulstrode N, Cugno S. *Plastic and Reconstructive Surgery: Approaches and Techniques*. Chichester: John Wiley & Sons (2015).
18. Robson MC, Krizek TJ. Predicting skin graft survival. *J Trauma* (1973) 13(3):213–7. doi:10.1097/00005373-197303000-00005
19. Ragnell A. The secondary contracting tendency of free skin grafts: an experimental investigation on animals. *Br J Plast Surg* (1952) 5(1):6–24. doi:10.1016/S0007-1226(52)80003-7
20. Corps BVM. The effect of graft thickness, donor site and graft bed on graft shrinkage in the hooded rat. *Br J Plast Surg* (1969) 22(2):125–33. doi:10.1016/S0007-1226(69)80053-6
21. Chaput B, de Bonnecaze G, Lopez R, Benjamin V, Garrido I, Grolleau JL. Modified keystone island flap design for lateral nasal defect: aesthetic subunit consideration. *Plast Reconstr Surg Glob Open* (2014) 2(9):e213. doi:10.1097/GOX.0000000000000143
22. Kostopoulos E, Casoli V, Agiannidis C, Konofaos P, Drimouras G, Dounavis A, et al. The keystone perforator island flap in nasal reconstruction: an alternative reconstructive option for soft tissue defects up to 2 cm. *J Craniofac Surg* (2015) 26(4):1374–7. doi:10.1097/SCS.0000000000001746
23. Kostopoulos E, Agiannidis C, Konofaos P, Kotsakis I, Champsas G, Frangoulis M, et al. Keystone perforator island flap as an alternative reconstructive option for partial thickness alar defects up to 1.5 centimeters. *J Craniofac Surg* (2016) 27(5):1256–60. doi:10.1097/SCS.0000000000002742
24. Shaw HM, McGovern VJ, Milton GW, Farago GA, McCarthy WH. Malignant melanoma: influence of site of lesion and age of patient in the female superiority in survival. *Cancer* (1980) 46(12):2731–5. doi:10.1002/1097-0142(19801215)46:12<2731::AID-CNCR2820461232>3.0.CO;2-2
25. Stone JP, Webb C, McKinnon JG, Dawes JC, McKenzie CD, Temple-Oberle CF. Avoiding skin grafts: the keystone flap in cutaneous defects. *Plast Reconstr Surg* (2015) 136(2):404–8. doi:10.1097/PRS.0000000000001449
26. Moncrieff MD, Bowen F, Thompson JF, Saw RPM, Shannon KF, Spillane AJ, et al. Keystone flap reconstruction of primary melanoma excision defects of the leg – the end of the skin graft? *Ann Surg Oncol* (2008) 15(10):2867–73. doi:10.1245/s10434-008-0018-8
27. Bajantri B, Bharathi RR, Sabapathy SR. Wound coverage considerations for defects of the lower third of the leg. *Indian J Plast Surg* (2012) 45(2):283–90. doi:10.4103/0970-0358.101299
28. Adkinson JM, Chung KC. Flap reconstruction of the elbow and forearm: a case-based approach. *Hand Clin* (2014) 30(2):153–63. doi:10.1016/j.hcl.2013.12.005
29. Zenn MR, Jones G. *Reconstructive Surgery: Anatomy, Technique, and Clinical Applications*. St. Louis, Missouri: Quality Medical Publishing, Inc (2012). 855 p.
30. Rao AL, Janna RK. Keystone flap: versatile flap for reconstruction of limb defects. *J Clin Diagn Res* (2015) 9(3):PC05–7. doi:10.7860/JCDR/2015/12595.5631

# 10

# Biologic Mesh Reconstruction of the Pelvic Floor after Extralevator Abdominoperineal Excision

*Nasra N. Alam[1], Sunil K. Narang[1], Ferdinand Köckerling[2], Ian R. Daniels[1] and Neil J. Smart[1]**

*[1] Exeter Surgical Health Services Research Unit (HeSRU), Royal Devon and Exeter Hospital, Exeter, Devon, UK, [2] Department of Surgery, Center for Minimally Invasive Surgery, Academic Teaching Hospital of Charité Medical School, Vivantes Hospital, Berlin, Germany*

**Introduction:** The aim of this review is to provide an overview of the evidence for the use of biologic mesh in the reconstruction of the pelvic floor after extralevator abdominoperineal excision of the rectum (ELAPE).

**Methods:** A systematic search of PubMed was conducted using the search terms: "ELAPE," "extralevator abdominoperineal excision of rectum," or "extralevator abdominoperineal resection." The search yielded 17 studies.

**Results:** Biologic mesh was used in perineal reconstruction in 463 cases. There were 41 perineal hernias reported but rates were not consistently reported in all studies. The most common complications were perineal wound infection ($n = 93$), perineal sinus and fistulae ($n = 26$), and perineal haematoma or seroma ($n = 11$). There were very few comparative studies, with only one randomized control trial (RCT) identified that compared patients undergoing ELAPE with perineal reconstruction using a biological mesh, with patients undergoing a conventional abdominoperineal excision of the rectum with no mesh. There was no significant difference in perineal hernia rates or perineal wound infections between the groups. Other comparative studies comparing the use of biologic mesh with techniques, such as the use of myocutaneous flaps, were of low quality.

**Conclusion:** Biologic mesh-assisted perineal reconstruction is a promising technique to improve wound healing and has comparable complications rates to other techniques. However, there is not enough evidence to support its use in all patients who have undergone ELAPE. Results from high-quality prospective RCTs and national/international collaborative audits are required.

**Keywords: ELAPE, extralevator abdominoperineal excision of rectum, extralevator abdominoperineal resection, pelvic floor reconstruction, biological mesh**

***Edited by:***
*Evangelos P. Misiakos, University of Athens School of Medicine, Greece*

***Reviewed by:***
*Scott R. Kelley, Mayo Clinic, USA*
*Juan Manuel Suárez-Grau, General Hospital of Riotinto, Spain*

****Correspondence:***
*Neil J. Smart*
*drneilsmart@hotmail.com*

***Specialty section:***
*This article was submitted to Visceral Surgery, a section of the journal Frontiers in Surgery*

## INTRODUCTION

Abdominoperineal excision of the rectum (APER) is used as a treatment modality in patients with rectal cancer where an anterior resection (AR) and an anastomosis cannot be performed (1). Extralevator abdominoperineal excision (ELAPE) involves the en bloc excision of the levator muscles and the rectum, in order to reduce the risk of tumor involvement in the circumferential resection margins (CRMs) and reduce the risk of tumor perforation intraoperatively. This method has been demonstrated as leading to a wider surgical margin and therefore fewer positive CRMs (2–5). Initially, the terminology used was "*cylindrical APER*" but with refinement and the use of MRI to highlight the area of risk of a positive CRM, the term ELAPE is more appropriate (4). The nomenclature surrounding the technique has been the source of much debate and confusion, with some authors noting that ELAPE is no different from the original description in English by Miles (6). Furthermore, what exactly constitutes "standard" surgery that allows differentiation of ELAPE has come under scrutiny (7).

Volumetric analysis has confirmed that ELAPE does remove more tissue (3), and the wider excision can, however, increase morbidity and wound complications and will require some form of perineal reconstruction (4). Perineal wound problems are reported in up to 57% of patients undergoing APER (8), although the precise rates following ELAPE are not yet known. Given that ELAPE produces a larger defect in the pelvic floor, leaving only the ischiorectal fat and skin to close the perineal wound; it is presumed that the perineal complication rate is higher. Furthermore, the changes in the proportion of patients having neoadjuvant (chemo)radiotherapy over the time course of ELAPE implementation are incompletely reported in individual studies and in national registries. If the wound fails to heal *via* primary intention, secondary wound healing can result in prolonged hospital stay that requires intensive wound care.

Various alternative techniques have been described to reconstruct the pelvic floor following ELAPE with the aim to reduce perineal wound complications and hernias. The optimal method of perineal reconstruction remains a matter of debate. Myocutaneous flaps, such as those derived from gluteus maximus (2, 4, 9), rectus abdominis, and latissimus dorsi muscles (4, 10), have been used but are associated with donor-site morbidity, flap necrosis, prolonged operative time, additional resources, and increased cost. Biologic mesh has recently been introduced as an alternative form of reconstruction in order to improve perineal wound healing and reduce perineal hernia rates (11). The mesh is usually placed as an inlay or bridge across the defect in the pelvic floor in close relation to the bony structures and sutured in 1-cm intervals to the origin of the levator muscles laterally (12). [**Figure 1** (13)] The mechanism by which the use of a bridging prosthesis reduces perineal wound problems is not clear. It has been suggested that biological mesh allows native cellular ingrowth and promotes tissue remodeling, which in turn reduces perineal wound problems (14, 15). Alternatively, the biologic mesh may act as a physical barrier, supporting the pelvic contents (omentum, small bowel, and uterus) and minimizing the pressure on the skin and ischiorectal fat as they heal.

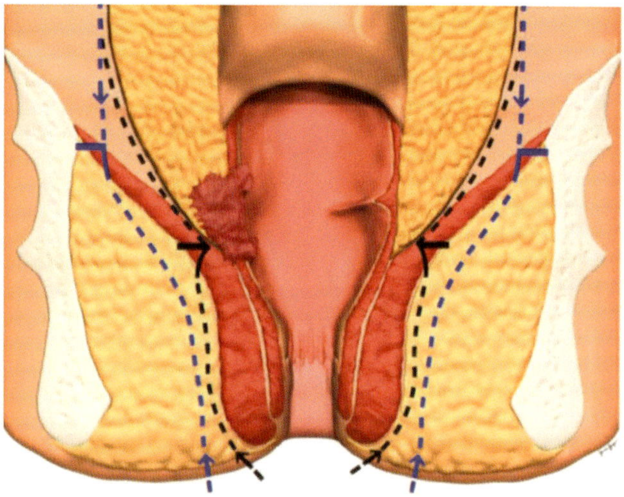

**FIGURE 1 | ELAPE technique (13).** Black line indicates dissection line of standard APE and blue line ELAPE. Horizontal line indicates meeting point of abdominal and perineal dissection.

Alternative methods for removing the pressure of small bowel that prolapses into the pelvis, directly on the perineum include the following:

(1) Omental pedicle flaps (16–18),
(2) Mobilization of the cecum (9),
(3) Retroversion of the uterus in female (19).

All of the above techniques are designed to close off the dead space in the pelvis, resulting from the removal of the rectum and to keep the small bowel out of the pelvis. Of these methods, the most widely established is the omental pedicle. However, these techniques largely related to an era of open surgery, and they have mostly been abandoned with the move to laparoscopic and other minimally invasive techniques and are not representative of contemporary practice. Omental pedicles are associated with perineal wound complication rates of 14–18% and decreased wound dehiscence in comparison to primary closure (16, 18) whereas others show no advantage to this technique (20). Mobilization of the cecum is uncommon and evidence is limited to case reports (9). Retroversion of the uterus involves retroverting the uterus and securing it to the bony pelvis at a level where it obliterates the pelvis, with the use of non-absorbable suture material (19). This can be achieved *via* the abdominal or perineal wound, although it has been associated with dyspareunia and positional menstruation (19).

The aim of this review is to provide an overview of the evidence for the use of biologic mesh in the reconstruction of the pelvic floor after extralevator abdominoperineal excision.

## METHODS

A systematic search of PubMed was conducted using the search terms: "ELAPE," "extralevator abdominoperineal excision of rectum," or "extralevator abdominoperineal resection" in order to identify studies evaluating the use of biologic mesh for reconstruction of the pelvic floor. Titles, abstracts, and full texts were analyzed for studies reporting on the use of biologic mesh for reconstruction of the pelvic floor. Inclusion criteria were studies that used biologic mesh for perineal reconstruction. Studies were excluded if only synthetic mesh was used or if there was no mention of a mesh. Furthermore, studies on patients under the age of 18 were excluded as well as non-English language studies, technical tips, conference abstracts, or duplicates series from the same research group. Overall, the search yielded 17 studies for analysis after the exclusion of review articles. The study characteristics are presented (**Table 1**).

## RESULTS

There were 15 case series, one randomized control trial (RCT), and one case report identified. A biologic mesh was used in perineal reconstruction in 463 cases. The different types of biologic mesh used were cross-linked porcine dermal collagen (Permacol™) in 206 cases, 44 using porcine intestinal submucosa (Surgisis©), 136 using human acellular dermal matrix, and 9 using a combination of Permacol™ and Surgisis©. Two studies did not specify the type of biologic mesh used.

### Perineal Hernia

There were 41 perineal hernias reported, but rates were not consistently reported in all studies. In those studies that did report perineal hernia rates, it was difficult to delineate whether hernias occurred in patients that had perineal reconstruction using a biological or synthetic mesh or a myocutaneous flap.

### Perineal Wound Infection/Healing Problems

Perineal wound infection was reported explicitly in 93 cases, whereas the overall rate of perineal problems was much higher. Perineal sinus and fistulae were reported in 26 cases, with a further 11 cases of perineal hematoma or seroma. Some studies have described "perineal wound complications" but not specified whether they were related to infection, dehiscence, hernia, or pain (**Table 1**).

The most common complications were perineal wound infection and perineal sinus. However, there are no standardized measures for reporting perineal outcomes of any type following ELAPE. Definitions of wound infection, wound healing problems, perineal herniation, pain measurement, and functional status assessment are inconsistent between studies, thus limiting comparisons.

There are very few studies comparing the use of biologic mesh for perineal reconstruction for ELAPE. Two case series compared biologic mesh with myocutaneous flaps and one series compared laparoscopic ELAPE with laparoscopic and open APER. However, they are all of low-level evidence (level 4). Only one RCT was identified that compared patients undergoing ELAPE with perineal reconstruction using a biological mesh, with patients undergoing a conventional APER with no mesh. There was no significant difference in perineal hernia rates or perineal wound infections between the two groups.

## DISCUSSION/SUMMARY

The use of ELAPE over conventional APER is becoming more widespread despite the reservations of some (13), and the optimal method of perineal wound closure remains a topic of discussion. The reported results of primary closure of the perineal defect are poor (34) and most surgeons performing ELAPE opt for an adjunct (35). The literature analyzed suggests that perineal closure using a biologic mesh produces wound infection and complication rates that are comparable to other methods of reconstruction, such as myocutaneous flaps. Myocutaneous flap reconstruction using a vertical rectus abdominis (VRAM), gracilis, or the gluteus maximus, however, has short-term disadvantages, such as longer operative times and the need for plastic surgical expertise, resulting in higher operative costs, flap necrosis, wound complications at the donor site, and longer bed rest (15). Longer term incisional hernias at the VRAM donor site and reduced abdominal wall strength have been reported (36). Biologic mesh reconstruction avoids all of these potential complications.

Synthetic non-absorbable mesh is associated with high infection rate in contaminated fields and consequently is considered by many to be contra-indicated for use in perineal reconstruction following ELAPE (37). The role of newer, absorbable synthetic meshes is, as yet, unclear. Biologic meshes are composed of an acellular collagen matrix that is believed to allow tissue regeneration, neovascularization, repopulation with fibroblasts, and therefore provides a scaffold for tissue incorporation (15, 23). This is thought to reduce the rate of infection. However, the overall volume and quality of evidence available regarding biologic mesh use for perineal reconstruction following ELAPE is poor, with observational retrospective studies predominating. There have been some attempts at comparative studies, but these too have been of low quality with a high risk of bias and confounding factors. Head-to-head randomized trials or high-quality prospective cohort studies comparing biological with synthetic mesh, types of biologic mesh, and biologic mesh with (myo)fasciocutaneous flaps are also lacking, partly because there is no consensus among surgeons as to the optimal biologic mesh or optimal tissue flap. Trials directly comparing any technical adjunct to primary closure alone as a control arm may be difficult to perform in light of the lack of equipoise among surgeons and possibly even unethical given the reported poor results of primary closure. Furthermore, there does not appear to be a consensus in the studies regarding perineal outcome reporting. There are a variety of different end points recorded across the studies, such as perineal defect size, blood loss, and operating time. There needs to be a focus on standardized definitions and reporting of perineal healing rates, perineal hernia, and functional outcomes following ELAPE (38).

Jensen et al. also examined the long-term follow-up for patients undergoing pelvic floor reconstruction with a biologic mesh following ELAPE (25). As well as low perineal hernia rates, there was no major restriction in movement or sitting. Chronic pain had resolved in all patients at a median of 8 months, and there was no major limitation to walking. However, other studies evaluating quality-of-life scores using validated tools (11) demonstrated a favorable comparison to the reference population of patients with colorectal cancer who had undergone a standard

**TABLE 1 | Reconstruction of the pelvic floor after ELAPE.**

| Reference | Study design | No. of pts | Age | Sex (M:F) | Patient characteristics | Material used | Intervention | Follow-up (months) | Complications | LoE |
|---|---|---|---|---|---|---|---|---|---|---|
| Christensen et al. (21) | Case series | 57 | FLAP: 67.8 (32.7–86.2)<br>MESH: 69.7 (48.7–84.5) | 11:22<br>10:14 | 52 primary rectal cancer<br>5 local recurrence<br>48 patients (84%) received neoadjuvant CRT | Gluteal flaps: 33<br>Permacol: 24 | ELAPE for low rectal cancer | Median follow-up: gluteal flap: 3.2 years (1.7– 4.3)<br>Biologic mesh: 1.7 (0.4 –2.2) years | Gluteal flap vs. biologic<br>Perineal hernia: 7 vs. 0, $P < 0.01$<br>Infectious complications: 2 (17%) vs. 4 (6%), $P < 0.26$<br>1 patient per group with a persistent perineal sinus | 4 |
| Dalton et al. (22) | Case series | 31 | Mean 66.8 ± SD 11.4 years | 8:23 | Neoadjuvant CRT: 14 | VRAM flap: 1<br>Permacol: 30 | Open ELAPE | Median: 20 (0–45) | Breakdown of perineal wound: 6<br>Skin paddle necrosis of a VRAM flap: 1<br>Perineal wound hematoma: 1<br>Minor wound discharge: 9 | 4 |
| Han et al. (23) | Case series | 12 | 68 (49–80) | 7:5 | Ultra low rectal cancer.<br>Neoadjuvant CRT: 3 | HADM | Cylindrical APR-open | Median: 8 (2–16) | Asymptomatic seroma: 1<br>Perineal wound infection: 1 | 4 |
| Han et al. (14) | Open label RCT | 67 | 63 median (44–81) | 20:15 | Neoadjuvant therapy: 10 | HADM | ELAPE: 35 | Median: 29 (12–48) | Bowel perforation: 2<br>Perineal wound infection: 4<br>Perineal seroma: 4<br>Peristomal hernia: 16<br>Abdominal wound infection: 2<br>Perineal herniation: 5 | 2 |
| | | | 68 (32–84) | 21:11 | Neoadjuvant therapy: 9 | None | APER: 32 | Median: 22 (14–46) | Bowel perforation: 5<br>Perineal wound infection: 6<br>Peristomal hernia: 13<br>Abdominal wound infection: 3<br>Perineal herniation: 4 | |
| Han et al. (24) | Multicenter prospective cohort study (case series) | 109 (102) | 61 years (27–78) | 60:42 | | HADM | Biological mesh: 83 (81.4%)<br>Primary closure: 19 (18.6%) | 44 median (18–68) | Biological mesh<br>Perineal wound complications: 15<br>Infection: 5<br>Seroma: 5<br>Hernia: 4<br>Abdominal wound infection: 3<br>Primary closure<br>Perineal wound complications: 9<br>Infection: 3<br>Seroma: 1<br>Hernia: 2<br>Wound dehiscence: 3<br>Chronic sinus: 1<br>Abdominal wound infection: 2 | 4 |

*(Continued)*

**TABLE 1** | Continued

| Reference | Study design | No. of pts | Age | Sex (M:F) | Patient characteristics | Material used | Intervention | Follow-up (months) | Complications | LoE |
|---|---|---|---|---|---|---|---|---|---|---|
| Jensen et al. (25) | Case series | 53 – 31 agreed to long-term f/u | 69 (33–83) median | 33:20 | Neoadjuvant CRT: 23 | Permacol | 6 planned open<br>47 laparoscopic of which 7 converted to open | Median: 36 (1–67) | Perineal hernia: 3<br>Fistuale: 11<br>Perineal abscess: 4<br>Superficial wound infections: 4<br>Removal of mesh: 1<br>Implantation of new mesh: 1 | 4 |
| Kipling et al. (26) | Case series | 28 | 70 (52–81 years) median | 20:8 | Neoadjuvant therapy<br>None: 9 (32%)<br>Short course: 2 (7%)<br>Long course: 17 (61%) | Permacol | Lap ELAPE, 5 conversions | Median 38 (23–66) | Bowel perforation: 1<br>Persistent perineal sinus at 6 months: 1<br>Delayed healing of the perineal wound: 1 | 4 |
| Peacock et al. (15) | Case series (comparative) | 15 | 68 median (48–74) | 4:1 | Long-course CT/RT: 4<br>Long-course RT: 1 | VRAM: 5 | Cylindrical APER | Median: 29 (23–35) | Perineal wound infection (wound dehiscence): 1<br>Flap necrosis: 1<br>Wound hematoma: 1 | 4 |
| | | | 57 median (47–68) | 9:1 | Long-course CT/RT: 6<br>Long-course RT: 2 (not suitable for CT): 2 | Surgisis: 10 | | 13 (3–27) | Perineal sinus: 1<br>Superficial perineal wound infection: 2<br>Abscess/collection: 3 | |
| Peacock et al. (27) | Case series | 34 | Median 62 years (40–77) | 27:7 | Long-course CRT: 26<br>Long-course RT (not suitable for CT): 2<br>Not required/declined: 6 | Surgisis: | Cylindrical APER | Median: 21 (1–54) | Perineal sinus: 5<br>Superficial perineal wound infection: 3<br>Abscess/collection: 3<br>Parastomal hernia: 1 | 4 |
| Vaughan-Shaw et al. (28) | Case series (case–control) | 16 | 71 (49–88) | 7:9 | Short-course RT: 7<br>Long-course CRT: 9 | 9 Permacol/ Surgisis (omentoplasty: 7) | Laparoscopic ELAPE: 14 (1 conversion)<br>Open: 2 | | Return to theater (<30 days): 2<br>Perineal wound complications: 2 | 4 |
| | | 10 | 72 (52–87) | 5:5 | Short-course RT: 7<br>Long-course CRT: 2 | | Lap APER: 10<br>Open APER: 10 | | Perineal wound complications: 5<br>Perineal hernia: 2<br>Infection: 1 | |
| | | 10 | 72.5 (46–89) | 8:2 | Short-course RT: 2<br>Long-course CRT: 5 | | | | Return to theater (<30 days): 1<br>In-hospital mortality: 1<br>Perineal wound complications: 2 | |
| Wille-Jørgensen et al. (29) | Case series | 11 | 63 median (51–77) | 7:4 | Neoadjuvant CRT: 6 | Permacol | Laparoscopic APER: 9 (2 conversions) Open APER: 2 | Median: 12 (3–18) | Mesh removal 2nd to infection: 1<br>Rectal perforation: 1<br>Long-lasting perineal pain: 6<br>Fistula: 1 | 4 |
| Chi et al. (30) | Case series | 6 | Mean: 69 | 4:2 | Neoadjuvant CRT 4 | HADM | | Mean: 5 (2–19) | Surgical site infection: 2 | 4 |

*(Continued)*

**TABLE 1** | Continued

| Reference | Study design | No. of pts | Age | Sex (M:F) | Patient characteristics | Material used | Intervention | Follow-up (months) | Complications | LoE |
|---|---|---|---|---|---|---|---|---|---|---|
| Palmer et al. (31) | Case series | 193 | 66 median (28–87) | 81:112 | Neoadjuvant CRT: 91<br>RT alone: 92<br>Locally advanced tumor on MRI (T4)-126 (65%) | Perineal closure<br>Gluteal flap: 99 (51)<br>Biological mesh: 66 (34)<br>Closure directly: 28 (15) | Pelvic exenteration: 25, extended resection with parts of other organs: 56<br>ELAPE alone: 112 | Median 31 (0–156) | Intra-operative perforation: 19<br>30-day postoperative mortality: 6 | 4 |
| West et al. (4) | Retrospective case series (multicenter) | 176 | 66 (58–73) Median | 116:54 6-unknown | Neoadjuvant RT<br>Yes: 135<br>No: 35<br>Unknown: 11<br>Neoadjuvant CT<br>Given: 84<br>Not given: 81<br>Unknown: 11 | Gluteus maximus: 60<br>Rectus abdominis: 12<br>Latissimus dorsi: 1<br>Permacol: 11 | ELAPE: 176<br>Open surgery: 122<br>Laparoscopic surgery: 19<br>Unknown: 35 | *NS* | Wound complications<br>Yes: 57<br>Infection/breakdown/sinus: 41<br>Perineal hernia: 5<br>Other: 11 | 4 |
| | | 124 | 68 (57–75) median | 87:37 | Neoadjuvant RT<br>Yes: 90<br>No: 24<br>Unknown: 10<br>Neoadjuvant CT<br>Given: 48<br>Not given: 66<br>Unknown: 10 | | APER: 124<br>Open surgery: 56<br>Laparoscopic surgery: 4<br>Unknown: 64 | *NS* | Wound complications<br>Yes: 11<br>Infection/breakdown/sinus: 7<br>Perineal hernia: 1<br>Other: 3<br>Unknown: 26 | |
| Harries et al. (32) | Prospective case series | 48 | Median: 63 (40–86) | 36:12 | Neoadjuvant treatment: 43 | Permacol | ELAPE<br>Lap: 28<br>Conversion: 7<br>Open: 23 | Median: 27 (1–85) | Specimen perforation: 3 (6.4%)<br>Unhealed at 6 months: 4 (8.3%)<br>Perineal sinus: 7<br>Abdominal wound dehiscence: 1<br>Ureteric injury: 1<br>Radiological drainage of pelvic collections: 2<br>Perineal wound infections: 9 | 4 |
| Kavanagh et al. (33) | Case report | 1 | 72 | 0:1 | Long-course CRT | Permacol | Lap ELAPE | 12 | NS | 4 |
| Sayers et al. (34) | Case series | 54 | Median: 69.5 (31–90) | 40:14 | Neoadjuvant CRT: 52 | Primary closure: 46<br>Bio: 2<br>FLAP: 6 (VRAM: 5 Gracilis: 1) | Lap ELAPE: 20<br>Open: 34 | Median: 38 (9–61) | Perineal complications: 24<br>Perineal hernia: 14<br>Perineal hematoma: 1<br>Infected myocutaneous flap: 1<br>Total dehiscence of the perineum: 1 | 4 |

*APER, abdominoperineal excision of the rectum; CRT, chemoradiotherapy; CT, chemotherapy; ELAPE, extralevator abdominoperineal excision; HADM, human acellular dermal matrix; LoE, level of evidence; RCT, randomized controlled trial; RT, radiotherapy; VRAM, vertical rectus abdominis muscle.*

APE, whereas patients who had undergone flap reconstruction had a lower quality of life score (11).

Of note, a number of studies from Beijing have been included for analysis. The three studies include patients managed over an approximately 3-year period, and there is overlap of the studies within the time period, therefore suggesting some replication. One study is classified as a case series (23), the second a RCT (14), and the third another case series (24). It is unclear as to whether these three studies are from the same patient group or three different cohorts.

## CONCLUSION

Overall, the use of a biologic mesh to close perineal defects has comparable complications rates to myocutaenous flaps but may offer advantages, such as shorter operating time and early mobilization, which results in a more cost-effective repair (15). Biologic mesh-assisted perineal reconstruction is a promising technique to improve wound healing, but there is not enough evidence to support its use in all patients who have undergone ELAPE. The results from high-quality prospective RCTs or national/international collaborative audits using statistical process control as a methodology of assessment of improvement are required.

## AUTHOR CONTRIBUTIONS

All authors listed have made substantial, direct, and intellectual contribution to the work and approved it for publication.

## REFERENCES


1. Perry WB, Connaughton JC. Abdominoperineal resection: how is it done and what are the results? *Clin Colon Rectal Surg* (2007) **20**(3):213–20. doi:10.1055/s-2007-984865
2. Holm T, Ljung A, Häggmark T, Jurell G, Lagergren J. Extended abdominoperineal resection with gluteus maximus flap reconstruction of the pelvic floor for rectal cancer. *Br J Surg* (2007) **94**(2):232–8. doi:10.1002/bjs.5489
3. West NP, Finan PJ, Anderin C, Lindholm J, Holm T, Quirke P. Evidence of the oncologic superiority of cylindrical abdominoperineal excision for low rectal cancer. *J Clin Oncol* (2008) **26**(21):3517–22. doi:10.1200/JCO.2007.14.5961
4. West NP, Anderin C, Smith KJ, Holm T, Quirke P. European Extralevator Abdominoperineal Excision Study Group. Multicentre experience with extralevator abdominoperineal excision for low rectal cancer. *Br J Surg* (2010) **97**(4):588–99. doi:10.1002/bjs.6916
5. Shihab OC, Heald RJ, Holm T, How PD, Brown G, Quirke P, et al. A pictorial description of extralevator abdominoperineal excision for low rectal cancer. *Colorectal Dis* (2012) **14**(10):e655–60. doi:10.1111/j.1463-1318.2012.03181.x
6. Miles WE. A method of performing abdomino-perineal excision for carcinoma of the rectum and of the terminal portion of the pelvic colon (1908). *CA Cancer J Clin* (1971) **21**(6):361–4. doi:10.3322/canjclin.21.6.361
7. Nicholls J. No more 'standard' abdominoperineal excision. *Colorectal Dis* (2013) **15**(11):1329–30. doi:10.1111/codi.12458
8. de Bruin AF, Gosselink MP, Wijffels NA, Coene PP, van der Harst E. Local gentamicin reduces perineal wound infection after radiotherapy and abdominoperineal resection. *Tech Coloproctol* (2008) **12**(4):303–7. doi:10.1007/s10151-008-0440-8
9. Habib K. Prevention of recurrent small bowel obstruction resulting from pelvic adhesions in patients who have previously undergone abdominoperineal excision of the rectum. *Tech Coloproctol* (2014) **18**(12):1179–80. doi:10.1007/s10151-014-1227-8
10. McMenamin DM, Clements D, Edwards TJ, Fitton AR, Douie WJ. Rectus abdominis myocutaneous flaps for perineal reconstruction: modifications to the technique based on a large single-centre experience. *Ann R Coll Surg Engl* (2011) **93**(5):375–81. doi:10.1308/003588411X572268
11. Foster JD, Pathak S, Smart NJ, Branagan G, Longman RJ, Thomas MG, et al. Reconstruction of the perineum following extralevator abdominoperineal excision for carcinoma of the lower rectum: a systematic review. *Colorectal Dis* (2012) **14**(9):1052–9. doi:10.1111/j.1463-1318.2012.03169.x
12. Svane M, Bulut O. Perineal hernia after laparoscopic abdominoperineal resection – reconstruction of the pelvic floor with a biological mesh (Permacol™). *Int J Colorectal Dis* (2012) **27**(4):543–4. doi:10.1007/s00384-011-1253-1
13. Prytz M, Angenete E, Ekelund J, Haglind E. Extralevator abdominoperineal excision (ELAPE) for rectal cancer – short-term results from the Swedish colorectal cancer registry. Selective use of ELAPE warranted. *Int J Colorectal Dis* (2014) **29**(8):981–7. doi:10.1007/s00384-014-1932-9
14. Han JG, Wang ZJ, Wei GH, Gao ZG, Yang Y, Zhao BC. Randomized clinical trial of conventional versus cylindrical abdominoperineal resection for locally advanced lower rectal cancer. *Am J Surg* (2012) **204**(3):274–82. doi:10.1016/j.amjsurg.2012.05.001
15. Peacock O, Pandya H, Sharp T, Hurst NG, Speake WJ, Tierney GM, et al. Biological mesh reconstruction of perineal wounds following enhanced abdominoperineal excision of rectum (APER). *Int J Colorectal Dis* (2012) **27**(4):475–82. doi:10.1007/s00384-011-1325-2
16. Hay JM, Fingerhut A, Paquet JC, Flamant Y. Management of the pelvic space with or without omentoplasty after abdominoperineal resection for carcinoma of the rectum: a prospective multicenter study. The French Association for Surgical Research. *Eur J Surg* (1997) **163**(3):199–206.
17. Moreaux J, Horiot A, Barrat F, Mabille J. Obliteration of the pelvic space with pedicled omentum after excision of the rectum for cancer. *Am J Surg* (1984) **148**(5):640–4. doi:10.1016/0002-9610(84)90342-8
18. Killeen S, Devaney A, Mannion M, Martin ST, Winter DC. Omental pedicle flaps following proctectomy: a systematic review. *Colorectal Dis* (2013) **15**(11):e634–45. doi:10.1111/codi.12394
19. Habib K. Uterus and extralevator abdominoperineal excision: a technique. *Dis Colon Rectum* (2013) **56**(9):1102–4. doi:10.1097/DCR.0b013e31829a2edc
20. O'Leary DP. Use of the greater omentum in colorectal surgery. *Dis Colon Rectum* (1999) **42**(4):533–9. doi:10.1007/BF02234183
21. Christensen HK, Nerstrøm P, Tei T, Laurberg S. Perineal repair after extralevator abdominoperineal excision for low rectal cancer. *Dis Colon Rectum* (2011) **54**(6):711–7. doi:10.1097/DCR.0b013e3182163c89
22. Dalton RS, Smart NJ, Edwards TJ, Chandler I, Daniels IR. Short-term outcomes of the prone perineal approach for extra-levator abdomino-perineal excision (elAPE). *Surgeon* (2012) **10**(6):342–6. doi:10.1016/j.surge.2011.10.001
23. Han JG, Wang ZJ, Gao ZG, Xu HM, Yang ZH, Jin ML. Pelvic floor reconstruction using human acellular dermal matrix after cylindrical abdominoperineal resection. *Dis Colon Rectum* (2010) **53**(2):219–23. doi:10.1007/DCR.0b013e3181b715b5
24. Han JG, Wang ZJ, Qian Q, Dai Y, Zhang ZQ, Yang JS, et al. A prospective multicenter clinical study of extralevator abdominoperineal resection for locally advanced low rectal cancer. *Dis Colon Rectum* (2014) **57**(12):1333–40. doi:10.1097/DCR.0000000000000235
25. Jensen KK, Rashid L, Pilsgaard B, Møller P, Wille-Jørgensen P. Pelvic floor reconstruction with a biological mesh after extralevator abdominoperineal excision leads to few perineal hernias and acceptable wound complication rates with minor movement limitations: single-centre experience including clinical examination and interview. *Colorectal Dis* (2014) **16**(3):192–7. doi:10.1111/codi.12492
26. Kipling SL, Young K, Foster JD, Smart NJ, Hunter AE, Cooper E, et al. Laparoscopic extralevator abdominoperineal excision of the rectum: short-term outcomes of a prospective case series. *Tech Coloproctol* (2014) **18**(5):445–51. doi:10.1007/s10151-013-1071-2
27. Peacock O, Simpson JA, Tou SI, Hurst NG, Speake WJ, Tierney GM, et al. Outcomes after biological mesh reconstruction of the pelvic floor following extra-levator abdominoperineal excision of rectum (APER). *Tech Coloproctol* (2014) **18**(6):571–7. doi:10.1007/s10151-013-1107-7
28. Vaughan-Shaw PG, Cheung T, Knight JS, Nichols PH, Pilkington SA, Mirnezami AH. A prospective case-control study of extralevator

abdominoperineal excision (ELAPE) of the rectum versus conventional laparoscopic and open abdominoperineal excision: comparative analysis of short-term outcomes and quality of life. *Tech Coloproctol* (2012) **16**(5):355–62. doi:10.1007/s10151-012-0851-4
29. Wille-Jørgensen P, Pilsgaard B, Møller P. Reconstruction of the pelvic floor with a biological mesh after abdominoperineal excision for rectal cancer. *Int J Colorectal Dis* (2009) **24**(3):323–5. doi:10.1007/s00384-008-0607-9
30. Chi P, Chen ZF, Lin HM, Lu XR, Huang Y. Laparoscopic extralevator abdominoperineal resection for rectal carcinoma with transabdominal levator transection. *Ann Surg Oncol* (2013) **20**(5):1560–6. doi:10.1245/s10434-012-2675-x
31. Palmer G, Anderin C, Martling A, Holm T. Local control and survival after extralevator abdominoperineal excision for locally advanced or low rectal cancer. *Colorectal Dis* (2014) **16**(7):527–32. doi:10.1111/codi.12610
32. Harries RL, Luhmann A, Harris DA, Shami JA, Appleton BN. Prone extralevator abdominoperineal excision of the rectum with porcine collagen perineal reconstruction (Permacol™): high primary perineal wound healing rates. *Int J Colorectal Dis* (2014) **29**(9):1125–30. doi:10.1007/s00384-014-1963-2
33. Kavanagh DO, Imran H, Almoudaris A, Ziprin P, Faiz O. Dynamic magnetic resonance imaging demonstrates the integrity of perineal reconstruction following cylindrical abdominoperineal excision with reconstruction of the pelvic floor using porcine collagen. *Case Rep Med* (2012) **2012**:752357. doi:10.1155/2012/752357
34. Sayers AE, Patel RK, Hunter IA. Perineal hernia formation following extralevator abdominoperineal excision. *Colorectal Dis* (2015) **17**(4):351–5. doi:10.1111/codi.12843
35. Dabbas N, Adams K, Chave H, Branagan G. Current practice in abdominoperineal resection: an email survey of the membership of the Association of Coloproctology. *Ann R Coll Surg Engl* (2012) **94**(3):173–6. doi:10.1308/003588412X13171221589973
36. Daigeler A, Simidjiiska-Belyaeva M, Drücke D, Goertz O, Hirsch T, Soimaru C, et al. The versatility of the pedicled vertical rectus abdominis myocutaneous flap in oncologic patients. *Langenbecks Arch Surg* (2011) **396**(8):1271–9. doi:10.1007/s00423-011-0823-6
37. Choi JJ, Palaniappa NC, Dallas KB, Rudich TB, Colon MJ, Divino CM. Use of mesh during ventral hernia repair in clean-contaminated and contaminated cases: outcomes of 33,832 cases. *Ann Surg* (2012) **255**(1):176–80. doi:10.1097/SLA.0b013e31822518e6
38. Haapamäki MM, Pihlgren V, Lundberg O, Sandzén B, Rutegård J. Physical performance and quality of life after extended abdominoperineal excision of rectum and reconstruction of the pelvic floor with gluteus maximus flap. *Dis Colon Rectum* (2011) **54**(1):101–6. doi:10.1007/DCR.0b013e3181fce26e

11

# Labral reconstruction: when to perform and how

*Brian J. White[1] and Mackenzie M. Herzog[2]**

[1] Western Orthopaedics, Denver, CO, USA, [2] Professional Research Institute for Sports Medicine, LLC, Chapel Hill, NC, USA

Over the past decade, the understanding of the anatomy and function of the hip joint has continuously evolved, and surgical treatment options for the hip have significantly progressed. Originally, surgical treatment of the hip primarily involved resection of damaged tissue. Procedures that maintain and preserve proper hip anatomy, such as labral repair and femoroacetabular impingement correction, have shown superior results, in terms of pain reduction, increased function, and ability to return to activities. Labral reconstruction is a treatment option that uses a graft to reconstruct the native labrum. The technique and outcomes of labral reconstruction have been described relatively recently, and labral reconstruction is a cutting edge procedure that has shown promising early outcomes. The aim of this article is to review the current literature on hip labral reconstruction. We will review the indications for labral reconstruction, surgical technique and graft options, and surgical outcomes that have been described to date. Labral reconstruction provides an alternative treatment option for challenging intra-articular hip problems. Labral reconstruction restores the original anatomy of the hip and has the potential to preserve the longevity of the hip joint. This technique is an important tool in the orthopedic surgeon's arsenal for hip joint treatment and preservation.

**Keywords: surgical techniques, hip arthroscopy, labral tear, labral reconstruction, labral pathology**

***Edited by:***
*Joshua David Harris,*
*Houston Methodist Orthopedics & Sports Medicine, USA*

***Reviewed by:***
*Claudia Di Bella,*
*St Vincent's Hospital, Australia*
*Nirav Kiritkumar Pandya,*
*University of California San Francisco, USA*

***Correspondence:***
*Mackenzie M. Herzog,*
*Professional Research Institute for Sports Medicine, LLC, PO Box 9522, Chapel Hill, NC 27515, USA*
*prismresearchconsulting@gmail.com*

***Specialty section:***
*This article was submitted to Orthopedic Surgery, a section of the journal Frontiers in Surgery*

## Background

Hip arthroscopy is a relatively new frontier in orthopedic surgery, with the first documented arthroscopy of the hip performed less than a century ago in 1931 (1, 2). Originally, arthroscopic treatment of the hip primarily involved diagnosis or, at most, irrigation, or simple resection of damaged tissue (1). Since that time, the understanding of the anatomy and function of the hip has continuously evolved, and surgical treatment options have significantly progressed to include a multitude of different procedures (1, 3).

Labral pathology is one of the most common diagnoses among adolescent and adult patients who present for treatment of hip pain (4, 5). The estimated prevalence of labral pathology is not well understood, but previous reports range from 22 to 55% in clinical population (4, 6, 7). Although the prevalence is not well understood, the understanding of the role of the acetabular labrum to biomechanical functioning of the hip has improved significantly in recent years. The labrum plays a crucial role in the stability, lubrication, and kinematics of the hip (8–15). Consequently, surgical procedures that maintain and preserve proper hip anatomy, such as labral repair (versus labral debridement) and FAI correction, have shown superior results in comparison, in terms of pain reduction, increased function, and ability to return to activities (5, 8–10, 16–19).

Labral reconstruction was first described in 2009 and is a treatment option that uses a graft to reconstruct the native labrum (20). The technique and outcomes of labral reconstruction have been described relatively recently, and labral reconstruction is a cutting edge procedure that has shown promising early outcomes. The aim of this article is to review the current literature on hip labral reconstruction. We will review the indications for labral reconstruction, surgical technique and graft options, and outcomes that have been described to date.

## Indications for Surgery

### Biomechanical Advantages

The labrum plays an important role in maintaining normal hip function. A previous cadaveric study indicated that partial labral resection resulted in loss of fluid pressurization and change of the hip seal (10). Labral reconstruction not only improved fluid pressurization, but maintained it over time, even better than labral repair in that study (10). While early biomechanical research supports labral reconstruction overall, one study does suggest that labral reconstruction may not prevent fluid efflux compared to labral repair or intact labral state (21).

The acetabular labrum also plays an important role in stabilization of the joint to distraction forces (9). Similar to the study of hip fluid pressurization, labral reconstruction was found to significantly improve stability to distractive forces compared to partial labral resection (9).

More recently, a cadaveric study assessed the contact area, contact pressure, and peak force in hips with labral pathology compared to hips with a reconstructed acetabular labrum (15). Hip contact pressure increased in the presence of labral resection but was reduced with labral reconstruction (15). In addition, labral reconstruction reduced peak forces in the hip compared to labral resection. These studies suggest that certain types of labral pathology may be indicated for labral reconstruction.

### Patient Characteristics

Arthroscopic labral repair has shown promising patient outcomes (22); however, there exists a population of patients in which labral repair is less optimal. The primary indications for labral reconstruction include irreparable labral tears or insufficient labral tissue (Table S1 in Supplementary Material) (8, 18, 20, 23–27). In these cases, a labral repair may not be feasible or adequate to restore the fluid seal of the hip joint (25, 26). When the tissue is too small, it lacks surface area to heal or the repair may not provide an adequate seal with the femoral head (9, 10). For this reason, a labrum <2–3 mm is considered an indication for labral reconstruction (28). On the contrary, when the tissue is too large, compression often cannot be achieved to allow the labrum to heal. Therefore, a labrum >8 mm is considered an indication for labral reconstruction, although this threshold has not been formally established in the literature. Labral tissue that is degenerative with intrasubstance cystic degeneration is also an indication for reconstruction. Revision procedures following previous labral debridement or resection often provide a challenging situation in which adequate labral tissue may not be available (18, 27). Labral reconstruction provides a viable alternative for maintaining and preserving labral function in patients with irreparable labral tears or insufficient labral tissue for repair.

Labral reconstruction may also be indicated for a variety of other reasons. In the presence of capsulolabral adhesions from previous surgery, it may not be possible to excise the scar tissue while preserving enough labral tissue to repair (25). Patients with rim ossification or global over coverage of the acetabulum may also benefit from labral reconstruction (8, 20, 23). Although contraindications for labral reconstruction have not been well-described, older patient age and preoperative joint space ≤2 mm have been proposed (Table S1 in Supplementary Material) (25). Overall, labral reconstruction should be considered in cases where the ability to maintain and preserve the native hip anatomy is compromised.

## Surgical Technique

### Open Technique

Sierra and Trousdale first reported hip labral reconstruction in 2009 (20). The original technique was described in association with an open surgical hip dislocation (20). Briefly, the technique described use of a ligamentum teres capitis autograft. The ligamentum teres was detached from the fovea and fixed to the acetabular rim in the same manner as labral refixation. In cases where the size of the ligamentum teres was not sufficient to adequately reconstruct the labrum, the ligament was opened longitudinally in order to lengthen the graft.

Open surgical dislocation remains an option for patients who meet indications for reconstruction. However, in recent years, hip arthroscopy has emerged as a new, less invasive treatment. While once considered the gold standard for surgical treatment of the hip, several recent studies have questioned the superiority of open surgical dislocation to arthroscopy (29–32). Although randomized comparative studies of open and arthroscopic techniques are lacking, hip arthroscopy has significantly fewer complications and re-operations versus open surgical dislocation (29–32).

### Arthroscopic Technique

Several arthroscopic techniques for labral reconstruction have been previously described (18, 27, 33–35). A modification of the original arthroscopic technique is presented here, including a front-to-back fixation technique (18, 28), and publication of the technique is currently in press (36). Briefly, the procedure is performed with the patient in a supine position on a fracture table. Combined general and spinal anesthesia is used, with an epidural anesthetic utilized in younger patients (<20 years). Rocuronium, a heavy paralytic agent, is employed at a loading dose of 1.5 mg per 1 kg. Total traction time does not exceed 90 min (in ≤45 min intervals).

Three arthroscopic portals are created for this procedure, including an anterolateral, mid anterior, and accessory portal. Three portals are necessary to maintain appropriate graft tension throughout the procedure. The anterolateral portal is located slightly anterior to the superior tip of the greater trochanter. The mid anterior portal is located 6 cm medial to the anterolateral portal and roughly 1 cm distal. The third, accessory portal is placed roughly 2–3 cm distal and 1–2 cm posterior to the mid anterior portal.

A femoral osteoplasty is performed to correct head-neck offset to eliminate any cam impingement and provide an excellent bleeding environment for graft incorporation. The acetabular rim is also reshaped in order to establish an improved anatomic shape, remove the pincer lesion, and expose a flat, congruent bleeding surface on the acetabular rim for graft incorporation. Torn and damaged labral tissue are fully excised from the low anterior portion of the acetabulum at the origin of the transverse acetabular ligament (7:30 on the left hip and 4:30 on right) to the posterior aspect of the acetabulum (typically 3:00 on the left hip and 9:00 on the right hip). No native labral tissue is retained in the anterior quadrant of the acetabulum because it is felt that loss of connection to the circumferential labrum leads to loss of hoop strength.

In preparation for graft placement, the labral defect is measured, and the graft length is overestimated to avoid the graft being too short. Anchors are placed close to the acetabular edge, without breeching the joint, roughly 11–14 mm apart. They are inserted from the distal accessory portal into the acetabular rim. The most antero-inferior anchor is placed as close to the origin of the anterior transverse acetabular ligament as possible.

For this technique, an iliotibial band allograft (AlloSource, Centennial, CO, USA and MTF Sports Medicine, Edison, NJ, USA), freeze dried or frozen, is preferred. The graft is prepared on the back table by soaking it in a 250 cc saline and 80 mg Gentamycin solution. Once thawed, the graft is measured and rolled to create a final tubularized graft measuring roughly 5–6 mm in diameter. The graft is folded into thirds and a 2-0 Vicryl suture is placed at each end of the graft using an accordion-type suture technique, where several small bites are taken across the end of the graft (**Figure 1A**). When tied, the tension bunches the graft and begins the tubularization process. Each suture is secured in the Graftmaster and another 2-0 absorbable Vicryl suture is run up and down the length of the graft to tubularize the graft (18).

The cannula is placed from the distal accessory portal through the intact antero-inferior capsule. The graft is then introduced into the joint, by fixing it to the non-post end of the first suture and pulling it into the joint with the post end. The suture is then tied with alternating half hitch sutures once the graft is provisionally placed in an appropriate position along the rim of the acetabulum. Circumferential sutures are tied from the distal accessory portal working from anterior to posterior. The second to last suture is passed but not tied to allow for mobility at the end of the graft. Excess graft is removed by cutting the graft with a beaver blade from the anterolateral portal, while maintaining tension with a grasper from the distal accessory portal. The most posterior suture is passed through the end of the graft with an ElitePass (Smith & Nephew, London, England) and then passed under and around the graft, creating a Mason-Allen type of suture construct. The graft is inspected after traction is taken down to ensure there is a complete, continuous seal between the graft and the femoral head (**Figures 1B,C**). Dynamic testing of the joint is done to assess the shape of the joint and to ensure there is no impingement. To complete the procedure, the anterior portion of the capsule is closed.

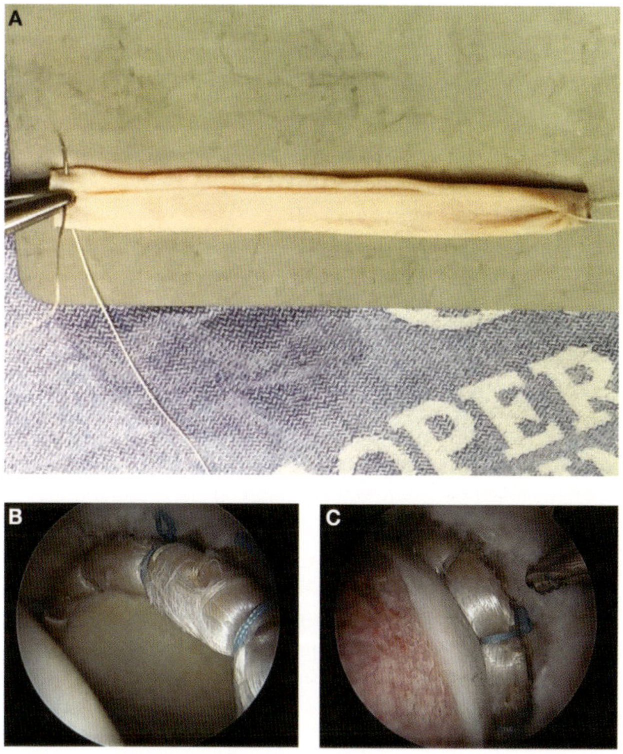


**FIGURE 1 | (A)** The iliotibial band allograft is measured and rolled to create a final tubularized graft, measuring roughly 5–6 mm in diameter. The graft is folded into thirds and a 2-0 Vicryl suture is placed at each end of the graft using an accordion-type suture technique, where several small bites are taken across the end of the graft. **(B)** After the labral reconstruction, this is a view of a left hip from the anterolateral portal, showing an 11 cm labral reconstruction using iliotibial band allograft and nine anchors in traction. **(C)** After the labral reconstruction, this is a view of a left hip from the anteromedial portal showing an 11 cm labral reconstruction using iliotibial band allograft and nine anchors. The joint is reduced with a view of the re-established seal between the reconstructed labrum and the femoral head.

## Graft Options

Several graft options for labral reconstruction have been previously proposed. Allograft tissue provides several benefits over autograft tissue, including the ability to control graft thickness, length, and consistency and the ability to eliminate donor site morbidity. In addition, allograft tissue is aneural, providing a potential benefit in pain reduction. In contrast, native labral tissue likely remains innervated during and following the repair process, which could lead to future pain. Other proposed graft options include iliotibal band autograft (18, 27), local capsular autograft (33), gracilis autograft (34), ligamentum teres capitis autograft (20), fascia lata autograft (23), and quadriceps tendon autograft (35). Advantages and disadvantages of these graft options have not been thoroughly explored in existing literature at this time; however, a recent study of comparing biomechanical properties of the native labrum to iliotibial band, gracilis, semitendinosus, and anterior tibialis grafts found similar biomechanical properties but differing levels of variability in elongation and geometry (37). Another recent study compared iliotibial band autograft to semitendinosus allograft and found no significant difference in contact area, contact pressure, or peak force (15).

## Postoperative Management

Rehabilitation for labral reconstruction is similar to that for labral repair; however, patients are cautioned regarding the aneural properties of their graft. Patients begin supervised physical therapy within 1 week of surgery. The focus of rehabilitation is gaining motion, strengthening the gluteus medius, rebalancing the hip musculature, and establishing a normal gait pattern. Weight bearing is typically restricted to 30% body weight for 4 weeks or 20% body weight for 6 weeks if a concomitant microfracture procedure is performed. Advanced rehabilitation focuses on building strength and returning to sport and activity. In our experience, full recovery typically occurs approximately 6 months postoperatively.

## Outcomes

### Open Labral Reconstruction Outcomes

Two published studies have analyzed the results of labral reconstruction performed during open surgical dislocation (**Table 1**) (20, 23). The first study of outcomes accompanied the original report of the open technique for labral reconstruction (20). The second published study was a case series of 20 hips that underwent labral reconstruction using ligamentum teres capitis or fascia lata autograft in conjunction with FAI treatment (23). The authors reported no complications in either study; however, at a minimum of 1-year follow-up (mean: 26.4 months), 13 hips (65%) underwent 19 subsequent operations, including removal of hardware ($n = 12$), lysis of adhesions ($n = 2$), iliopsoas release ($n = 1$), unspecified arthroscopy ($n = 1$), and THA ($n = 3$) (23).

### Arthroscopic Labral Reconstruction Outcomes

Promising patient-reported outcomes and low revision rate have been achieved with arthroscopic labral reconstruction. The lead author has performed over 1,000 labral reconstructions to date (July 2009–March 2015) and, overall, has found superior results with reconstruction compared to repair or debridement in patients with complex intra-articular pathology. Minimum 2-year outcomes from allograft labral reconstruction by the authors are currently in press (38). Among 152 allograft reconstructions, 118 hips were primary reconstructions and 34 were revision reconstructions. One hundred and thirty-one hips were available for follow-up (86%). Thirteen hips (10%) converted to THA and five hips (4%) underwent revision hip arthroscopy at mean 28 months follow-up. Patients who underwent subsequent surgery were found to have significantly lower preoperative MHHS and LEFS, higher VAS pain scores, and were more likely to have undergone previous open dislocation procedure. Of the remaining hips that did not undergo subsequent procedure ($n = 113$), there was significant improvement in MHHS, LEFS, and VAS for pain at rest, with ADLs, and with athletic activities (**Table 1**) ($p < 0.0001$). Overall patient-reported satisfaction was 9 on a VAS scale from 1 to 10 (10, extremely satisfied). Future studies will identify outcome in specific patient subsets, compare procedures, and report long-term outcome.

A recent literature review identified five additional published reports of outcomes from arthroscopic labral reconstruction (**Table 1**) (18, 24–26, 39). The original report of arthroscopic labral reconstruction in 2010 included early outcomes following arthroscopic labral reconstruction with iliotibial band autograft (18, 28). The study reported promising early outcomes (**Table 1**). No complications were reported, and four hips (9%) progressed to THA at a mean follow-up of 18 months. Continued promising clinical results were reported in this patient population at a mean of 49 months (minimum 3 years) postoperatively (**Table 1**) (25). The proportion of hips that converted to THA increased to 24% ($n = 18$), with one additional hip converting to resurfacing. Identified patient factors associated with conversion to THA were patient age and preoperative joint space $\leq 2$ mm (18, 25). In an additional report in an elite athlete population, the authors found that 18 of 21 athletes were able to return to the elite playing level following surgery, and 17 of those athletes returned to their previous level of performance or better (24).

Outcomes of arthroscopic labral reconstruction with gracilis autograft have also been reported (26, 39). The first study compared a cohort of eight patients who underwent labral reconstruction to a cohort of 46 patients who underwent labral refixation (26). A second study compared a cohort of 11 patients who underwent labral reconstruction to a cohort of 22 matched patients who underwent arthroscopic segmental labral resection (39). No major complications were reported in either study, but two patients who underwent labral reconstruction had pudendal nerve neuropraxias that resolved within 3 months (26). There were no conversions to THA reported (26, 39). Overall, the labral reconstruction group appeared to have better outcomes than both the labral refixation group and the labral resection group (**Table 1**) (26, 39).

## Conclusion

Labral reconstruction provides an alternative treatment option for challenging intra-articular hip problems. The primary indications for labral reconstruction are irreparable labral tears or insufficient labral tissue. Labral reconstruction provides several biomechanical advantages as a treatment option for labral pathology, including improved fluid pressurization, stabilization of the hip to distractive forces, and reduced contact pressure in the hip joint (9, 10, 15). Labral reconstruction should be considered in cases where the ability to maintain and preserve the native hip anatomy is compromised.

Several surgical techniques and graft options have been proposed for labral reconstruction, including open surgical dislocation and arthroscopic techniques and autograft and allograft options (18, 20, 27, 33–36). The lead author prefers the arthroscopic front-to-back surgical technique for labral reconstruction with iliotibial band allograft. The technique described here differs from other arthroscopic techniques in that previous techniques fix the graft in the front and back first, followed by fixation in between. The success of that technique relies on creation of the perfectly sized graft, which can be challenging. The front-to-back technique described here allows the surgeon to make a graft that is 1–2 cm longer than necessary and cut excess graft after front-to-back fixation. The resulting graft is correct size, and the procedure is reproducible; however, it is important to note that the procedure is also technically demanding. Some tips for the "experienced hip arthroscopist" but "novice labral

**TABLE 1 | Published open and arthroscopic labral reconstruction outcomes.**

| Study | Open vs arthroscopic/ graft | *n* | Sex | Age | Follow-up | Convert to THA | Preoperative outcome | Postoperative outcome |
|---|---|---|---|---|---|---|---|---|
| Sierra and Trousdale (20) | Open/ ligamentum teres capitis autograft | 5 | 3 M, 2 F | 33 (19–50) years | 10 (5–20) months | 1 (20%) | –3 "severe pain"<br>–2 "moderately severe pain"<br>–UCLA:5 (2–6) | –3 "no pain"<br>–1 "moderate pain"<br>–1 "same pain as preoperatively"<br>–UCLA: 8 (6–10) |
| Walker et al. (23) | Open/ ligamentum teres capitis autograft or fascia lata autograft | 20 | 5 M, 14 F | 29 (16–50) years | 26 (12–56) months | 3 (15%) | Not reported | –UCLA: 8.5 (5–10) |
| White et al. (38) | Arthroscopic/ iliotibial band allograft | 152 | 64 M, 78 F | 39 (16–58) years | 28 (24–39) months | 13 (10%) | –MHHS: 54<br>–LEFS: 41<br>–VAS rest: 5<br>–VAS ADLs: 6<br>–VAS sport: 8 | –MHHS: 88<br>–LEFS: 68<br>–VAS rest: 2<br>–VAS ADLs: 2<br>–VAS sport: 3<br>–Satisfaction: 9/10 |
| Philippon et al. (18) | Arthroscopic/ iliotibial band autograft | 47 | 32 M, 15 F | 37 (18–55) years | 18 (12–32) months | 4 (9%) | –MHHS: 62 | –MHHS: 85<br>–Satisfaction: 8/10 |
| Geyer et al. (25) | Arthroscopic/ iliotibial band autograft | 76 | 42 M, 33 F | 39 (18–64) years | 49 (36–70) months | 18 (24%) + 1 (1%) resurface | –MHHS: 59<br>–HOS-ADL: 69<br>–HOS-Sport: 41<br>–SF-12 physical:42<br>–SF-12 mental:55 | –MHHS: 83<br>–HOS-ADL: 81<br>–HOS-Sport: 67<br>–SF-12 physical: 50<br>–SF-12 mental: 53<br>–Satisfaction: 8/10 |
| Boykin et al. (24) | Arthroscopic/ iliotibial band autograft | 21 | 19 M, 0 F | 28 (19–41) years | 41 (20–74) months | 2 (10%) | –MHHS: 67<br>–HOS-ADL: 77<br>–HOS-Sport: 56<br>–SF-12 physical: 44<br>–SF-12 mental: 49 | –MHHS: 84<br>–HOS-ADL: 85<br>–HOS-Sport: 77<br>–SF-12 physical: 51<br>–SF-12 mental: 54<br>–Satisfaction: 8/10<br>–Returned to play: 18 (86%) |
| Matsuda and Burchette (26) | Arthroscopic/ gracilis autograft | 8 | 7 M, 1 F | 35 (18–58) years | 30 (24–37) months | 0 (0%) | –NAHS: 42 | –NAHS: 92<br>–Satisfaction: 7 "high,"1 "moderate" |
| Domb et al. (39) | Arthroscopic/ gracilis tendon autograft | 11 | 7 M, 4 F | 33 (18–45) years | 26 (24–32) months | 0 (0%) | –NAHS: 53<br>–HOS-ADL: 59<br>–HOS-Sport: 39<br>–MHHS: 55<br>–VAS: 7 | –NAHS: 78<br>–HOS-ADL: 80<br>–HOS-Sport: 60<br>–MHHS: 82<br>–VAS: 3<br>–Satisfaction: 8/10 |

[a]*Data are expressed as count (%) or mean (range).*
*MHHS, modified harris hip score; HOS-ADL, hip outcome score-activities of daily living; HOS-sport, hip outcome score-sports-specific subscale; SF-12 physical, short form-12 physical component; SF-12 mental, short form-12 mental component; NAHS, non-arthritic hip score; VAS, visual analog scale for pain; ADLs, activities of daily living.*

reconstructionist" are provided in Table S2 in Supplementary Material. Adequate training and practice in hip arthroscopy and labral reconstruction are necessary in order to ensure proficiency in placing the anchors in the most anterior and posterior position on the acetabular rim and being able to manage and appropriately fix the graft to obtain a perfect seal with the femoral head.

Long-term outcomes are necessary to determine the longevity of this procedure, but promising early outcomes of have been achieved (18, 20, 23–26, 38, 39). The published literature indicates few complications, improved subjective patient scores, and a low revision rate. Short-term improvement in patient symptomology and function were appreciated with both open and arthroscopic labral reconstruction. Labral repair remains an option in the young, healthy patient with healthy labral tissue; however, labral reconstruction should be considered in patients who do not meet these criteria.

Overall, labral reconstruction increases function, decreases pain, leads to a high level of patient satisfaction, and allows patients to return to activities of daily living and athletics. Labral reconstruction restores the original anatomy of the hip and has the potential to preserve the longevity of the hip joint. This technique is an important tool in the orthopedic surgeon's arsenal for hip joint preservation.

## Acknowledgments

Thank you to Tara Hawkes, Clinical Research Coordinator at Western Orthopaedics Research & Education Foundation, for her assistance with compiling data.

## References

1. Glick JM, Valone F III, Safran MR. Hip arthroscopy: from the beginning to the future – an innovator's perspective. *Knee Surg Sports Traumatol Arthrosc* (2014) **22**:714–21. doi:10.1007/s00167-014-2859-y
2. Burman MS. Arthroscopy or the direct visualization of joints: an experimental cadaver study. 1931. *Clin Orthop Relat Res* (2001) **390**:5–9. doi:10.1097/00003086-200109000-00003
3. Ayeni OR, Levy BA, Musahl V, Safran MR. Current state-of-the-art of hip arthroscopy. *Knee Surg Sports Traumatol Arthrosc* (2014) **22**:711–3. doi:10.1007/s00167-014-2866-z
4. Reiman MP, Goode AP, Cook CE, Holmich P, Thorborg K. Diagnostic accuracy of clinical tests for the diagnosis of hip femoroacetabular impingement/labral tear: a systematic review with meta-analysis. *Br J Sports Med* (2014) **49**:811. doi:10.1136/bjsports-2014-094302
5. Krych AJ, Kuzma SA, Kovachevich R, Hudgens JL, Stuart MJ, Levy BA. Modest mid-term outcomes after isolated arthroscopic debridement of acetabular labral tears. *Knee Surg Sports Traumatol Arthrosc* (2014) **22**:763–7. doi:10.1007/s00167-014-2872-1
6. McCarthy JC, Noble PC, Schuck MR, Wright J, Lee J. The Otto E. Aufranc award: the role of labral lesions to development of early degenerative hip disease. *Clin Orthop Relat Res* (2001) **393**:25–37. doi:10.1097/00003086-200112000-00004
7. Narvani AA, Tsiridis E, Kendall S, Chaudhuri R, Thomas P. A preliminary report on prevalence of acetabular labrum tears in sports patients with groin pain. *Knee Surg Sports Traumatol Arthrosc* (2003) **11**:403–8. doi:10.1007/s00167-003-0390-7
8. Ayeni OR, Alradwan H, de Sa D, Philippon MJ. The hip labrum reconstruction: indications and outcomes – a systematic review. *Knee Surg Sports Traumatol Arthrosc* (2014) **22**:737–43. doi:10.1007/s00167-013-2804-5
9. Nepple JJ, Philippon MJ, Campbell KJ, Dornan GJ, Jansson KS, LaPrade RF, et al. The hip fluid seal – part II: the effect of an acetabular labral tear, repair, resection, and reconstruction on hip stability to distraction. *Knee Surg Sports Traumatol Arthrosc* (2014) **22**:730–6. doi:10.1007/s00167-014-2875-y
10. Philippon MJ, Nepple JJ, Campbell KJ, Dornan GJ, Jansson KS, LaPrade RF, et al. The hip fluid seal – part I: the effect of an acetabular labral tear, repair, resection, and reconstruction on hip fluid pressurization. *Knee Surg Sports Traumatol Arthrosc* (2014) **22**:722–9. doi:10.1007/s00167-014-2874-z
11. Ferguson SJ, Bryant JT, Ganz R, Ito K. An in vitro investigation of the acetabular labral seal in hip joint mechanics. *J Biomech* (2003) **36**:171–8. doi:10.1016/S0021-9290(02)00365-2
12. Ferguson SJ, Bryant JT, Ganz R, Ito K. The influence of the acetabular labrum on hip joint cartilage consolidation: a poroelastic finite element model. *J Biomech* (2000) **33**:953–60. doi:10.1016/S0021-9290(00)00042-7
13. Crawford MJ, Dy CJ, Alexander JW, Thompson M, Schroder SJ, Vega CE, et al. The 2007 Frank Stinchfield Award. The biomechanics of the hip labrum and the stability of the hip. *Clin Orthop Relat Res* (2007) **465**:16–22. doi:10.1097/BLO.0b013e31815b181f
14. Greaves LL, Gilbart MK, Yung AC, Kozlowski P, Wilson DR. Effect of acetabular labral tears, repair and resection on hip cartilage strain: a 7T MR study. *J Biomech* (2010) **43**:858–63. doi:10.1016/j.jbiomech.2009.11.016
15. Lee S, Wuerz TH, Shewman E, McCormick FM, Salata MJ, Philippon MJ, et al. Labral reconstruction with iliotibial band autografts and semitendinosus allografts improves hip joint contact area and contact pressure: an in vitro analysis. *Am J Sports Med* (2015) **43**:98–104. doi:10.1177/0363546514553089
16. Larson CM, Giveans MR. Arthroscopic debridement versus refixation of the acetabular labrum associated with femoroacetabular impingement. *Arthroscopy* (2009) **25**:369–76. doi:10.1016/j.arthro.2008.12.014
17. Larson CM, Giveans MR, Stone RM. Arthroscopic debridement versus refixation of the acetabular labrum associated with femoroacetabular impingement: mean 3.5-year follow-up. *Am J Sports Med* (2012) **40**:1015–21. doi:10.1177/0363546511434578
18. Philippon MJ, Briggs KK, Hay CJ, Kuppersmith DA, Dewing CB, Huang MJ. Arthroscopic labral reconstruction in the hip using iliotibial band autograft: technique and early outcomes. *Arthroscopy* (2010) **26**:750–6. doi:10.1016/j.arthro.2009.10.016
19. Larson CM, Giveans MR. Arthroscopic management of femoroacetabular impingement: early outcomes measures. *Arthroscopy* (2008) **24**:540–6. doi:10.1016/j.arthro.2007.11.007
20. Sierra RJ, Trousdale RT. Labral reconstruction using the ligamentum teres capitis: report of a new technique. *Clin Orthop Relat Res* (2009) **467**:753–9. doi:10.1007/s11999-008-0633-5
21. Cadet ER, Chan AK, Vorys GC, Gardner T, Yin B. Investigation of the preservation of the fluid seal effect in the repaired, partially resected, and reconstructed acetabular labrum in a cadaveric hip model. *Am J Sports Med* (2012) **40**:2218–23. doi:10.1177/0363546512457645
22. Ayeni OR, Adamich J, Farrokhyar F, Simunovic N, Crouch S, Philippon MJ, et al. Surgical management of labral tears during femoroacetabular impingement surgery: a systematic review. *Knee Surg Sports Traumatol Arthrosc* (2014) **22**:756–62. doi:10.1007/s00167-014-2886-8
23. Walker JA, Pagnotto M, Trousdale RT, Sierra RJ. Preliminary pain and function after labral reconstruction during femoroacetabular impingement surgery. *Clin Orthop Relat Res* (2012) **470**:3414–20. doi:10.1007/s11999-012-2506-1
24. Boykin RE, Patterson D, Briggs KK, Dee A, Philippon MJ. Results of arthroscopic labral reconstruction of the hip in elite athletes. *Am J Sports Med* (2013) **41**:2296–301. doi:10.1177/0363546513498058
25. Geyer MR, Philippon MJ, Fagrelius TS, Briggs KK. Acetabular labral reconstruction with an iliotibial band autograft: outcome and survivorship analysis at minimum 3-year follow-up. *Am J Sports Med* (2013) **41**:1750–6. doi:10.1177/0363546513487311
26. Matsuda DK, Burchette RJ. Arthroscopic hip labral reconstruction with a gracilis autograft versus labral refixation: 2-year minimum outcomes. *Am J Sports Med* (2013) **41**:980–7. doi:10.1177/0363546513482884
27. Deshmane PP, Kahlenberg CA, Patel RM, Han B, Terry MA. All-arthroscopic iliotibial band autograft harvesting and labral reconstruction technique. *Arthrosc Tech.* (2013) **2**:e15–9. doi:10.1016/j.eats.2012.10.001
28. Ejnisman L, Philippon MJ, Lertwanich P. Acetabular labral tears: diagnosis, repair, and a method for labral reconstruction. *Clin Sports Med* (2011) **30**:317–29. doi:10.1016/j.csm.2010.12.006
29. Bedi A, Chen N, Robertson W, Kelly BT. The management of labral tears and femoroacetabular impingement of the hip in the young, active patient. *Arthroscopy* (2008) **24**:1135–45. doi:10.1016/j.arthro.2008.06.001
30. Ng VY, Arora N, Best TM, Pan X, Ellis TJ. Efficacy of surgery for femoroacetabular impingement: a systematic review. *Am J Sports Med* (2010) **38**:2337–45. doi:10.1177/0363546510365530
31. Botser IB, Smith TW Jr, Nasser R, Domb BG. Open surgical dislocation versus arthroscopy for femoroacetabular impingement: a comparison of clinical outcomes. *Arthroscopy* (2011) **27**:270–8. doi:10.1016/j.arthro.2010.11.008
32. Domb BG, Stake CE, Botser IB, Jackson TJ. Surgical dislocation of the hip versus arthroscopic treatment of femoroacetabular impingement: a

prospective matched-pair study with average 2-year follow-up. *Arthroscopy* (2013) **29**:1506–13. doi:10.1016/j.arthro.2013.06.010

33. Domb BG, Gupta A, Stake CE, Hammarstedt JE, Redmond JM. Arthroscopic labral reconstruction of the hip using local capsular autograft. *Arthrosc Tech.* (2014) **3**:e355–9. doi:10.1016/j.eats.2014.02.004
34. Matsuda DK. Arthroscopic labral reconstruction with gracilis autograft. *Arthrosc Tech.* (2012) **1**:e15–21. doi:10.1016/j.eats.2011.12.001
35. Park SE, Ko Y. Use of the quadriceps tendon in arthroscopic acetabular labral reconstruction: potential and benefits as an autograft option. *Arthrosc Tech.* (2013) **2**:e217–9. doi:10.1016/j.eats.2013.02.003
36. White BJ, Herzog MM. Arthroscopic labral reconstruction of the hip using iliotibial band allograft and front-to-back fixation technique. *Arthrosc Tech* (2015) (in press).
37. Ferro FP, Philippon MJ, Rasmussen MT, Smith SD, LaPrade RF, Wijdicks CA. Tensile properties of the human acetabular labrum and hip labral reconstruction grafts. *Am J Sports Med* (2015) **43**:1222–7.
38. White BJ, Stapleford AB, Hawkes TK, Finger MJ, Herzog MM. Allograft use in arthroscopic labral reconstruction of the hip: minimum 2-year follow-up with front-to-back fixation technique. *Arthroscopy* (2015) (in press).
39. Domb BG, El Bitar YF, Stake CE, Trenga AP, Jackson TJ, Lindner D. Arthroscopic labral reconstruction is superior to segmental resection for irreparable labral tears in the hip: a matched-pair controlled study with minimum 2-year follow-up. *Am J Sports Med* (2014) **42**:122–30. doi:10.1177/0363546513508256

# 12

# Preoperative Radiotherapy and Wide Resection for Soft Tissue Sarcomas: Achieving a Low Rate of Major Wound Complications with the Use of Flaps. Results of a Single Surgical Team

*Lester Wai Mon Chan[1,2]*, Jungo Imanishi[1], Damien Glen Grinsell[3] and Peter Choong[1,4]*

[1] *Department of Orthopaedics, St. Vincent's Hospital, Melbourne, VIC, Australia,* [2] *Department of Orthopaedic Surgery, Tan Tock Seng Hospital, Singapore, Singapore,* [3] *Department of Plastic Surgery, St Vincent's Hospital, Melbourne, VIC, Australia,* [4] *Department of Surgery, University of Melbourne, Melbourne, VIC, Australia*

***Edited by:***
*Iain Stuart Whitaker, Swansea University, United Kingdom*

***Reviewed by:***
*David J. Hunter-Smith, Monash University Plastic and Reconstructive Surgery Group, Australia*
*Thomas David Dobbs, Swansea University, United Kingdom*

****Correspondence:***
*Lester Wai Mon Chan*
*drlesterchan@gmail.com*

***Specialty section:***
*This article was submitted to Reconstructive and Plastic Surgery, a section of the journal Frontiers in Surgery*

**Background:** Surgery in combination with radiotherapy (RT) has become the standard of care for most soft tissue sarcomas. The choice between pre- and postoperative RT is controversial. Preoperative RT is associated with a 32–35% rate of major wound complications (MWC) and 16–25% rate of reoperation. The role of vascularized soft tissue "flaps" in reducing complications is unclear. We report the outcomes of patients treated with preoperative RT, resection, and flap reconstruction.

**Patients and methods:** 122 treatment episodes involving 117 patients were retrospectively reviewed. All patients were treated with 50.4 Gy of external beam radiation. Surgery was performed at 4–8 weeks after completion of RT by the same combination of orthopedic oncology and plastic reconstructive surgeon. Defects were reconstructed with 64 free and 59 pedicled/local flaps.

**Results:** 30 (25%) patients experienced a MWC and 17 (14%) required further surgery. 20% of complications were exclusively related to the donor site. There was complete or partial loss of three flaps. There was no difference in the rate of MWC or reoperation for complications with respect to age, sex, tumor site, previous unplanned excision, tumor grade, depth, and type of flap. Tumor size ≥8 cm was associated with a higher rate of reoperation (11/44 vs 6/78; $P = 0.008$) but the rate of MWC was not significant (16/44 vs 14/78; $P = 0.066$).

**Conclusion:** The use of soft tissue flaps is associated with a low rate of MWC and reoperation. Our results suggest that a high rate of flap usage may be required to observe a reduction in complication rates.

**Keywords: soft tissue sarcoma, preoperative radiotherapy, wound complication, reconstructive surgery, flap reconstruction**

## INTRODUCTION

Surgery in combination with radiotherapy (RT) has become the standard of care for soft tissue sarcomas (STSs) of the extremity and trunk (1–3), however, the choice between preoperative vs postoperative RT continues to be controversial (4, 5). Preoperative RT is delivered to well-oxygenated, undisrupted tissues, allowing lower doses to be administered to a smaller field and resulting in reduced rates of long-term radiation toxicity with similar rates of local control (5, 6). The main disadvantage of preoperative RT is the high rate of postoperative wound complications. The reported rates are variable and partially dependent on the definition used; the rate of major wound complications (MWCs) as defined by the Canadian Clinical Trials Group is around 32–35% with 16–25% of patients requiring further surgery for complications (4, 7–13).

On principle, the requirements for predictable wound healing are low wound tension, minimization of dead space, and well-vascularized tissue. All three factors are negatively affected in the preoperatively irradiated sarcoma wound. Theoretically, all these factors can be improved with the use of vascularized soft tissue flaps (14). While flaps are commonly used for the closure of soft tissue defects, only one historical series has demonstrated a reduction in the rate of wound complications (15) with the majority of the literature reporting no difference in outcomes (10, 11, 13, 16–19).

Preoperative RT followed by wide surgical resection is the preferred management of STSs at our center (16). In 2002, we published the results of our STS protocol. At that time, free and pedicled flaps were used in only 35% of cases. 44% of patients developed postoperative wound complications and 23% required further surgery. Since that time, we have increased our utilization of soft tissue flaps in an attempt to achieve more predictable wound healing. We currently employ flaps in 79% of cases (source: 2011–2015 data. Decision Support Unit, St. Vincent's Hospital, Melbourne).

The aim of this study is to report the wound complication outcomes of a strategy of preoperative RT, resection, and flap reconstruction.

## PATIENTS AND METHODS

This was a retrospective study of consecutive cases performed by the same combination of orthopedic oncology surgeon (PC) and plastic surgery reconstructive surgeon (DG). Institutional review board approval was obtained prior to the study (HREC number: QA106/15). Subjects were identified from the institution database. Inclusion criteria were patients with STSs and other locally aggressive soft tissue tumors treated with a standard protocol of preoperative RT, surgical resection and soft tissue reconstruction with a flap. Only patients operated on by the two senior authors were included. The cohort included patients from the private and public hospital systems. Inpatient and outpatient hospital medical records and electronic medical records from private consulting rooms were reviewed for complications. Patients who were closed without a flap and those with missing data were excluded.

Patients underwent surgery between April 2008 and June 2015. During the study period, there were 512 episodes of definitive surgery for STS identified from our institution database. Of these, 129 episodes were performed by the two senior authors. Three episodes were excluded as closure was achieved without a flap and four episodes were excluded because of missing data. In total, there were 122 treatment episodes involving 117 patients that were eligible for review. Five patients were included twice with soft tissue metastases distant to the original resection site that were treated with a separate course of preoperative RT, wide resection, and flap reconstruction.

The patient and disease characteristics are shown in **Table 1**.

After confirmation of diagnosis at our sarcoma multidisciplinary meeting, patients were treated with 50.4 Gy of external beam radiation delivered in 28 fractions over five and a half weeks. Surgery was performed at 4–8 weeks post completion of RT to allow subsidence of inflammation. We have previously reported our protocol and experience with preoperative RT (16, 20).

The definition of MWC was that of the NCI Canadian Clinical Trials Group (21). This included any of the following criteria occurring within 120 days of surgery: a secondary operation under general or regional anesthesia for wound repair, an invasive procedure without general or regional anesthesia (mainly aspiration of seroma), readmission for wound care such as intravenous

**TABLE 1** | Patient characteristics.

| Parameter | No. (%), $n = 122$ |
|---|---|
| **Mean age** | 58 years (range: 15–89) |
| **Sex** | |
| Male | 64 (52) |
| Female | 58 (48) |
| **Diagnosis** | |
| Undifferentiated pleomorphic sarcoma | 39 (32) |
| Liposarcoma | 26 (21) |
| Myxofibrosarcoma | 18 (15) |
| Synovial sarcoma | 9 (7) |
| Leiomyosarcoma | 6 (5) |
| Solitary fibrous tumor | 5 (4) |
| Fibromyxoid sarcoma | 4 (3) |
| MPNST | 4 (3) |
| Clear cell sarcoma | 3 (2) |
| Others | 8 (7) |
| **FNCLCC grade** | |
| I/borderline malignancy | 19 (16) |
| II | 44 (36) |
| III | 59 (48) |
| **Tumor size** | |
| <8 cm | 78 (64) |
| ≥8 cm | 44 (36) |
| **Tumor depth** | |
| Superficial | 32 (26) |
| Deep | 90 (74) |
| **Tumor site** | |
| Upper limb | 19 (16) |
| Lower limb | 85 (70) |
| Axial | 18 (15) |
| **Previous surgery to tumor bed** | |
| None | 62 (51) |
| Intralesional/marginal | 54 (44) |
| Wide margin | 7 (6) |

*MPNST, Malignant Peripheral Nerve Sheath Tumor; FNCLCC, Fédération Nationale des Centres de Lutte Contre le Cancer.*

antibiotics, and wound packing deep to dermis in an area >2 cm with or without prolonged dressings >6 weeks from wound breakdown.

## Statistical Analysis

Statistical analysis was performed using JMP® version 10 (SAS Institute Inc., Cary, NC, USA). The association of factors with MWC and reoperation for complications were analyzed using chi-squared or Fisher's exact test. $P < 0.05$ was regarded as statistically significant.

# RESULTS

There were 64 free flap and 59 pedicled or local flaps utilized in 122 treatment episodes. One patient had reconstruction with a combination of two flaps. The types of free and pedicled or local flaps employed are shown in **Tables 2** and **3** respectively.

A summary of MWCs is shown in **Figure 1**. A total of 30 patients (25%) experienced a MWC; 17 patients (14%) required surgery for correction of complications. MWCs affected the irradiated resection site in 24 patients and the donor site in seven patients (one patient had complications affecting the donor and resection site).

**TABLE 2** | Type of free flap used.

| Free flap type | No. |
|---|---|
| Anterolateral thigh | 18 |
| Latissimus dorsi | 11 |
| Gracilis | 12 |
| Parascapula/scapula | 10 |
| Rectus | 5 |
| Groin | 3 |
| Tensor fasciae latae | 2 |
| Anteromedial thigh | 1 |
| Radial artery forearm | 1 |
| Fibula osteocutaneous | 1 |
| **Total** | **64** |

**TABLE 3** | Type of pedicled/local flap.

| Pedicled/local type | No. |
|---|---|
| Anterolateral thigh | 14 |
| Latissimus dorsi | 10 |
| Rectus | 8 |
| Gluteal perforator | 4 |
| Gastrocnemius/soleus | 3 |
| Parascapular/scapula | 3 |
| Pectoralis major | 2 |
| Sartorius | 2 |
| Thoracodorsal artery perforator | 2 |
| Medial thigh perforator | 2 |
| Radial artery forearm | 1 |
| Medial arm | 1 |
| Superficial inferior epigastric artery | 1 |
| Internal mammary artery perforator | 1 |
| Lumbar artery perforator | 1 |
| Local deepithelialized skin | 2 |
| Random pattern skin flap | 2 |
| **Total** | **59** |

For patients requiring further surgery, the average number of additional surgical procedures was 1.5 (range 1–3). An analysis of the association of MWC with patient and disease variables is shown in **Table 4**. There was no difference in the rate of MWC or reoperation for age, sex, site of tumor, previous unplanned excision, FNCLCC grade, tumor depth, and type of flap. Tumor size ≥8 cm was associated with an increased rate of reoperation ($P = 0.008$) but no significant difference in MWC ($P = 0.066$).

There were four patients who required complex revision surgery. Two patients had methicillin-resistant *Staphylococcus aureus* infection with complete or partial necrosis of free flaps. One required debridement of 40% of a free anterolateral thigh flap and the remaining defect was adequately covered with a pedicled medial arm flap and a split skin graft; the second required complete removal of a free gracilis flap that was revised to a pedicled latissimus dorsi flap. Another patient had bleeding from the anastomosis for an innervated latissimus dorsi flap. This was revised once but a further episode of severe bleeding necessitated emergency flap removal. The fourth patient was readmitted for a delayed presentation of a leaking superficial femoral artery vein graft on postoperative day 61. This was resolved with revision of the graft. All severe complications occurred in elderly patients (mean age 82, range 74–89) who had undergone free flap reconstruction.

The remaining 13 patients who underwent secondary surgery required relatively simple procedures; surgery was at the resection site in nine cases and the donor site in four. Resection site procedures included closure of wound dehiscences, skin edge debridements, and open drainage of collections. Donor site complications were typically mild. Three patients had simple wound dehiscences that were debrided and resutured and one patient had a hematoma that was evacuated and closed over a surgical drain.

There were 13 complications not requiring surgery (see **Figure 1**). Of these, there were five patients requiring percutaneous needle drainage of seromas, four patients with prolonged dressings, and four patients who were admitted to hospital for intravenous antibiotics. All patients with prolonged dressings went on to complete wound healing.

We performed a subgroup analysis of early vs late cases (see **Table 5**). There were no significant differences in age, sex, size, previous unplanned excision, FNCLCC grade MWC, or reoperation. A higher proportion of free flaps were performed in the early part of the study (free/pedicled-local; 37/23 vs 26/35, $P = 0.036$).

# DISCUSSION

Preoperative RT for STSs is associated with a high rate of postoperative wound complications. In 1992, Barwick et al. reported a series of 82 patients, comparing their use of vascularized tissue transfer with direct closure in irradiated wounds. Direct closure was used early in their series and the authors noted a high rate of wound complications. This caused them to adopt a practice of routine plastic surgical consultation before surgery, which led to an increased utilization of flaps. They showed a lower complication rate (19 vs 51%) and fewer secondary procedures (10 vs

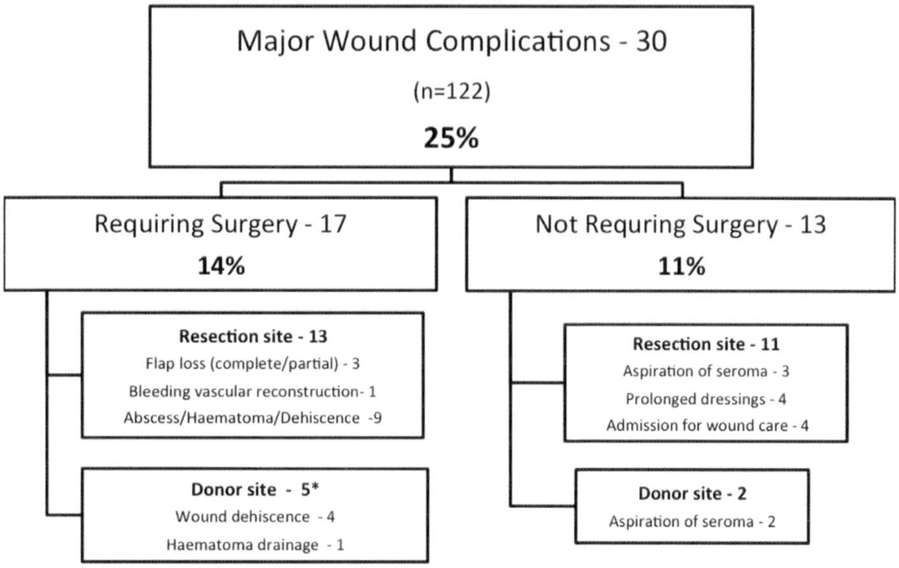


**FIGURE 1** | Summary of major wound complications*. One patient had resection and donor site complications.

**TABLE 4** | Association of MWC and reoperations with patient and disease variables.

| Variable | Major wound complication (MWC), no. (%) | *P*-value | Reoperation, no. (%) | *P*-value |
|---|---|---|---|---|
| **Age** | | | | |
| ≥60 | 12/56 (21.4) | 0.46 | 9/66 (13.6) | 0.91 |
| <60 | 18/66 (27.3) | | 8/56 (14.3) | |
| **Sex** | | | | |
| M | 16/64 (25) | 0.91 | 9/64 (14.1) | 0.97 |
| F | 14/58 (24.1) | | 8/58 (13.8) | |
| **Site** | | | | |
| Upper limb | 6/19 (31.6) | 0.24 | 3/19 (15.8) | 0.47 |
| Lower limb | 22/85 (25.9) | | 13/85 (15.3) | |
| Axial | 2/18 (11.1) | | 1/18 (5.6) | |
| **Size** | | | | |
| ≥8 cm | 16/44 (36.4) | 0.066 | **11/44 (25)** | **0.008** |
| <8 cm | 14/78 (17.9) | | **6/78 (7.7)** | |
| **Previous unplanned excision** | | | | |
| Y | 11/54 (20.4) | 0.33 | 7/54 (13.0) | 0.78 |
| N | 19/68 (27.9) | | 10/68 (14.7) | |
| **FNCLCC grade** | | | | |
| 0 and 1 | 3/19 (15.8) | 0.40 | 1/19 (5.3) | 0.47 |
| 2 and 3 | 27/103 (26.2) | | 16/103 (15.5) | |
| **Deep/superficial** | | | | |
| Deep | 25/90 (27.7) | 0.17 | 13/90 (14.4) | 0.78 |
| Superficial | 5/32 (15.6) | | 4/32 (12.5) | |
| **Type of flap** | | | | |
| Free flap | 19/63 (30.2) | 0.33 | 11/63 (17.5) | 0.26 |
| Pedicled/local | 11/58 (19.0) | | 6/58 (10.3) | |

*FNCLCC, Fédération Nationale des Centres de Lutte Contre le Cancer.*
*The bold text indicates a statistically significant result P < 0.05.*

**TABLE 5** | Subgroup analysis of early vs late cases.

| Variable | Early (61) | Late (61) | *P*-value |
|---|---|---|---|
| **Age** | | | |
| ≥60 | 33 | 33 | 1 |
| <60 | 28 | 28 | |
| **Sex** | | | |
| M | 32 | 32 | 1 |
| F | 29 | 29 | |
| **Size** | | | |
| ≥8 cm | 26 | 18 | 0.13 |
| <8 cm | 35 | 43 | |
| **Previous unplanned excision** | | | |
| Y | 29 | 25 | 0.33 |
| N | 32 | 36 | |
| **FNCLCC grade** | | | |
| 0 and 1 | 8 | 11 | 0.62 |
| 2 and 3 | 53 | 50 | |
| **Type of flap** | | | |
| Free flap | 37 | 26 | 0.036 |
| Pedicled/local | 23 | 35 | |
| **MWC** | | | |
| Yes | 11 | 19 | 0.09 |
| No | 50 | 42 | |
| **Reoperation** | | | |
| Yes | 6 | 11 | 0.30 |
| No | 55 | 50 | |

*FNCLCC, Fédération Nationale des Centres de Lutte Contre le Cancer.*

35%) with flap reconstruction. The overall flap rate in their study was 52% (15). Since this report more than 20 years ago multiple authors have failed to show a lower complication rate with the use of flaps (4, 10, 11, 13, 16, 17, 19). There are no randomized trials evaluating the use of flaps for sarcoma wounds and retrospective studies suffer from inherent bias against advanced reconstruction techniques; wounds at high risk of failure tend to be treated with flaps whereas small low risk wounds are treated by direct closure, therefore masking any positive effect of flaps.

The present study is a single armed series of recent (2008–2015) STS cases treated with vascularized soft tissue flap reconstruction.

It demonstrates a low rate of MWC (25%) and secondary operations (14%) compared to other reports (see **Table 6**) and suggest that the use of "flaps" may be useful in reducing the rate of wound complications. This series represents modern microsurgical practice and does not include any previously published data on this topic. It also represents a change in reconstructive philosophy compared to that of a previous study conducted at our center in 2002. At that time, flaps were used in 35% of patients; 44% developed a wound complication and 23% required an additional surgical procedure. In an effort to reduce our complication rate, we began routine preoperative consultation with our plastic surgeons. This led to an increase in our utilization of flaps such that we now use them in 79% of cases (16).

We note that the rate of flap use is low in most series evaluating pre-operative RT for sarcomas (13–40%). We consider this to reflect a difference in philosophy where flaps are used to achieve wound closure rather than to reduce wound complications. By contrast, the indication for flaps at our center is not purely to achieve wound closure; but rather to reduce tension, dead space, and introduce vascularized tissue into wounds that we previously may have closed primarily (14, 16). This was also the intent of flaps reported by Barwick et al. (15). We, therefore, emphasize the difference between wounds that *can* be closed primarily vs wounds that *should* be closed. By reducing our threshold for the use of flaps both Barwick et al. and the current study have been able to achieve lower rate of wound complications.

For the purpose of comparison, we used the Canadian Trials Group definition of MWCs as our primary endpoint; however, we recognize that the definition is broad and includes severe wound complications requiring extensive additional surgery alongside milder complications such as seromas requiring needle aspiration or admissions for intravenous antibiotics alone. In order to better define severity, we also reported the number of patients requiring further surgery as a second endpoint. While this is an imperfect surrogate measure of severity (the same wound breakdown might be treated with surgery or dressings according to the practice of the treating surgeon), it is objective and simple to record and compare.

We found that the type of complications in our series reflected the nature of flap surgery with one-fifth of complications being exclusively related to the donor site. We found complications at the non-irradiated donor site generally straightforward to

**TABLE 6** | Summary of recent papers investigating complications of preoperative radiation for soft tissue sarcomas (STSs).

| Reference | Description | Outcome measure | Complication rate | Reoperation rate | Use of vascularized flaps |
|---|---|---|---|---|---|
| O'Sullivan et al. (4) | Randomized control trial of pre- vs postoperative RT for STS | Canadian Trials group | 35% preoperative, 17% postoperative[a] | Not reported | 28% |
| Virkus et al. (7) | Retrospective study of preoperative RT | Moderate or major wound complications (MWCs). Seroma aspiration, IV antibiotics not included as complications | 22% preoperative[b] | Not reported | 13% Flap or split-thickness skin graft |
| Kunisada et al. (16) | Retrospective study of preoperative RT | Complication—not stated. MWC—requiring a second procedure | 44% preoperative | 23% | 35% |
| Tseng et al. (19) | Preoperative RT. Retrospective analysis of impact of plastic surgical closure | Canadian Trials group | 32% (plastics closure 32%)[a] | Not reported | 40% |
| Cannon et al. (9) | Retrospective analysis of factors influencing wound complications | Similar to Canadian trials group but included "mild" complications not requiring specific intervention | 34% preoperative, 16% postoperative | Not reported | 22% |
| Townley et al. (17) | Retrospective analysis of free flap reconstruction in patients with preoperative RT vs postoperative/non-RT control group | Wound complication—not specified. Microsurgical flap complications | 50% preoperative, 14% control, 12.5% flap complications | Not reported | 100%—only free flap cases reviewed |
| Baldini et al. (10) | Preoperative RT. Retrospective analysis of predictors of wound complications | Canadian Trials group | 35% preoperative[a] | **25%** | 27% |
| Schwartz et al. (12) | Retrospective analysis of wound complications following resection of sarcomas. Included patients with preoperative RT + brachytherapy/IntraopRT | Requiring secondary flap | 15% preoperative, 11% postoperative | Not reported | 0%—primary flap closure excluded |
| Rosenberg et al. (13) | Preoperative RT. Retrospective analysis of impact of plastics closure | Canadian Trials group | 32% (plastics closure 28%)[a] | **16% (11%)** | 22% |
| Moore et al. (11) | Retrospective analysis of risk factors for WC after sarcoma resection | Surgical intervention or outpatient debridement and negative pressure wound therapy. Seroma aspiration, IV antibiotics not included. | 23.8% preoperative[b], 11.9 postoperative | | Unknown |
| Chan (2017) (Current series) | Preoperative RT with flap reconstruction. Retrospective analysis of complications | Canadian Trials group | 25% preoperative RT with flap closure[a] | **15%** | 79% |

[a]*Canadian Trial Group criteria highlighted in bold.*
[b]*The definition of wound complication for Virkus and Moore did not include aspiration of seroma or admission for IV antibiotics. The comparative wound complication rate in our study was 17%.*

rectify. In this way, flap surgery may trade-off more challenging complications at the resection site for "simple" wound issues at the donor site. The original definition of MWC does not specifically mention donor site complications; for the purpose of this study they were included as MWCs. If donor site complications were excluded, the MWC rate for the irradiated wound would be 20%.

There were three complications related to the microvascular anastomosis in elderly patients with free flaps, this included one case of life threatening bleeding. While neither age nor type of flap was significantly associated with MWC or reoperation, this finding raises some caution for this subgroup.

There were two patients who suffered complete flap necrosis and were subsequently closed with a pedicled flap and direct closure, respectively; both these patients could have been closed initially without a free flap, however, as mentioned previously, the indications for flaps in our series and the choice of flap was made on the basis of reasons other than closure alone (filling of dead space, introduction of vascularized tissue, reduction of wound tension) and influenced by factors, including the size and suitability of donor tissue and potential donor site morbidity. In the first case, a free gracilis was felt to be a more suitable donor for an anterior arm defect with lower donor morbidity than the pedicled latissimus dorsi that was subsequently required for salvage; in the second case, a free latissimus dorsi was used to fill the dead space in a large posterior thigh defect that eventually had to be closed directly. Unfortunately neither of these patients benefited from the theoretical advantages of their flaps.

Previous authors have shown an association of complications with larger, high-grade tumors and lower extremity location (7, 9–13, 19). We did not find any significant differences in MWC or reoperation rates for any of the factors reviewed with the exception of size ≥8 cm. The reasons for this are uncertain; however, a lower rate of complications of itself may make statistical significance more difficult to achieve.

Late complications and functional outcomes were not assessed as part of this study. While this is consistent with the majority of the contemporary literature, a recent study by Miller et al. examined the pattern and timing of MWC in 102 patients with STS treated with multimodal therapy and noted that 45% of MWC occurred after 120 days post resection; of note, 8 out of 10 late complications occurred in patients who were treated with post-operative RT and the authors did not comment on the type and severity of late complications (22). In the present study, all MWCs occurred within 120 days from surgery and we did not detect any new MWCs after this period. We postulate that late complications may be of greater significance in studies involving post-operative RT where wound complications may be induced to occur later, during the post-RT period, rather than in the earlier post-operative period.

Microsurgical flap reconstruction is technically demanding, particularly in the context of pre-operative RT. Previous authors have demonstrated that good outcomes can be achieved in irradiated wounds and that flap outcomes are not adversely affected in experienced hands (17, 23, 24). We attempted to review the effect of experience on MWC and reoperation, however, a subgroup analysis of early vs late cases with respect to MWC, reoperations showed no significant difference in the rate of MWC or reoperation. There was, however, an increase in the use of pedicled/local flaps in the latter half of the study. We postulate that this difference could be due to a clinically but not statistically significant difference in tumor size. Smaller tumors in the latter part of the study ($P = 0.13$) may have resulted in wounds more amenable to pedicled flap closure. This difference in tumor size may also represent a reduction in threshold for flap during the study period, although we are cautious in drawing conclusions based on this non-statistically significant result.

This study was limited by its design as a retrospective, observational, single armed study with no comparison group. The patient cohort was operated on by a specific experienced surgical team with a subspecialist interest in sarcoma surgery. Results may vary according to surgical expertise and experience. Potential selection bias and possible shifts in clinical practice during the study period confound our ability to make definitive recommendations regarding the indications for flaps.

## CONCLUSION

This study demonstrates a low rate of MWCs and reoperation for irradiated sarcoma wounds reconstructed with soft tissue flaps by a single surgical team. Flap reconstruction is resource intensive with potential for flap related morbidity. Further prospective studies are required to confirm the utility of flaps, the generalizability of the approach and to clearly define the indications for free and pedicled soft tissue transfer.

## AUTHOR CONTRIBUTIONS

LC contributed to the design of the study, collected and analyzed data and prepared the manuscript. JI assisted in analysis of data and preparation of the manuscript. DG and PC provided clinical cases, contributed to the design of the study, and assisted in preparation of the manuscript. All authors agreed to be accountable for the content of the work.

## ACKNOWLEDGMENTS

The authors would like to thank Ms. Deborah May (Orthopaedic Oncology Research Nurse) for her assistance in obtaining cases from the St. Vincent's Hospital Bone and Soft Tissue Sarcoma Database.

## REFERENCES

1. Rosenberg SA, Tepper J, Glatstein E, Costa J, Baker A, Brennan M, et al. The treatment of soft-tissue sarcomas of the extremities: prospective randomized evaluations of (1) limb-sparing surgery plus radiation therapy compared with amputation and (2) the role of adjuvant chemotherapy. *Ann Surg* (1982) 196(3):305–15. doi:10.1097/00000658-198209000-00009
2. Pisters P, Harrison L, Leung D, Woodruff J, Casper E, Brennan M. Long-term results of a prospective randomized trial of adjuvant brachytherapy in soft tissue sarcoma. *J Clin Oncol* (1996) 14(3):859–68. doi:10.1200/JCO.1996.14.3.859

3. Yang J, Chang A, Baker A, Sindelar W, Danforth D, Topalian S, et al. Randomized prospective study of the benefit of adjuvant radiation therapy in the treatment of soft tissue sarcomas of the extremity. *J Clin Oncol* (1998) 16(1):197–203. doi:10.1200/JCO.1998.16.1.197
4. O'Sullivan B, Davis A, Turcotte R, Bell R, Catton C, Chabot P, et al. Preoperative versus postoperative radiotherapy in soft-tissue sarcoma of the limbs: a randomised trial. *Lancet* (2002) 359(9325):2235–41. doi:10.1016/S0140-6736(02)09292-9
5. Davis A, O'Sullivan B, Turcotte R, Bell R, Catton C, Chabot P, et al. Late radiation morbidity following randomization to preoperative versus postoperative radiotherapy in extremity soft tissue sarcoma. *Radiother Oncol* (2005) 75(1):48–53. doi:10.1016/j.radonc.2004.12.020
6. Al-Absi E, Farrokhyar F, Sharma R, Whelan K, Corbett T, Patel M, et al. A systematic review and meta-analysis of oncologic outcomes of pre- versus postoperative radiation in localized resectable soft-tissue sarcoma. *Ann Surg Oncol* (2010) 17(5):1367–74. doi:10.1245/s10434-009-0885-7
7. Virkus W, Mollabashy A, Reith J, Zlotecki R, Berrey B, Scarborough M. Preoperative radiotherapy in the treatment of soft tissue sarcomas. *Clin Orthop Relat Res* (2002) 397:177–89. doi:10.1097/00003086-200204000-00022
8. Kuklo T, Temple H, Owens B, Juliano J, Islinger R, Andejeski Y, et al. Preoperative versus postoperative radiation therapy for soft-tissue sarcomas. *Am J Orthop (Belle Mead NJ)* (2005) 34(2):75–80.
9. Cannon C, Ballo M, Zagars G, Mirza A, Lin P, Lewis V, et al. Complications of combined modality treatment of primary lower extremity soft-tissue sarcomas. *Cancer* (2006) 107(10):2455–61. doi:10.1002/cncr.22298
10. Baldini EH, Lapidus MR, Wang Q, Manola J, Orgill DP, Pomahac B, et al. Predictors for major wound complications following preoperative radiotherapy and surgery for soft-tissue sarcoma of the extremities and trunk: importance of tumor proximity to skin surface. *Ann Surg Oncol* (2013) 20(5):1494–9. doi:10.1245/s10434-012-2797-1
11. Moore J, Isler M, Barry J, Mottard S. Major wound complication risk factors following soft tissue sarcoma resection. *Eur J Surg Oncol* (2014) 40(12):1671–6. doi:10.1016/j.ejso.2014.10.045
12. Schwartz A, Rebecca A, Smith A, Casey W, Ashman J, Gunderson L, et al. Risk factors for significant wound complications following wide resection of extremity soft tissue sarcomas. *Clin Orthop Relat Res* (2013) 471(11):3612–7. doi:10.1007/s11999-013-3130-4
13. Rosenberg LA, Esther RJ, Erfanian K, Green R, Kim HJ, Sweeting R, et al. Wound complications in preoperatively irradiated soft-tissue sarcomas of the extremities. *Int J Radiat Oncol Biol Phys* (2013) 85(2):432–7. doi:10.1016/j.ijrobp.2012.04.037
14. Kane J, Gibbs J, McGrath B, Loree T, Kraybill W. Large, deep high-grade extremity sarcomas: when is a myocutaneous flap reconstruction necessary? *Surg Oncol* (1999) 8(4):205–10. doi:10.1016/S0960-7404(99)00046-8
15. Barwick WJ, Goldberg JA, Scully SP, Harrelson JM. Vascularized tissue transfer for closure of irradiated wounds after soft tissue sarcoma resection. *Ann Surg* (1992) 216(5):591–5. doi:10.1097/00000658-199211000-00011
16. Kunisada T, Ngan SY, Powell G, Choong PFM. Wound complications following pre-operative radiotherapy for soft tissue sarcoma. *Eur J Surg Oncol* (2002) 28(1):75–9. doi:10.1053/ejso.2001.1213
17. Townley W, Mah E, O'Neill A, Wunder J, Ferguson P, Zhong T, et al. Reconstruction of sarcoma defects following pre-operative radiation: free tissue transfer is safe and reliable. *J Plast Reconstr Aesthet Surg* (2013) 66(11):1575–9. doi:10.1016/j.bjps.2013.06.029
18. Temple C, Ross D, Magi E, DiFrancesco L, Kurien E, Temple W. Preoperative chemoradiation and flap reconstruction provide high local control and low wound complication rates for patients undergoing limb salvage surgery for upper extremity tumors. *J Surg Oncol* (2007) 95(2):135–41. doi:10.1002/jso.20629
19. Tseng JF, Ballo MT, Langstein HN, Wayne JD, Cormier JN, Hunt KK, et al. The effect of preoperative radiotherapy and reconstructive surgery on wound complications after resection of extremity soft-tissue sarcomas. *Ann Surg Oncol* (2006) 13(9):1209–15. doi:10.1245/s10434-006-9028-6
20. Hui A, Ngan S, Wong K, Powell G, Choong P. Preoperative radiotherapy for soft tissue sarcoma: the Peter MacCallum Cancer Centre experience. *Eur J Surg Oncol* (2006) 32(10):1159–64. doi:10.1016/j.ejso.2006.04.003
21. Davis AM, O'Sullivan B, Bell RS, Turcotte R, Catton CN, Wunder JS, et al. Function and health status outcomes in a randomized trial comparing preoperative and postoperative radiotherapy in extremity soft tissue sarcoma. *J Clin Oncol* (2002) 20(22):4472–7. doi:10.1200/JCO.2002.03.084
22. Miller E, Mo X, Andonian N, Haglund K, Martin D, Liebner D, et al. Patterns of major wound complications following multidisciplinary therapy for lower extremity soft tissue sarcoma. *J Surg Oncol* (2016) 114:385–91. doi:10.1002/jso.24313
23. Choi S, Schwartz DL, Farwell DG, Austin-Seymour M, Futran N. Radiation therapy does not impact local complication rates after free flap reconstruction for head and neck cancer. *Arch Otolaryngol Head Neck Surg* (2004) 130:1308–12. doi:10.1001/archotol.130.11.1308
24. Chao AH, Chang DW, Shuaib SW, Hanasono MM. The effect of neoadjuvant versus adjuvant irradiation on microvascular free flap reconstruction in sarcoma patients. *Plast Reconstr Surg* (2012) 129(3):675–82. doi:10.1097/PRS.0b013e3182412a39

# 13

# Soft Tissue Sarcomas of the Arm – Oncosurgical and Reconstructive Principles within a Multimodal, Interdisciplinary Setting

*Georgios Koulaxouzidis[1], Filip Simunovic[1] and Holger Bannasch[1,2]**

*[1] Department of Plastic and Hand Surgery, University of Freiburg Medical Center, Freiburg, Germany, [2] Section for Plastic-Reconstructive Tumor Surgery, University of Freiburg Medical Center, Freiburg, Germany*

Soft tissue sarcomas of the upper extremity represent a severe threat for the patient and a difficult task for the treatment team. Due to the complex anatomy of the arm, most sarcomas involve valuable functional structures. Nonetheless, a large portion of the patients can be treated in a limb-sparing manner, and surgery is the mainstay of local tumor control. This review gives an overview of the disease entities and their epidemiology, on necessary patient work-up, staging, and imaging modalities, as well as the importance of interdisciplinary decision-making. The surgical therapies and principles of tumor excision are outlined, as well as reconstructive options. Furthermore, adjuvant treatments are discussed with a special focus on the various application techniques for radiation therapy. In spite of established treatment algorithms, each case is an individual challenge and individually tailored therapy is required. This aspect is illustrated by presenting three comprehensive cases demonstrating useful strategies. A summary of the relevant literature is given.

**Keywords: soft tissue sarcoma, plastic-reconstructive surgery, upper extremity reconstruction**

***Edited by:***
*Adrien Daigeler,*
*BG-University Hospital Bergmannsheil, Germany*

***Reviewed by:***
*Wanda Petz,*
*European Institute of Oncology, Italy*
*Rutie Yin,*
*West China Second University Hospital, China*

****Correspondence:***
*Holger Bannasch*
*holger.bannasch@uniklinik-freiburg.de*

***Specialty section:***
*This article was submitted to Surgical Oncology, a section of the journal Frontiers in Surgery*

## INTRODUCTION

Soft tissue sarcomas (STS) are a heterogeneous group of rare malignant mesenchymal tumors representing <1% of newly diagnosed solid tumors a year (1). They have an annual incidence of two to three cases per 100,000 (2). Although sarcomas can occur throughout the body, 60% of STS in adults occur in the limbs (15% in the upper extremity and 45% in the lower extremity) (3). One-fifth of all STS occur in the upper extremity (4). Therefore, this condition is very rare, and consequently, the literature is limited to small case series (5–9). Compared to the lower extremity, where liposarcoma and myxoid sarcoma are commonly encountered; synovial sarcoma, epithelioid sarcoma, and fibrosarcoma are relatively more common in the upper extremity (10).

Treatment of upper extremity STS presents a major challenge as the complex anatomy and high functional demands compete with oncological safety demands. Until the 1970s, extremity STS often required limb amputation due to high rates of local recurrence (11, 12). Nowadays, limb-sparing surgery can be performed in more than 90% of the patients without compromise in local recurrence rates or survival rates (8, 13). This development reflects the success of a modern treatment concept with a multidisciplinary team approach (7, 14–18). However, surgical resection remains the cornerstone of treatment, and surgical resection margins are the main prognostic factor for local and systemic tumor control (6, 8, 19). In this review, we highlight key principles of oncological and reconstructive surgery of the upper extremity with focus on the upper arm and the forearm.

## DIAGNOSTIC AND STAGING WORK-UP

Patients usually present with a subcutaneous tumor discovered by palpation. STS of the upper extremity are more readily noticed by the patient compared to the lower extremity. The estimation of duration and progression of the tumor is often uncertain, and there is no association to traumatic injury. The clinical behavior of STS is mostly misleading as they are characterized by slow growth, few physical complaints, and harmless appearance in cross-sectional imaging (20). However, due to the anatomic proximity of functional and neurovascular structures at the upper extremity complains of nerve involvement or functional impairment at first presentation are more common than in the lower extremity. Due to these circumstances, tumors of the upper extremity tend to be smaller at the time of presentation. In any case, every refractory swelling that is not recurrent after 4 weeks should initiate diagnostic work-up, as described and discussed in this article and elsewhere (21).

It is generally recommended that STS should be treated in tumor centers (16, 22–28). However, given the rarity and diversity of these tumors, it is not surprising that excisions are often performed without preoperative suspicion of malignancy and adequate preoperative diagnostic and staging work-up (22, 26, 29). Tumors of the upper extremity are twice as likely to undergo unplanned excision, probably because of their smaller size and more superficial location (30). In our own patient collectively, more than 50% of the patients are referred after such a procedure for further treatment. As shown, resection margins and histopathological assessments from referring institutions are often unreliable and unsuitable for further treatment planning. Moreover, especially in the upper extremity, the risk for residual tumor after unplanned primary excision is high. Although tumors are usually smaller than in the lower extremity, complex regional anatomy may be the reason for close margins or positive margins, necessitating more frequently postoperative radiotherapy. There is significantly more frequent residual disease and local recurrence in the upper extremity, especially around the elbow (10). Completion of diagnostic and staging work-up followed by re-excision is required in this patient group.

Contrast-enhanced MRI represents the standard procedure of diagnostic imaging, as it provides a detailed three-dimensional anatomic presentation of the tumor. With this information, tumor biopsy and excision can be planned (20, 31). A diagnosis can only be achieved by histopathological examination of a representative tumor sample. Therefore, excisional (only for small, superficial tumors) or incisional/punch biopsy has to be performed, as described elsewhere (21, 32). Second opinion reference-center pathology should be indicated generously.

Additionally, before a definitive treatment plan is established, completion of the clinical staging is mandatory. The assessment of tumor size, nodal status, and presence of metastasis has to be performed (TNM status) (33). A spiral CT of the thorax is indicated, as STS are primarily characterized by pulmonary metastasis. However, at the time of diagnosis, only 10% of the patients present with pulmonary metastasis (34). Only rarely, adult type STS metastasize to regional lymph nodes. Nevertheless, there are some sarcoma subtypes (synovial sarcoma, vascular sarcomas, rhabdomyosarcomas, and epithelioid and clear cell sarcomas) with a higher probability of lymphatic spread. However, the role of sentinel lymph node biopsy in these sarcoma subtypes is still unclear (35, 36). Although positron emission tomography (FDG–PET) has not been yet established as standard imaging modality, it has some relevant advantages. As a functional imaging procedure, FDG–PET provides, besides the metastatic situation of the whole body, data on tumor activity and treatment response after neoadjuvant treatment. However, limited experience, availability, and examination costs are actually restricting factors for standardized use (37).

## TUMOR BOARD REVIEW

Categorization of the patients takes place according to the American Joint Committee on Cancer/International Union against Cancer classification (33, 38). A thorough treatment plan is determined in an interdisciplinary tumor board setting, including oncosurgical, reconstructive, neoadjuvant, and adjuvant treatment options.

## PROGNOSTIC FACTORS

Complete tumor resection is the most important prognostic factor for local and distant disease control (8, 9). If local tumor control is not achieved, there can be no successful treatment. Similarly, the general patient outcome is strongly correlated to distant metastasis. In case of insufficient primary excision and evidence of residual tumor, maximum effort should be made to achieve complete resection by re-excision. Re-excision has to include all previous incisions and drainage exit sites as well as every anatomic compartment suspicious for contamination. Furthermore, the presentation status, whether it is a primary or recurrent tumor, as well as the tumor size (<5 or >5 cm), tumor grading, and extracompartimental location are relevant prognostic factors (8, 9). The specific anatomic tumor location is also a relevant factor: for example, tumor location at the shoulder girdle hampers limb-sparing surgery (39–41). As previously stated, residual disease and recurrence are more common in the upper extremity. Besides anatomical factors, this is also due to the fact that histological entities, which are more common in the upper extremity (angiosarcoma, malignant peripheral nerve sheath tumor), are associated with a higher risk of recurrence (42) that more frequent tumors of the lower extremity, such as low grade liposarcoma.

## ONCOSURGICAL RESECTION

The extent of surgical margins is subject of discussion, as there is no solid evidence. The trend during the past decades has been directed toward reduction of the margins (43, 44). The most frequent type of excision is termed "wide excision," signifying that the tumor is to be removed within healthy tissue, in the manner that the tumor is not seen by the surgeon. Contrastingly, the so-called "marginal excision" (excision at the level of the tumor capsule) is not adequate since it does not include a macroscopic layer of uninvolved tissue, which is required by the pathologist in order to certify an R0 status. Resection of the entire compartment, involving all muscles from their origin to the insertion is largely historical and is rarely required. Recently, the type of connective tissue involved was a topic of interest, as sarcomas grow along, rather than transverse, major fascial planes. This enables preservation of major nerves, bones, and muscles with <1 cm resection margin, when fascial planes can be included in the resection (45). Microsurgical techniques enable us to maintain the balance between radical resection and preservation of function. Tumor invasion of nerves is a rare occurrence. In case of close proximity to the tumor, epineural dissection is a safe option (46). Furthermore, neoadjuvant, intraoperative (IORT), or adjuvant radiotherapy treatment modalities additionally contributed to the reduction of resection margins. However, when neurovascular or functional structures cannot be preserved, the oncosurgical defects have to be incorporated into the reconstructive plan.

In cases of advanced disease and extensive infiltration, amputation of the limb is required. Also in these cases, there are useful reconstructive options, such as composite-tissue elbow transfer for reconstruction of the shoulder silhouette (41). In order to offer consultation to these patients, the surgeon also needs to be aware of the current advances in bionic prosthetics, which is a rapidly evolving field offering good solutions. The resected specimen should be clearly marked with sutures and the corresponding sites in the tumor bed with clips. An intraoperative biopsy examination is generally not recommended.

## RECONSTRUCTION

Whenever possible, reconstruction should be achieved as a one-step procedure during tumor excision. Otherwise, wound closure by vacuum-assisted closure can be an alternative, especially when resection margins are uncertain.

The goal of reconstruction is to provide reconstruction of every resected tissue and the related function and to achieve primary wound healing in the interest of timely rehabilitation and adjuvant therapy. In modern reconstructive surgery, it is not sufficient to merely achieve wound closure. It is just as important to strive for optimal functional and esthetic results. For example, split-thickness skin grafts can be transplanted on vital muscle tissue with success. However, this will not lead to an esthetically pleasing result, and it can possibly cause extensive wound healing problems, especially if tendons are exposed. In our patients, almost 70% of the patients with upper extremity sarcoma require reconstructive surgery, compared to 50% at the lower extremity. Reconstructive techniques are more often required in the distal parts of an extremity. In most of these patients, the whole reconstructive armamentarium has to be utilized (16, 18). Due to small case numbers, there is no evidence supporting the use of individual reconstructive techniques, so that the plastic surgeons use the traditional "reconstructive-ladder" when devising the treatment plan. It is, however, common for experienced surgeons, especially in the light of increasing expertise and confidence in free-flap surgery, to skip one or more ladders in the decision-making process.

Several authors have reported that local or regional flaps are associated with higher complication rates and have inferior functional results compared to free flaps (7, 47), which is also our own experience. Some authors found that free-flap reconstruction after soft tissue sarcoma excision at the upper extremity is associated with increased morbidity but better local control (48). Others found that functional outcome achieved satisfactory levels with both pedicled and free flaps (49).

Proximal upper extremity can be successfully treated with traditional random-pattern flaps or axial-pattern flaps originating from the extremity (lateral upper arm flap) or the shoulder (subscapular vascular territory). Axial flaps, such as dorsal interosseous flap, can be used on the forearm. Local flaps that compromise one of the major vessels, such as the pedicled radial artery flap, are not recommended any more due to extensive donor-site morbidity.

There are several free-flap options with minimal donor-site issues, which are used routinely. Since there is no advantage in using a muscle flap and since there are several good perforator flaps available, the perforator flaps have become the mainstay of modern reconstructive surgery. The workhorse flap for extremity reconstruction is the anterolateral thigh (ALT) flap (17), which enables a two-team parallel approach in the supine position. The parascapular flap is another good alternative, requiring surgery in the lateral position. The thoracodorsal artery perforator (TDAP) flap or the musculocutaneous latissimus-dorsi (LD) flap is available for larger defects.

Functional reconstruction of nerve defects (commonly using sural nerve grafting) or blood vessel interposition is also performed at this stage. If there is a tendon defect and the muscle can be preserved, free tendon transplants are performed, usually using the palmaris longus or plantaris tendon. If the muscle has to be sacrificed, the first-line solutions available are the classical tendon transfers, e.g., radial nerve palsy tendon transfer (50). Functional free flaps are rarely required. In this case, free functional gracilis transfer is the primary option, e.g., for reconstruction of finger flexion, as shown in case 3.

## ADJUVANT THERAPY

### Radiation Therapy

Radiation therapy is almost always used as neoadjuvant therapy. The only indication for radiation monotherapy is rare cases that are deemed inoperable because of significant comorbidities. Using the combination of surgical and radiation therapy, 90–95% rates of limb salvage can be achieved. Radiation is usually administered as adjuvant therapy, in a combined dosage of 60–66 Gy with conventional fractionation. The field of radiation includes the tumor bed, margin of safety, as well as scars from previous operations and drainage exit sites. In this way, an improvement of local control for G2 and G3 STS can be achieved. Radiation for G1 tumors is not indicated after R0 resection. Adjuvant radiation can negatively influence complex reconstruction, so that high-grade sarcoma requiring extensive surgery should preferably be treated

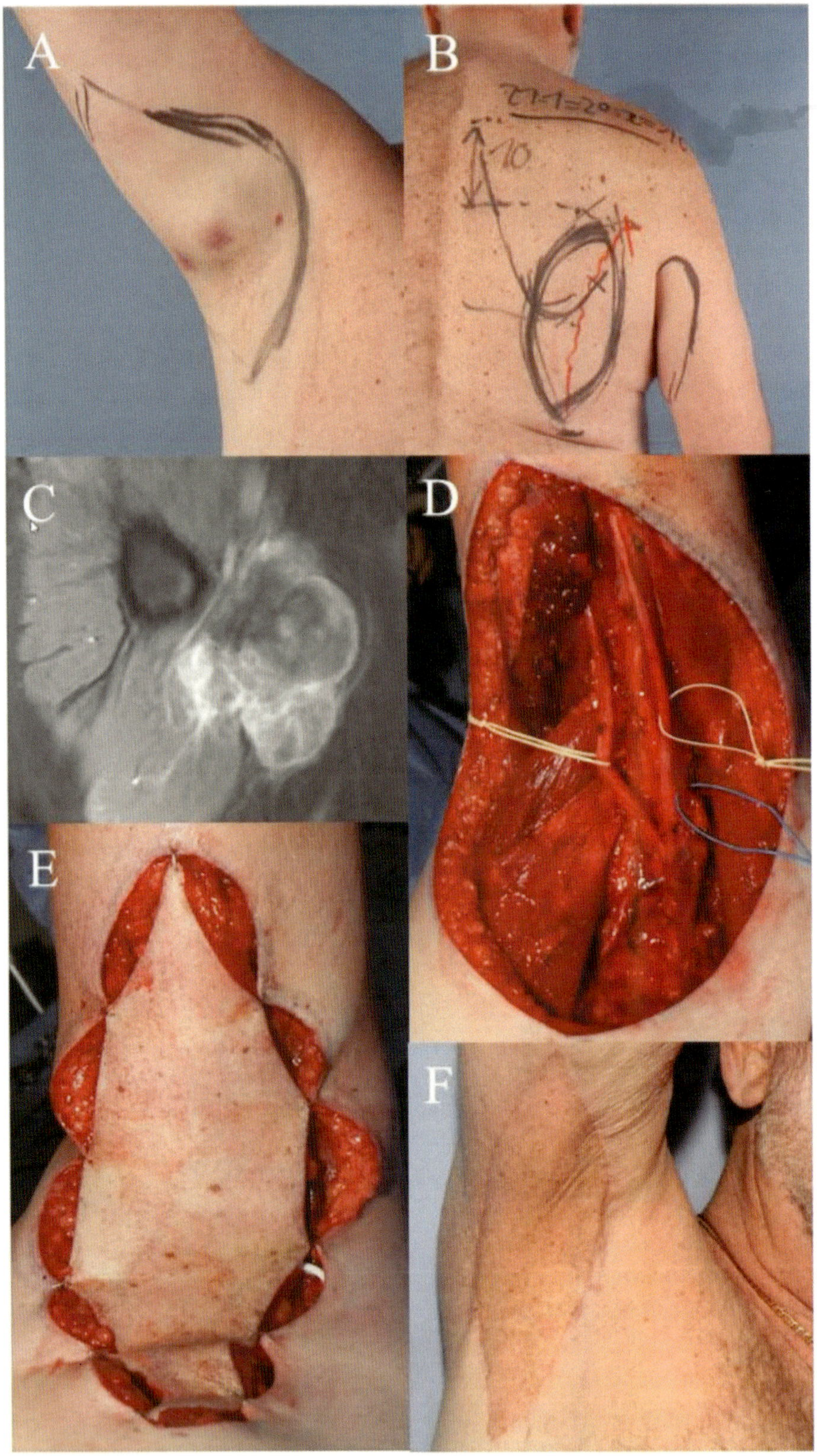


**FIGURE 1** | **Case 1: (A) clinical visible mass in the right axilla, pre-OP drawing of the wide resection margins**. **(B)** Pre-OP drawing demonstrates planned pedicled parascapular fasciocutaneous flap. **(C)** Pre-OP MRI of the right axilla. **(D)** Intraoperative situation after wide en-bloc excision of tumor. Deep margins were achieved by epineurectomy and adventitiectomy. **(E)** Pedicled parascapular flap inset reconstructs the defect. **(F)** Clinical appearance 5 years after surgery and external post-OP radiation therapy.

with neoadjuvant radiation (51). Neoadjuvant radiation has comparable effects on local disease control as adjuvant therapy. The advantages are that the field of radiation can be kept smaller, and the dosage required (50 Gy) is lower. The often discussed severe postoperative wound healing complications after neoadjuvant radiotherapy are much more frequent in the lower extremity (52). Thus in the upper extremity, this strategy can be applied more liberally by taking advantage of the smaller irradiation field and dose. Intraoperative radiation therapy is always used in addition to neoadjuvant radiation therapy, the dosage of which can be reduced accordingly. Usually, 12–15 Gy are administered to the tumor bed (case 2).

## Chemotherapy

Most types of STS are not very sensitive to chemotherapy, with exception of small-round-blue-cell tumors, extraosseous Ewing sarcoma, rhabdomyosarcoma, primitive neuroectodermal tumor, and desmoplastic small-round-cell tumor. Despite an increase in experimental data, there is still limited application of molecular-targeted therapy for treatment of STS. Two examples of successful targeted therapy are the use of imatinib in treatment of dermatofibrosarcoma protuberans and the use of sorafenib in treatment of angiosarcoma. The use of standard chemotherapeutics, such as anthracyclines or ifosfamide after R0 resection, is not generally recommended.

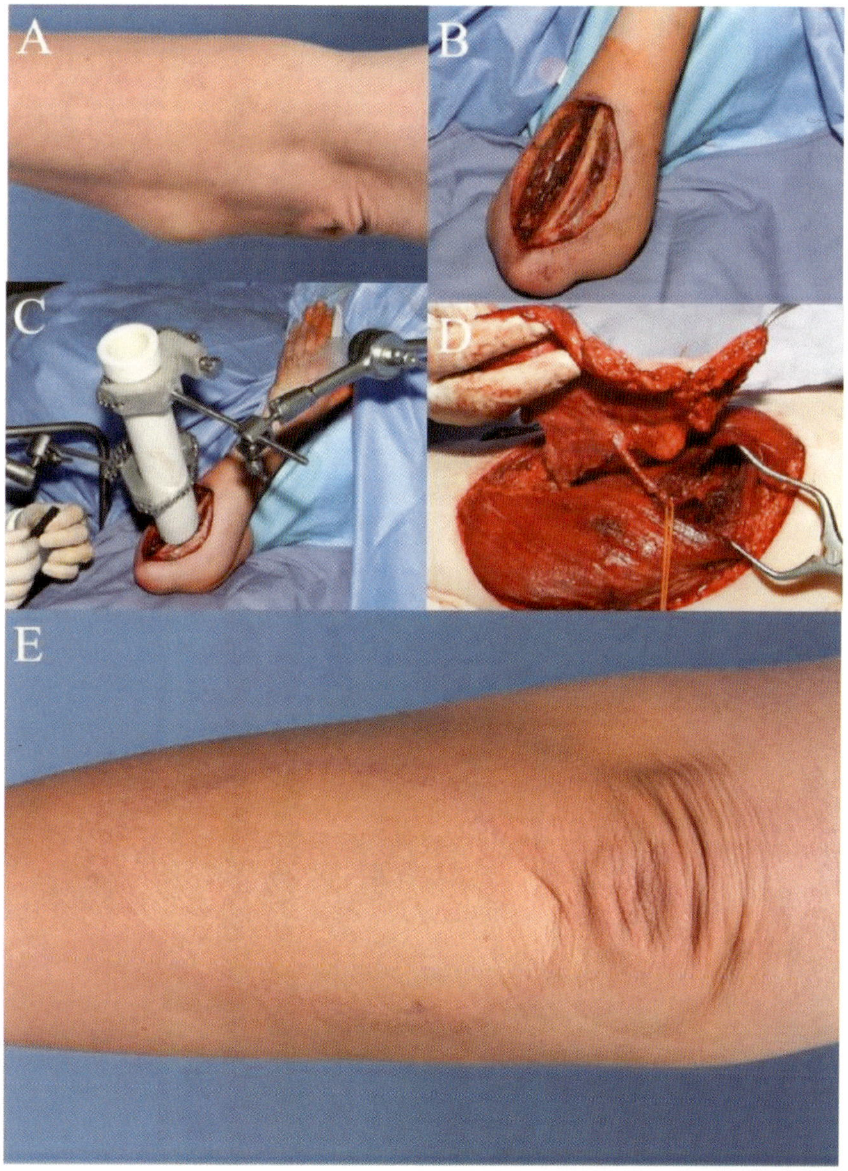


**FIGURE 2** | **Case 2: (A) pre-OP picture shows mass in the proximal forearm. (B)** Intra-OP situation after wide en-bloc excision. **(C)** Intra-OP application of radiation therapy in the wound bed close to the ulna (15 Gy). **(D)** Raised anterolateral thigh flap from the left leg for microvascular reconstruction. **(E)** Clinical appearance of the reconstructed forearm 1 year after additional external radiation therapy (50.4 Gy).

## Hyperthermia and Isolated Limb Perfusion

The combination of neoadjuvant or adjuvant chemotherapy and regional hyperthermia, possibly with additional radiation therapy, can improve local disease control in locally advanced tumors. Isolated limb perfusion with tumor necrosis factor alpha or melphalan can be considered in tumors, which cannot be resected with R0 margins, or when surgical excision would lead to mutilating loss of function.

# CONCLUSION

To achieve optimal outcomes, treatment of STS of the upper extremity should be carried out at experienced institutions where

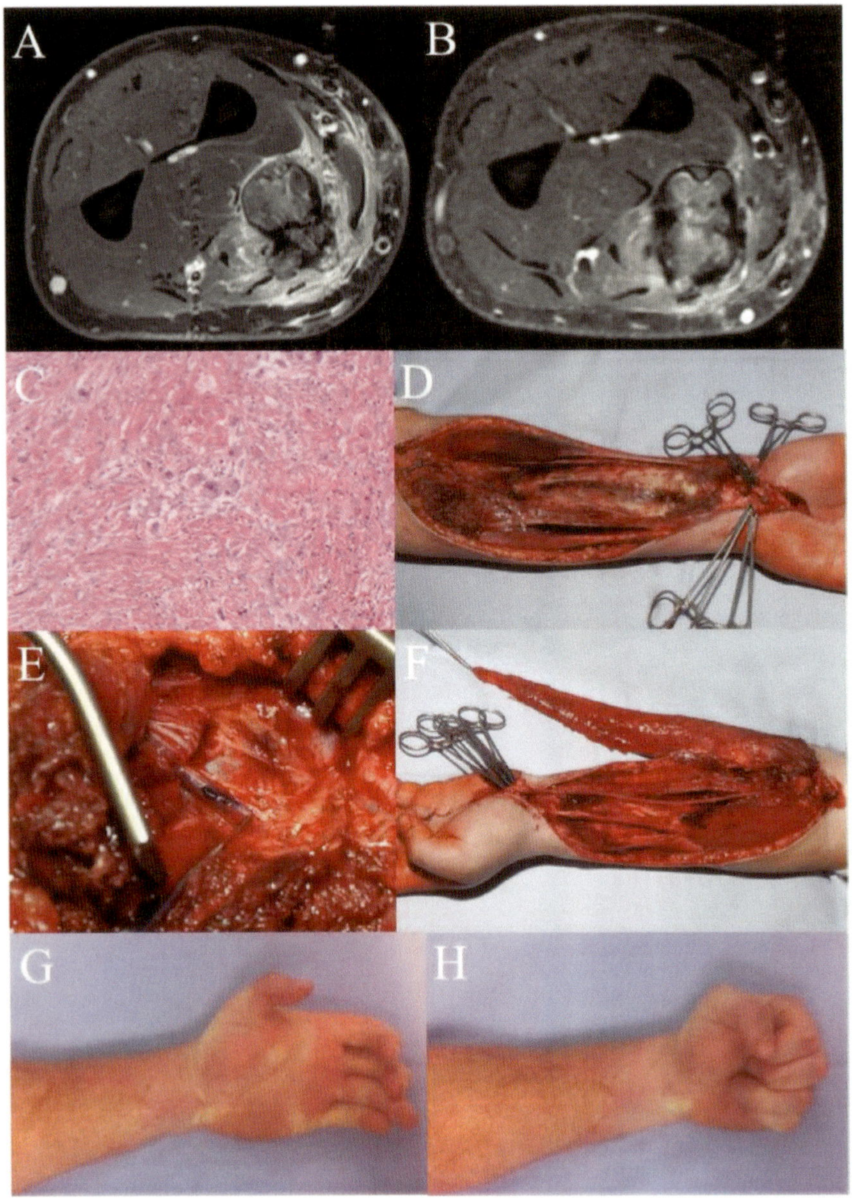


**FIGURE 3** | **Case 3: (A) MRI left forearm before radiation**. **(B)** MRI left forearm post radiation. **(C)** H&E specimen showing only few scattered remaining tumor cells as a result of the preoperative radiotherapy. **(D)** Intraoperative situation after en-bloc excision of the flexor compartment. **(E)** Intraoperative detail photography of the transected median nerve. The blue marking shows the motor branch to the deep flexors, later used for nerve coaptation to the obturator branch of the transferred gracilis muscle. **(F)** Gracilis muscle after microvascular transfer and motor nerve coaptation. After defining the proper tension, the muscle will be fixed to the deep flexor tendons (II–V). Flexor pollicis longus function was reconstructed using a brachioradial tendon transfer. **(G,H)** Clinical result 5 years after therapy. There is a remaining extension deficit, but a full finger flexion with a strong grip could be achieved. Patient is in complete remission and rehabilitated in his original job as a truck driver.

all relevant disciplines are represented. Each sarcoma has its specific histopathological phenotype, grading, size, and, importantly, specific anatomical localization within the complex anatomy of the arm.

Nevertheless, widely accepted treatment principles exist that can be adapted to the individual situation. Prior to treatment, it is mandatory to discuss the case in a multidisciplinary conference defining the use and the sequence of treatment modalities. The mainstay of local tumor control – the prerequisite for curing the patient – is surgery. A radical oncosurgical approach in the upper extremity requires plastic-reconstructive procedures in more than 70% of the cases. The continuously expanding plastic-surgical options for reconstruction of surface, volume, and function enable surgeons to customize the oncosurgical procedure and to preserve the upper extremity with a good oncological and functional result in most of the cases.

## CASE DEMONSTRATIONS

Case 1 (**Figure 1**) demonstrates the case of a 64-year-old male patient suffering from a high-grade pleomorphic sarcoma in the right axilla (T2b, N0, M0, G3). A wide excision was planned and carried out with sufficient removal of skin and subcutaneous tissue due to the extracompartimental localization of the sarcoma. Margins to the deep structures of the axilla could be achieved by thorough dissection of the nerve and vessel sheaths. The transfer of a pedicled parascapular flap was performed in the same operation. Noteworthy, we dissect the pedicle completely back through the medial axillary gap, ligating the osseous branches of the circumflex scapular artery. The flap can be advanced through this tunnel, allowing a completely tension-free placement in the axilla. The patient is shown 5 years after surgery and post-OP radiation therapy with an excellent functional result. The parascapular flap delivers sufficient pliable soft tissue coverage avoiding functional impairment of shoulder movement (53–55).

Case 2 (**Figure 2**) shows a 47-year-old female patient with fast recurrence of an incompletely resected high-grade sarcoma of the left forearm (pleomorphic sarcoma, initially T1b, N0, M0, G3). She had underwent the so-called "whoops procedure" – a term referring to an unplanned sarcoma resection where no malignancy had been suspected. A wide resection was performed with partial removal of the ulnar periosteum. The deep tumor bed was treated with an internal radiation therapy with the application of 15 Gy, thus reducing the post-OP dose from 65 to 50 Gy. Distal to the elbow, large defects are difficult to cover with local tissue transfer. The transfer of a free-flap offers an elegant option to avoid additional morbidity in proximity to the tumor region. The demonstrated ALT flap is one of the "work-horse" microvascular flaps in reconstructive tumor surgery of the extremities (17).

Case 3 (**Figure 3**) shows a 29-year-old patient with an epithelioid cell sarcoma (T2b, N0, M0, G3) of the left forearm within the flexor compartment. Crucial structures (flexor muscles, median nerve, and radial artery) are involved. When complex functional reconstruction of those structures is necessary, postoperative radiation therapy should be avoided, which is why preoperative radiation therapy (50 Gy) was conducted in this case. The MRI pre- and postradiation do not differ much in tumor size, but a significant reduced contrast enhancement can be demonstrated. Histology reflects good response to radiation therapy with only few vital, scattered tumor cells. Radical resection was carried out with en-bloc removal of all flexors (except FCU), the median nerve, and the radial artery. Sensory reconstruction was performed *via* multiple sural nerve cable grafts, which resulted in recovery of protection sensation. Functional reconstruction for the flexors was achieved with a free microvascular, functional gracilis muscle transfer, covered with a split-thickness skin graft (56). The patient has recovered quite well from this radical approach and is rehabilitated in his former job as truck driver. In the upper extremity, much less wound healing complications arise from this sequence of treatment modalities, especially when free tissue transfer is performed. In the lower extremity, there is a higher occurrence of severe wound healing complications after preoperative radiation.

## AUTHOR CONTRIBUTIONS

GK: data acquisition, literature search, manuscript preparation, and final approval. FS: data acquisition, critical manuscript review, literature search, and final approval. HB: data acquisition, case reports, critical manuscript review, and final approval.

## ACKNOWLEDGMENTS

The authors thank Dr. Philipp Kurz (Department of Pathology, University Medical Center Freiburg) for the histological slide in case 3.

## REFERENCES

1. Jemal A, Tiwari RC, Murray T, Ghafoor A, Samuels A, Ward E, et al. Cancer statistics, 2004. *CA Cancer J Clin* (2004) **54**:8–29. doi:10.3322/canjclin.54.1.8
2. Jane MJ, Hughes PJ. Disease incidence and results of extremity lesion treatment: Mersey region soft tissue sarcomas (1975-1985). *Sarcoma* (1998) **2**:89–96. doi:10.1080/13577149878046
3. Lahat G, Lazar A, Lev D. Sarcoma epidemiology and etiology: potential environmental and genetic factors. *Surg Clin North Am* (2008) **88**:451–81. doi:10.1016/j.suc.2008.03.006
4. Gustafson P, Arner M. Soft tissue sarcoma of the upper extremity: descriptive data and outcome in a population-based series of 108 adult patients. *J Hand Surg Am* (1999) **24**:668–74. doi:10.1053/jhsu.1999.0406
5. Muller M, Bickert B, Germann G, Sauerbier M. [Soft-tissue sarcoma of the forearm and hand. Plastic surgical management]. *Chirurg* (2008) **79**:682–8. doi:10.1007/s00104-008-1529-3
6. Muramatsu K, Ihara K, Doi K, Hashimoto T, Taguchi T. Sarcoma in the forearm and hand: clinical outcomes and microsurgical reconstruction for limb salvage. *Ann Plast Surg* (2009) **62**:28–33. doi:10.1097/SAP.0b013e3181743a11
7. Barner-Rasmussen I, Popov P, Bohling T, Blomqvist C, Tukiainen E. Microvascular reconstructions after extensive soft tissue sarcoma

resections in the upper limb. *Eur J Surg Oncol* (2010) **36**:78–83. doi:10.1016/j.ejso.2009.08.003
8. Lehnhardt M, Hirche C, Daigeler A, Goertz O, Ring A, Hirsch T, et al. [Soft tissue sarcoma of the upper extremities. Analysis of factors relevant for prognosis in 160 patients]. *Chirurg* (2012) **83**:143–52. doi:10.1007/s00104-011-2124-6
9. Baroudi MR, Ferguson PC, Wunder JS, Isler MH, Mottard S, Werier JA, et al. Forearm soft tissue sarcoma: tumors characteristics and oncologic outcomes following limb salvage surgery. *J Surg Oncol* (2014) **110**:676–81. doi:10.1002/jso.23686
10. Gerrand CH, Bell RS, Wunder JS, Kandel RA, O'Sullivan B, Catton CN, et al. The influence of anatomic location on outcome in patients with soft tissue sarcoma of the extremity. *Cancer* (2003) **97**:485–92. doi:10.1002/cncr.11076
11. Cantin J, Mcneer GP, Chu FC, Booher RJ. The problem of local recurrence after treatment of soft tissue sarcoma. *Ann Surg* (1968) **168**:47–53. doi:10.1097/00000658-196807000-00005
12. Hoekstra HJ, Thijssens K, Van Ginkel RJ. Role of surgery as primary treatment and as intervention in the multidisciplinary treatment of soft tissue sarcoma. *Ann Oncol* (2004) **15**(Suppl 4):iv181–6. doi:10.1093/annonc/mdh924
13. Canter RJ, Beal S, Borys D, Martinez SR, Bold RJ, Robbins AS. Interaction of histologic subtype and histologic grade in predicting survival for soft-tissue sarcomas. *J Am Coll Surg* (2010) **210**(191–198):e192. doi:10.1016/j.jamcollsurg.2009.10.007
14. Clark MA, Fisher C, Judson I, Thomas JM. Soft-tissue sarcomas in adults. *N Engl J Med* (2005) **353**:701–11. doi:10.1056/NEJMra041866
15. Gronchi A, Olmi P, Casali PG. Combined modalities approach for localized adult extremity soft-tissue sarcoma. *Expert Rev Anticancer Ther* (2007) **7**:1135–44. doi:10.1586/14737140.7.8.1135
16. Bannasch H, Haivas I, Momeni A, Stark GB. Oncosurgical and reconstructive concepts in the treatment of soft tissue sarcomas: a retrospective analysis. *Arch Orthop Trauma Surg* (2009) **129**:43–9. doi:10.1007/s00402-008-0576-z
17. Momeni A, Kalash Z, Stark GB, Bannasch H. The use of the anterolateral thigh flap for microsurgical reconstruction of distal extremities after oncosurgical resection of soft-tissue sarcomas. *J Plast Reconstr Aesthet Surg* (2011) **64**:643–8. doi:10.1016/j.bjps.2010.08.005
18. Penna V, Iblher N, Momeni A, Stark GB, Bannasch H. Free tissue transfer in reconstruction following soft tissue sarcoma resection. *Microsurgery* (2011) **31**:434–40. doi:10.1002/micr.20895
19. Gronchi A, Lo Vullo S, Colombo C, Collini P, Stacchiotti S, Mariani L, et al. Extremity soft tissue sarcoma in a series of patients treated at a single institution: local control directly impacts survival. *Ann Surg* (2010) **251**:506–11. doi:10.1097/SLA.0b013e3181cf87fa
20. Berger F, Winkler EC, Ruderer C, Reiser MF. [Imaging of soft tissue sarcomas: standard approaches and new strategies]. *Chirurg* (2009) **80**:175–85. doi:10.1007/s00104-008-1594-7
21. Bannasch H, Eisenhardt SU, Grosu AL, Heinz J, Momeni A, Stark GB. The diagnosis and treatment of soft tissue sarcomas of the limbs. *Dtsch Arztebl Int* (2011) **108**:32–8. doi:10.3238/arztebl.2011.0032
22. Noria S, Davis A, Kandel R, Levesque J, O'Sullivan B, Wunder J, et al. Residual disease following unplanned excision of soft-tissue sarcoma of an extremity. *J Bone Joint Surg Am* (1996) **78**:650–5.
23. Davis AM, Kandel RA, Wunder JS, Unger R, Meer J, O'Sullivan B, et al. The impact of residual disease on local recurrence in patients treated by initial unplanned resection for soft tissue sarcoma of the extremity. *J Surg Oncol* (1997) **66**:81–7. doi:10.1002/(SICI)1096-9098(199710)66:2<81::AID-JSO2>3.0.CO;2-H
24. Rydholm A. Improving the management of soft tissue sarcoma. Diagnosis and treatment should be given in specialist centres. *BMJ* (1998) **317**:93–4. doi:10.1136/bmj.317.7151.93
25. Siebenrock KA, Hertel R, Ganz R. Unexpected resection of soft-tissue sarcoma. More mutilating surgery, higher local recurrence rates, and obscure prognosis as consequences of improper surgery. *Arch Orthop Trauma Surg* (2000) **120**:65–9.
26. Bhangu AA, Beard JA, Grimer RJ. Should soft tissue sarcomas be treated at a specialist centre? *Sarcoma* (2004) **8**:1–6. doi:10.1080/13577140410001679185
27. Gutierrez JC, Perez EA, Moffat FL, Livingstone AS, Franceschi D, Koniaris LG. Should soft tissue sarcomas be treated at high-volume centers? An analysis of 4205 patients. *Ann Surg* (2007) **245**:952–8. doi:10.1097/01.sla.0000250438.04393.a8
28. Lehnhardt M, Daigeler A, Homann HH, Hauser J, Langer S, Steinstrasser L, et al. [Importance of specialized centers in diagnosis and treatment of extremity-soft tissue sarcomas. Review of 603 cases]. *Chirurg* (2009) **80**:341–7. doi:10.1007/s00104-008-1562-2
29. Giuliano AE, Eilber FR. The rationale for planned reoperation after unplanned total excision of soft-tissue sarcomas. *J Clin Oncol* (1985) **3**:1344–8.
30. Korah MP, Deyrup AT, Monson DK, Oskouei SV, Weiss SW, Landry J, et al. Anatomic tumor location influences the success of contemporary limb-sparing surgery and radiation among adults with soft tissue sarcomas of the extremities. *Int J Radiat Oncol Biol Phys* (2012) **82**:933–9. doi:10.1016/j.ijrobp.2010.11.020
31. Misra A, Mistry N, Grimer R, Peart F. The management of soft tissue sarcoma. *J Plast Reconstr Aesthet Surg* (2009) **62**:161–74. doi:10.1016/j.bjps.2008.08.018
32. Megerle K, Sauerbier M. Reconstructive treatment of soft tissue sarcoma of the upper extremity. *J Hand Surg Am* (2011) **36**:1241–7. doi:10.1016/j.jhsa.2011.04.017
33. Greene FL; American Joint Committee on Cancer. *AJCC Cancer Staging Atlas*. New York, NY: Springer (2006).
34. Dadia S, Grimer R. Characteristics, diagnosis and treatment of bone and soft tissue sarcomas. *Br J Hosp Med (Lond)* (2007) **68**:589–93. doi:10.12968/hmed.2007.68.11.27680
35. Tunn PU, Andreou D, Illing H, Fleige B, Dresel S, Schlag PM. Sentinel node biopsy in synovial sarcoma. *Eur J Surg Oncol* (2008) **34**:704–7. doi:10.1016/j.ejso.2007.07.014
36. Maduekwe UN, Hornicek FJ, Springfield DS, Raskin KA, Harmon DC, Choy E, et al. Role of sentinel lymph node biopsy in the staging of synovial, epithelioid, and clear cell sarcomas. *Ann Surg Oncol* (2009) **16**:1356–63. doi:10.1245/s10434-009-0393-9
37. Schuetze SM. Utility of positron emission tomography in sarcomas. *Curr Opin Oncol* (2006) **18**:369–73. doi:10.1097/01.cco.0000228744.49294.12
38. Lahat G, Tuvin D, Wei C, Anaya DA, Bekele BN, Lazar AJ, et al. New perspectives for staging and prognosis in soft tissue sarcoma. *Ann Surg Oncol* (2008) **15**:2739–48. doi:10.1245/s10434-008-9970-6
39. Litasova EE. [Three operations of intrascapulo-thoracic amputation for sarcoma of the shoulder girdle]. *Vestn Khir Im I I Grek* (1957) **79**:127–8.
40. Marinescu S, Giuglea C, Mihai R, Oporanu A, Manea S, Florescu IP. Forequarter amputation (upper limb and shoulder girdle) in a synovial sarcoma case – case report. *J Med Life* (2010) **3**:444–8.
41. Koulaxouzidis G, Simunovic F, Stark GB. Shoulder silhouette and axilla reconstruction with free composite elbow tissue transfer following interscapulothoracic amputation. *J Plast Reconstr Aesthet Surg* (2014) **67**:81–6. doi:10.1016/j.bjps.2013.10.040
42. Collin C, Hajdu SI, Godbold J, Friedrich C, Brennan MF. Localized operable soft tissue sarcoma of the upper extremity. Presentation, management, and factors affecting local recurrence in 108 patients. *Ann Surg* (1987) **205**:331–9. doi:10.1097/00000658-198704000-00001
43. Dickinson IC, Whitwell DJ, Battistuta D, Thompson B, Strobel N, Duggal A, et al. Surgical margin and its influence on survival in soft tissue sarcoma. *ANZ J Surg* (2006) **76**:104–9. doi:10.1111/j.1445-2197.2006.03615.x
44. Tunn PU, Kettelhack C, Durr HR. Standardized approach to the treatment of adult soft tissue sarcoma of the extremities. *Recent Results Cancer Res* (2009) **179**:211–28. doi:10.1007/978-3-540-77960-5_13
45. Daigeler A, Harati K, Goertz O, Hirsch T, Steinau HU, Lehnhardt M. [Prognostic factors and surgical tactics in patients with locally recurrent soft tissue sarcomas]. *Handchir Mikrochir Plast Chir* (2015) **47**:118–27. doi:10.1055/s-0034-1394425
46. Clarkson PW, Griffin AM, Catton CN, O'Sullivan B, Ferguson PC, Wunder JS, et al. Epineural dissection is a safe technique that facilitates limb salvage surgery. *Clin Orthop Relat Res* (2005) **438**:92–6. doi:10.1097/01.blo.0000180057.22712.53
47. Vinals JM, Rodrigues TA, Sildenikova DP, Payro JM, Porte JA, Sune CH, et al. Indications of microsurgery in soft tissue sarcomas. *J Reconstr Microsurg* (2012) **28**:619–25. doi:10.1055/s-0032-1326740
48. Kang S, Han I, Kim S, Lee YH, Kim MB, Kim HS. Outcomes after flap reconstruction for extremity soft tissue sarcoma: a case-control study using propensity score analysis. *Eur J Surg Oncol* (2014) **40**:1101–8. doi:10.1016/j.ejso.2014.05.004

49. Payne CE, Hofer SO, Zhong T, Griffin AC, Ferguson PC, Wunder JS. Functional outcome following upper limb soft tissue sarcoma resection with flap reconstruction. *J Plast Reconstr Aesthet Surg* (2013) **66**:601–7. doi:10.1016/j.bjps.2013.01.034
50. Koulaxouzidis G, Stark GB, Lampert FM. [Motor replacement surgery via tendon transfer in radial nerve palsy]. *Oper Orthop Traumatol* (2015) **27**:47–62. doi:10.1007/s00064-014-0322-3
51. Townley WA, Mah E, O'Neill AC, Wunder JS, Ferguson PC, Zhong T, et al. Reconstruction of sarcoma defects following pre-operative radiation: free tissue transfer is safe and reliable. *J Plast Reconstr Aesthet Surg* (2013) **66**:1575–9. doi:10.1016/j.bjps.2013.06.029
52. O'Sullivan B, Davis AM, Turcotte R, Bell R, Catton C, Chabot P, et al. Preoperative versus postoperative radiotherapy in soft-tissue sarcoma of the limbs: a randomised trial. *Lancet* (2002) **359**:2235–41. doi:10.1016/S0140-6736(02)09292-9
53. Kim PS, Lewis VL Jr. Use of a pedicled parascapular flap for anterior shoulder and arm reconstruction. *Plast Reconstr Surg* (1985) **76**:942–4. doi:10.1097/00006534-198512000-00029
54. Klinkenberg M, Fischer S, Kremer T, Hernekamp F, Lehnhardt M, Daigeler A. Comparison of anterolateral thigh, lateral arm, and parascapular free flaps with regard to donor-site morbidity and aesthetic and functional outcomes. *Plast Reconstr Surg* (2013) **131**:293–302. doi:10.1097/PRS.0b013e31827786bc
55. Sachs C, Lehnhardt M, Daigeler A, Goertz O. [Free fasciocutaneous parascapular flap. Coverage of extensive skin and soft tissue defects]. *Unfallchirurg* (2015) **118**:881–4. doi:10.1007/s00113-014-2686-0
56. Ihara K, Shigetomi M, Kawai S, Doi K, Yamamoto M. Functioning muscle transplantation after wide excision of sarcomas in the extremity. *Clin Orthop Relat Res* (1999) (358):140–8.

14

# Decision making in double-pedicled DIEP and SIEA abdominal free flap breast reconstructions: an algorithmic approach and comprehensive classification

*Charles M. Malata[1,2]* and Nicholas G. Rabey[2,3]*

[1] Postgraduate Medical Institute, Faculty of Health Sciences, Anglia Ruskin University, Cambridge and Chelmsford, UK, [2] Cambridge Breast Unit, Plastic and Reconstructive Surgery Department, Cambridge University Hospitals NHS Foundation Trust, Cambridge, UK, [3] Department of Plastic and Reconstructive Surgery, Salisbury District Hospital, Salisbury, UK

**Edited by:**
Michel Saint-Cyr,
Mayo Clinic, USA

**Reviewed by:**
Furkan Erol Karabekmez,
Kecioren Training and Research Hospital, Turkey
Sydney Ch'Ng,
Royal Prince Alfred Hospital, Australia

***Correspondence:**
Charles M. Malata,
Addenbrooke's Hospital, Cambridge University Hospitals NHS Foundation Trust, Cambridge CB2 2QQ, UK
cmalata@hotmail.com

**Specialty section:**
This article was submitted to Reconstructive and Plastic Surgery, a section of the journal Frontiers in Surgery

**Introduction:** The deep inferior epigastric artery perforator free flap is the gold standard for autologous breast reconstruction. However, using a single vascular pedicle may not yield sufficient tissue in patients with midline scars or insufficient lower abdominal pannus. Double-pedicled free flaps overcome this problem using different vascular arrangements to harvest the entire lower abdominal flap. The literature is, however, sparse regarding technique selection. We therefore reviewed our experience in order to formulate an algorithm and comprehensive classification for this purpose.

**Methods:** All patients undergoing unilateral double-pedicled abdominal perforator free flap breast reconstruction (AFFBR) by a single surgeon (CMM) over 40 months were reviewed from a prospectively collected database.

**Results:** Of the 112 consecutive breast free flaps performed, 25 (22%) utilised two vascular pedicles. The mean patient age was 45 years (range = 27–54). All flaps, but one (which used the thoracodorsal system), were anastomosed to the internal mammary vessels using the rib-preservation technique. The surgical duration was 656 min (range = 468–690 min). The median flap weight was 618 g (range = 432–1275 g) and the mastectomy weight was 445 g (range = 220–896 g). All flaps were successful and only three patients requested minor liposuction to reduce and reshape their reconstructed breasts.

**Conclusion:** Bipedicled free abdominal perforator flaps, employed in a fifth of all our AFFBRs, are a reliable and safe option for unilateral breast reconstruction. They, however, necessitate clear indications to justify the additional technical complexity and surgical duration. Our algorithm and comprehensive classification facilitate technique selection for the anastomotic permutations and successful execution of these operations.

**Levels of evidence:** Therapeutic level IV.

**Keywords: Bipedicled free flaps, double-pedicle free flaps, stacked free flaps, breast reconstruction, abdominal free flaps, DIEP and SIEA breast free flaps, intra-flap and extra-flap microvascular anastomoses, rib sparing internal mammary vessel exposure**

## Introduction

The free single-pedicled deep inferior epigastric artery perforator (DIEP) flap is the gold standard for autologous breast reconstruction. However, its harvest based on one vascular pedicle may not provide enough viable abdominal tissue in patients who are slim, nulliparous, post massive-weight loss, have midline abdominal scars, or possess minimal abdominal tissue with comparatively large breasts. Double-pedicled abdominal free flaps are designed to overcome this deficit by utilizing most of the lower abdominal tissue for unilateral breast reconstruction. While single-pedicled free TRAM flaps may perfuse more tissue than a single-pedicled DIEP flap they carry a higher donor site morbidity and do not consistently or reliably perfuse Hartrampf Zone 4, which is necessary to harvest a larger flap.

Bipedicled or double-pedicled abdominal perforator flaps are so-named because they are supplied by two anatomically distinct vascular pedicles, thereby increasing the total tissue volume with a Hartrampf Zone I type perfusion (1, 2). Harvesting the entire lower abdomen on two vascular pedicles was pioneered by Arnez and Scamp in 1992 using their bipedicled free TRAM flap design (3). Blondeel and Boecyx, however, were the first to apply this concept to free abdominal perforator flaps in their 1994 description of a DIEP flap (4). Several series have since shown the reliability of bipedicled free DIEP flaps (5–8). However, there are multiple flap configurations and arrangements of the vascular anastomoses (**Table 1**).

The blood supply of bipedicled free abdominal flaps may originate from the deep inferior epigastric arteries (DIEAs), superficial inferior epigastric arteries (SIEAs), DIEP perforators, or a combination of these. These options were first classified by Hamdi et al. according to the named vessel and vascular configuration employed (6). Various authors have since utilized similar or different anatomical vascular arrangements (5–8, 14, 15). Hitherto there has, however, been no comprehensive classification. In general the anastomoses of the two pedicles

**TABLE 1 | Published reports on the abdominal bipedicled flap for breast reconstruction.**

| Study | Number of cases | Indications | Flap tissue arrangement | Vascular arrangements | Complications |
|---|---|---|---|---|---|
| (4) | 1 | Midline abdominal scar | Single layer | Primary DIEA to IMV<br>Secondary DIEA to inferior continuity of primary DIEA | Nil |
| (9) | 1 | Large contralateral breast, midline abdominal scar | Stacked | Primary DIEA to subscapular artery<br>Secondary DIEA to inferior continuity of primary DIEA | Re-exploration needing vein anastomosis and graft |
| (6) | 16 | Previous liposuction (19%), abdominal scars (31%), insufficient tissue volume (50%) | Single layer, folded if required | DIEA/DIEA flaps (43.8%)<br>DIEA/SIEA flaps (43.8%)<br>DIEA/perforator flaps (12.5%)<br>All primary pedicle anastomosis to IMV, secondary pedicle to primary DIEA (81.3%), secondary pedicle to TDAs (18.8%) | • Scar correction (25%)<br>• Donor wound dehiscence (19%)<br>• Fat necrosis (6%)<br>• Lipofilling (6%) |
| (10) | 1 | Midline abdominal scar | Stacked | Primary: DIEA to TDA<br>Secondary: SIEA to inferior continuity of DIEA | Nil |
| (5) | 14 | Thin abdominal wall (21%), large contralateral breast (C cup or above 57%) | Single layer | DIEA/DIEA (42.9%)<br>DIEA/MS-TRAM (57.1%)<br>Donor vessels<br>• TDA and serratus (21.4%)<br>• TDA and IMV (71.4%)<br>• IMVs anterograde and retrograde (7.1%) | • Cellulitis (7%)<br>• Delayed healing (7%)<br>• Hypertrophic scar (7%)<br>• Local recurrence (7%)<br>• Contralateral mastopexy 14%<br>• Abdominal bulge (7%)<br>• Blood transfusion (21%) |
| (11) | 5 | Infraumbilical vertical abdominal scar (100%) | Single layer | Primary DIEA pedicle to IMV. Secondary DIEA pedicle to superior continuity of primary pedicle | Minor fat necrosis (40%) |
| (7) | 96 | Previous abdominal scars (31.9%) including midline abdominal scars (25.7%) | Single layer | All used IMVs for primary DIEA pedicle anastomoses. For secondary DIEA pedicle<br>• Superior continuity: 43.7%<br>• Inferior continuity end-to-end: 30.2%<br>• Inferior continuity artery end-to-side: 24.0%<br>• Extra-flap anterograde/retrograde: 2% | • Total Flap Loss – 1.8%<br>• Partial flap loss – 0.9%<br>• Re-exploration – 6.2%<br>• Breast fat necrosis – 10.6%<br>• Abd wound infection: 2.7%<br>• Abdominal bulge (0.9%) |
| (12) | 1 | Large contralateral breast | Folded | DIEA/DIEA to IMV extra-flap anterograde/ retrograde. | Nil |
| (13) | 55 | Insufficient abdominal volume | Folded and stacked | Primary DIEA pedicle (superficial) to IMVs, secondary DIEA pedicle (deep) intra-flap anastomosis to primary pedicle | Hematoma (5.4%) |

may take the form of an *intraflap* ("in-series") arrangement as described by Hamdi et al., an *extraflap* ("in-parallel") arrangement or a *combined intraflap–extraflap* arrangement using the internal mammary vessels (IMVs) in combination with the thoracodorsal or other vessels (9, 10, 16, 17). In the *extraflap* arrangement the two pedicles are independently anastomosed to the IMVs for the primary flap and to the thoracodorsal vessels (TDVs) or retrograde IMVs or other vessels for the secondary flap (6, 10). The *combined intraflap–extraflap* arrangement employs an arterial anastomosis of the secondary flap pedicle to an intraflap site and the venous anastomosis to an extraflap site or vice versa.

Despite the proven efficacy of abdominal bipedicled free flaps (**Table 1**), the literature is sparse regarding the choice of vessel configuration and flap inset. We therefore deemed it useful to present an algorithm for technique selection and propose a comprehensive classification. This was based on a single surgeon's experience with 25 consecutive bipedicled free flap breast reconstructions. We predict our algorithm will optimize patient outcomes for this complex microvascular procedure.

## Patients and Methods

All patients undergoing unilateral bipedicled abdominal free flap breast reconstruction were identified from a prospective database of microsurgical procedures carried out at Cambridge University Hospital, UK. All procedures were performed over a 40-month period from November 2010 to March 2014 by a single surgeon (CMM).

Data collected included indications, microvascular anastomotic details and flap outcomes. In addition, patient demographics, breast size, previous adjuvant therapy, co-morbidities, inter-rib space type and width were recorded. Collation of the patient demographics, BMI, mastectomy weights, flap weights, inter-rib space distances, surgery duration and flap ischemia times was carried out using Microsoft Excel™ Software.

### Flap Selection: Bipedicled DIEP Versus Unipedicled DIEP

Patients requiring autologous tissue reconstruction based on their need for adjuvant radiotherapy or refusal to accept implant-based reconstructions were considered for abdominal tissue reconstruction. The decision to perform a bipedicled flap rather than a standard unipedicled flap was based on clinical assessment of the donor abdomen by the senior author (CMM). This was based on an estimate that three quarters of the lower abdominal tissue (which can be reliably perfused by one set of deep inferior epigastric vessels) would not be sufficient to reconstruct the required breast size. This took into account increasing the abdominal tissue available by schamfering the harvest while enabling safe closure of the donor site. An underlying assumption was (the nearly universally held view) that DIEP flaps are preferable to free TRAM flaps in view of the donor site morbidity. No intraoperative tests, such as clamping of the one set of perforators, were undertaken to determine the horizontal extent of the flap perfusion.

### Flap Harvest

All patients were marked up the day before surgery. The perforators were located using an 8 MHz Doppler probe. Later in the series, all patients ($n = 15$) underwent CT angiography of the abdominal wall vessels (DIEP and SIEA). The flap was raised in a standard fashion from lateral to medial then inferior to superior and then superior to inferior carefully identifying and preserving the perforators. The SIEA pedicle was utilized if the artery was deemed suitable with good pulsatility and a diameter of >1 mm (3). The dissection end point of the SIEA pedicle was at the femoral vessel junction, beyond the artery bifurcation. This is important in ensuring a large enough artery and minimizing discrepancy with the recipient arteries.

For DIEP flaps, the perforators were exposed by carefully incising the rectus sheath with a size 15 blade without excising any of the sheath. The perforator course was then followed through the muscle up to the main pedicle carefully ligating the side branches. At least 2 cm of vessel was preserved at the superior continuity and inferior continuity of the DIE vascular pedicles in case these were needed for *intraflap* anastomoses.

The pedicle was dissected toward its origin from the external iliac vessels aiming beyond the confluence of the venae commitantes. This was repeated on the opposite side.

The side with the best perforators became the primary flap and anastomosed anterograde to the internal mammary vessels. In the entire series, one flap was divided into two hemiflaps and rotated 90° to lie vertically adjacent to each other in the breast pocket (in order to increase its width).

### Recipient Vessel Preparation

This utilized the total rib-preservation technique detailed in the author's previous publication (15). The IMVs were exposed in the second intercostal space (ICS) without cartilage sacrifice but removal of the intercostal muscles. Occasionally, the third ICS was exposed in order to try and identify veins proximal to any confluence.

### Rectus Sheath Closure

When required, the opening(s) in the rectus sheath was closed using looped "0" nylon over-and-over continuous sutures in two layers. If the flap configuration utilized two DIE vascular pedicles repair of the two incisions in the sheaths was performed simultaneously by two surgeons to avoid unequal distribution of tension and facilitate closure of the second side. Mesh reinforcement was not used in any of the patients.

### Vessel Selection for Anastomoses

This is detailed in the algorithm (*vide infra*).

## Results

Over the 40-month period, a total of 112 free abdominal flaps were performed in 98 consecutive patients by one surgeon. 25 (22%) had a bipedicled vascular configuration (**Table 2**). The mean patient age was 45 years (27–54). The median BMI was 23.7 kg/m$^2$ (20.2–28.7). The bra cup sizes were 2 As, 3 Bs, 9 Cs, 7 Ds, 2 Es, and 2 Gs. The indications for surgery were (alone or in combination): inadequate abdominal tissue for one breast,

**TABLE 2 | Bipedicled abdominal free flap patient summary.**

| Case no. | Age | BMI | Cup size | Immediate (I)/ delayed (D) | Flap configuration | Ischemia duration (min) | Surgery duration (min) | Rib space width (mm) | Adjuvant postoperative radiotherapy | Complications |
|---|---|---|---|---|---|---|---|---|---|---|
| 1 | 26 | 24.9 | 34B/C 32DD | I | DIEA/DIEA extraflap | 104 | 770 | 14.5 | No | |
| 2 | 43 | 23.4 | 34B/C | I | III b | 98 | 744 | 20 | Yes | |
| 3 | 38 | 23.1 | 32A/B | I | II b | 83 | 780 | 24 | Yes | Requested liposuction |
| 4 | 45 | 26 | 36B | I | III a | 91 | 690 | 19 | Yes | |
| 5 | 51 | 25.3 | 34C | I | DIEA/DIEA extraflap | 90 | 600 | 26 | No | |
| 6 | 43 | 24 | 36B/C | Salvage | III a | 110 | 790 | 21 | No | |
| 7 | 43 | 24.7 | 34D | I | DIEA/DIEA extraflap | 65 | 600 | 26 | No | |
| 8 | 46 | 20.2 | 36C | I | II b | 115 | 748 | 27 | No | Requested liposuction |
| 9 | 50 | 22.8 | 34B/C | I | DIEA/DIEA extraflap | 81 | 716 | 15 | No | |
| 10 | 42 | 22.9 | 36D | I | II a | 82 | 690 | 15 | Yes | Small area fat necrosis |
| 11 | 47 | 20.3 | 34C | I | III a | 190 | 675 | 16 | Yes | Requested liposuction |
| 12 | 40 | 22.5 | 36B | I | DIEA/DIEA extraflap | 76 | 654 | 19 | Yes | Abdominal wound dehiscence |
| 13 | 46 | 23.9 | 36B | I | DIEA/DIEA extraflap | 125 | 650 | 23 | Yes | |
| 14 | 44 | 21.3 | 32D | I | III b | 101 | 554 | 20 | Yes | |
| 15 | 54 | 23.9 | 32D | I | DIEA/DIEA extraflap | 106 | 572 | 26 | Yes | |
| 16 | 53 | 23.4 | 34D | I | DIEA/DIEA extraflap | 130 | 647 | 26 | No | |
| 17 | 53 | 25.2 | 32G | I | DIEP-DIEA extraflap | 157 | 554 | 17 | Yes | |
| 18 | 46 | 23 | 32E | I | SIEA/SIEA extraflap | 118 | 622 | 20 | Yes | |
| 19 | 34 | 18.7 | 34D | I | DIEP–DIEP extraflap | 129 | 693 | 14 | Yes | |
| 20 | 48 | 28.8 | 34E | Delayed | II b | 55 | 535 | 14 | Yes. Pre-op | |
| 21 | 50 | 26.2 | 32D | I | DIEA–DIEA extraflap | 87 | 670 | 24 | No | |
| 22 | 45 | 24.3 | 36AA | Delayed | DIEA–DIEA extraflap | 107 | 582 | 22 | Yes | |
| 23 | 48 | 25 | 32G | I | DIEA–DIEA extraflap | 182 | 691 | 18 | No | |
| 24 | 49 | 23.5 | 36C | I | DIEP–SIEA extraflap | 92 | 702 | 19 | No | |
| 25 | 26 | 26 | 36C | Salvage | DIEP–DIEP extraflap | 60 | 468 | 22 | Yes. Pre-op | |

refusal of implant-based reconstruction, small breast volume or planned postoperative radiotherapy (**Figures 1–3**). Two patients had failed prosthetic reconstructions salvaged with bipedicled free flaps. No patients had midline abdominal scars.

The median mastectomy weight was 445 g (range = 220–896) with a median flap weight of 618 g (range = 432–1275). The microvascular anastomoses used (**Table 3**) were DIEA/DIEA extraflap in 15 patients (**Figures 1** and **4**), DIEA/DIEA intraflap in four (two superior and two inferior "continuities") (**Figure 2**), DIEA/SIEA extraflap in one, DIEA/SIEA intraflap in four (two superior and two inferior "continuities") (**Figure 5**) and SIEA/SIEA in one patient (**Figure 3**).

The median surgery duration was 670 min (468–790) with flap ischemia time of 103 min (24–190). Twenty-one reconstructions

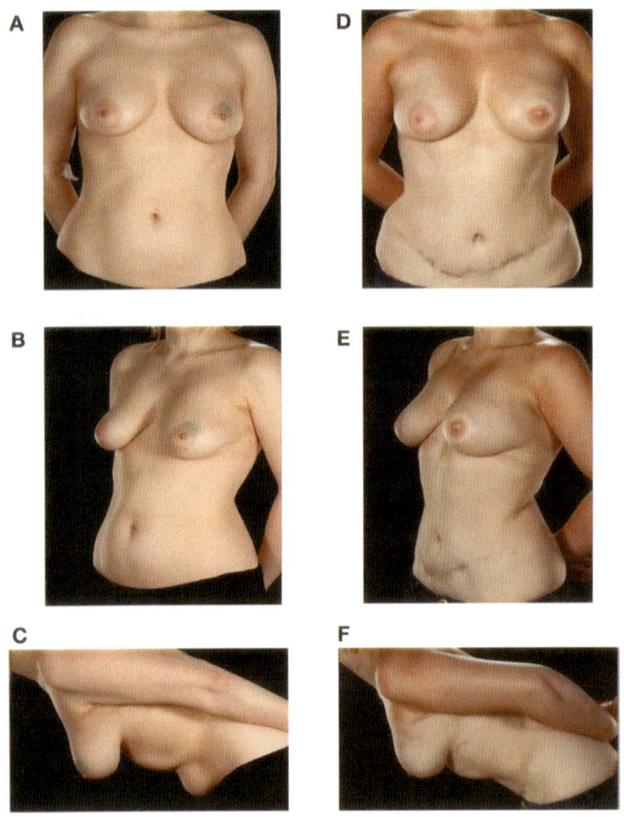

**FIGURE 1 | Preoperative (A–C) and postoperative (D–F) appearances of a 26-year-old patient with size D cup breasts**. She received an extraflap configuration DIEP–DIEP bipedicled free flap breast reconstruction.

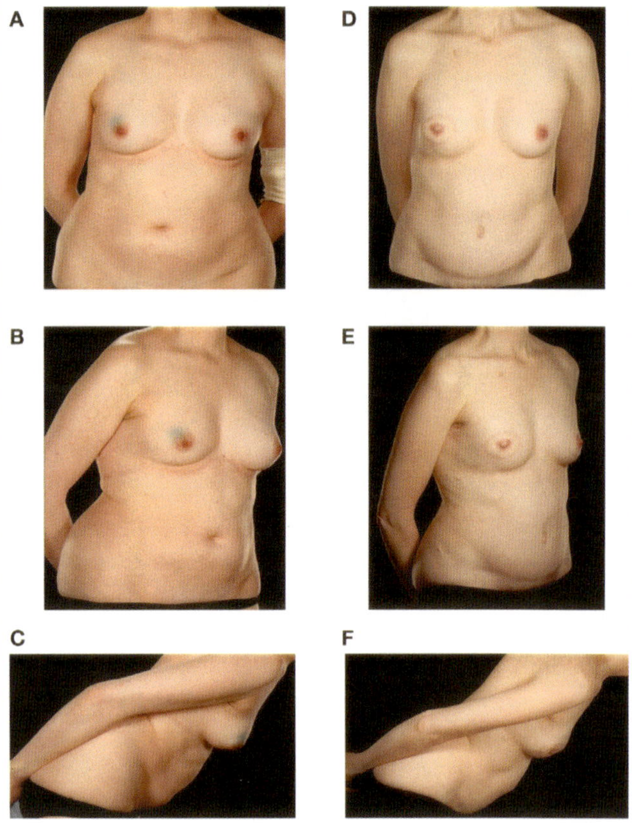

**FIGURE 2 | Preoperative (A–C) and postoperative (D–F) appearances of a 43-year-old nulliparous patient with size B cup breasts who required postoperative radiotherapy and refused to countenance the idea of an implant-based reconstruction**. She underwent a Type IIIb DIEP–DIEP bipedicled flap reconstruction.

were immediate, two were delayed and two were salvage (tertiary). All patients used the total ipsilateral rib-preservation method of IMV harvest. The second ICS was used in 17 patients and both second and third spaces in 8 patients. The widths for the ICSs ranged from 14 to 27 mm for the second space and 11 to 25 mm for the third.

The arterial anastomoses were all performed end-to-end using interrupted 9/0 monofilament nylon (S&T®). The venous anastomoses were undertaken with a venous coupler in 45 anastomoses (83%) and with 9/0 MFN continuous suture in eight (17%). The vein of the second flap was anastomosed to the bifurcated anterograde IMV vein in 6 cases (24%), its retrograde limb in 14 (56%), intraflap superior continuity 5 (20%), intraflap inferior continuity 3 (12%) and to the thoracodorsal vein in 1 (4%) (**Table 4**). The intercostal perforators and the pectoral vein were not used. The secondary pedicle arterial anastomoses were the retrograde IM artery in 16 cases (64%) with identical figures for the superior and inferior "continuities" and the TDVs. There were no anterograde internal mammary secondary pedicle arterial anastomoses [as these would have to be end-to-side (ETS) on the same IMA used as the recipient for the primary pedicle].

All flap reconstructions were successful with no partial flap losses and no re-explorations. One patient needed on-table revision of the primary arterial anastomosis whilst another two required venous anastomoses revision due to coupler device malfunction. Where indicated ($n = 14$) the immediate reconstructions received adjuvant radiotherapy post-operatively without delay. One patient developed a 2-cm area of fat necrosis laterally on the SIEA flap side and this was managed conservatively. Another patient experienced exacerbation of a pre-existing lower abdominal bulge currently being treated conservatively. She also had minor dehiscence of her abdominal incision possibly due to smoking history. There have been no complaints of herniation or symptomatic abdominal wall tightness after a median follow up of 18.5 months (1–40). Three patients requested liposuction to reshape their reconstructed breasts.

## Discussion

Bipedicled free abdominal flaps widen the pool of patients who can benefit from the advantages of autologous tissue breast reconstruction. This series shows that the technique of transferring the entire lower abdominal flap on two vascular pedicles is reliable whilst being associated with minimal morbidity. The indications for double-pedicled flaps in the present series were usually a combination of factors which included the patient's body habitus (relative size of the breast versus the lower abdomen) and their preference for totally autologous reconstruction. This was

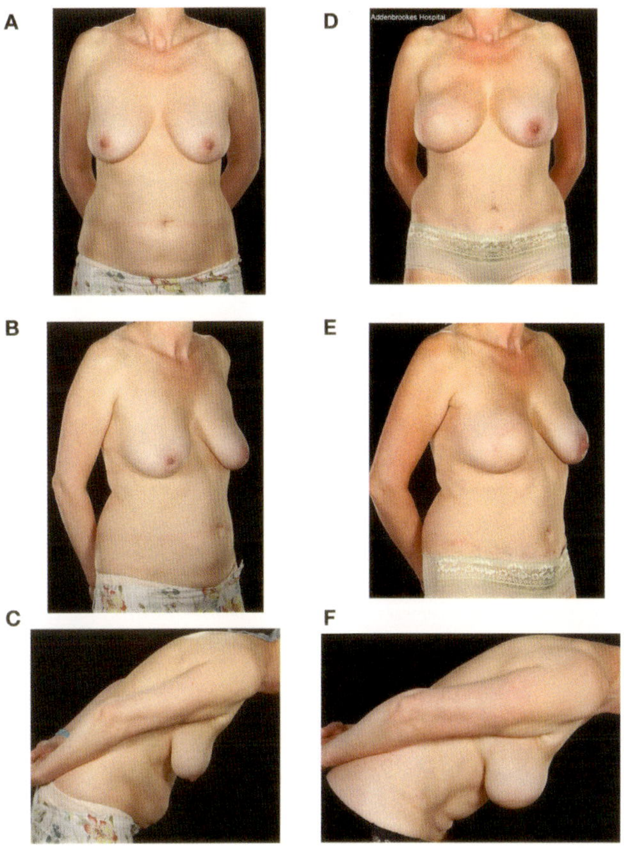

**FIGURE 3 | Preoperative (A–C) and two-year postoperative (D–F) and post-radiation appearances of a 46-year-old nulliparous patient with large breasts (size E cup) and a relatively small abdomen.** She underwent a Type 1 SIEA-SIEA double-pedicled free flap breast reconstruction at the time of her therapeutic mastectomy. She has hitherto declined nipple reconstruction.

**TABLE 3 | Summary of the vessel constructs used in this bipedicled abdominal free flap series.**

| Name of construct | DIEP/DIEP | DIEP/SIEA | SIEA/SIEA |
|---|---|---|---|
| Inferior continuity | 2 | 2 | – |
| Superior continuity | 2 | 2 | – |
| Extraflap anastomoses | 15 | 1 | 1 |
| Totals | 19 | 5 | 1 |

especially when adjuvant radiotherapy was planned. The decision whether to undertake a unipedicled or bipedicled DIEP flap was a clinical one made preoperatively in the outpatient clinic.

Previous published series have discussed various options for the arrangement of transferred tissue and microvascular configurations (**Table 1**). There are four described flap arrangements once the abdominal tissue is transferred onto the chest wall (5–10, 14–17). In the "*stacked*" variety the flap is split into two and positioned one on top of the other. The "*coned*" variant contours the horizontally orientated flap to various degrees. In a third option the bipedicled flap is rotated 90° to be vertical and "*folded*" over. This is useful for narrow breasts. The fourth type splits the flap into two, rotates each hemiflap 90° toward each other then arranges them vertically "*adjacent*" to each other. These arrangements are designed to maximize volume but must not be viewed in isolation from the microvascular anastomotic permutations.

The anastomoses for the second vascular pedicle can be performed *intraflap*, *extraflap*, or rarely both *intraflap–extraflap* (**Table 4**; **Figure 6**). The *intraflap* configurations consist of anastomosing the secondary vascular pedicle to branches of the primary flap's vascular pedicle as detailed by Hamdi et al. (**Figure 7**).

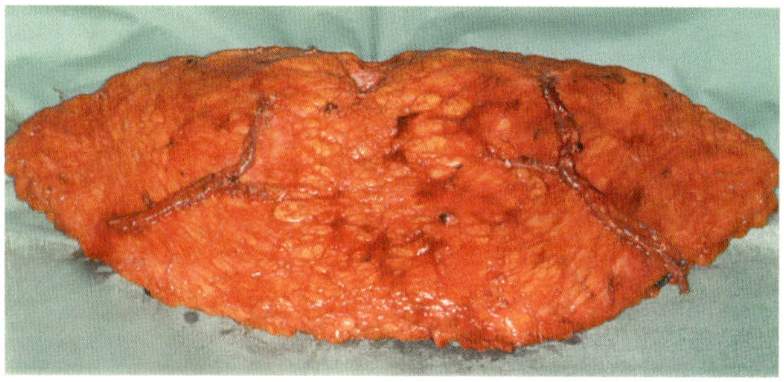

**FIGURE 4 | An intraoperative photograph of a bipedicled DIEP–DIEP flap after harvest prior to micro-anastomoses.** Each hemiflap is based on two perforators.

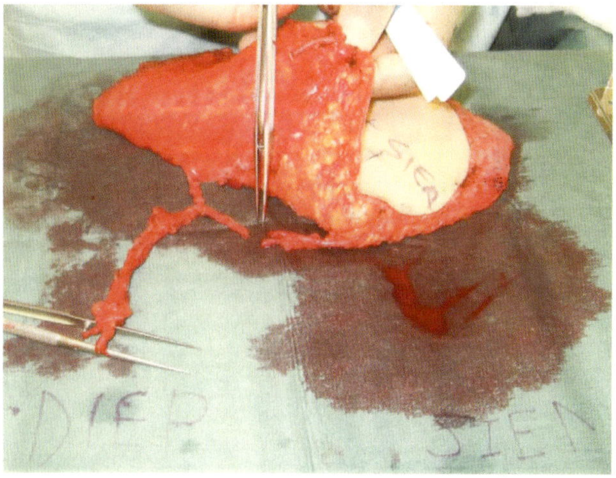



**FIGURE 5 | An intraoperative photograph of a DIEP–SIEA showing the ease of anastomoses of the SIEA second pedicle to the superior continuity of the DIEP primary vascular pedicle.**

**TABLE 4 | Summary of recipients used for venous and arterial anastomoses for the secondary flap.**

| Recipient vessels | Venous number (%) | Arterial number (%) |
|---|---|---|
| Retrograde IM vessel | 11 (44) | 16 (64) |
| Anterograde IM vessel | 6 (24) | 0 (0) |
| Superior pedicle continuity | 5 (20) | 5 (20) |
| Inferior pedicle continuity | 3 (12) | 3 (12) |
| Thoracodorsal vessel | 1 (4) | 1 (4) |
| Intercostal perforator | 0 (0) | 0 (0) |
| Pectoral vein | 0 (0) | 0 (0) |

In the *extraflap* arrangement the secondary flap's vessels are separately anastomosed retrogradely to the internal mammary vessels or anterogradely to the TDVs or other chest wall vessels (5–10, 14–17) (**Table 1**). Although all these articles report good outcomes, there is a wide variability in the microvascular configurations used. From our experience we have identified two points in the procedure when careful consideration of the arrangement to use for the microvascular anastomoses is critical. The first is the selection of pedicle design during flap harvest (**Figure 8**), and the second is the combination of recipient vessels for anastomoses (**Figure 9**), especially when an *extraflap* configuration for two pedicles is required. We have found that preoperative CT angiography can assist our vessel selection.

Intra-operatively we therefore make the following considerations. The superficial inferior epigastric (SIE) vessels are evaluated initially for pulsatility, size and location (**Figure 8**). This pedicle should be explored first because it is easier and quicker to dissect and gives less donor site morbidity. The SIEA vascular pedicle may provide good flap perfusion whilst avoiding trauma to the rectus abdominis muscle and fascia, such as that required for the raising of a DIE pedicle (3). However, occasionally the SIE vessels may have been injured in previous abdominal surgery, so care needs to be taken over their selection. If both arteries have a good caliber of >1 mm and display good pulsatility and orientation, then they are determined to be adequate and a bilateral SIEA Hamdi type I flap can be fashioned. If not, then the DIEAs must be considered next.

In our experience the easier and faster-to-dissect lateral row perforators can be used preferentially as an adequate basis of the bipedicled DIEP flap as there is sufficient perfusion of Hartrampf zones IV or III across the flap midline. This is in contrast to the situation in a unipedicled DIEP free flap where the more centrally located medial row perforators are to be preferred. Usually the medial row perforators are larger than lateral row ones and single (medial row) perforator unilateral DIEP pedicles are commonplace. When based on the lateral row we prefer to use at least two perforators in unipedicled flaps to be assured of overall flap perfusion and especially venous drainage. However, if two DIEA pedicles are being used then one lateral row perforator on each side should be adequate.

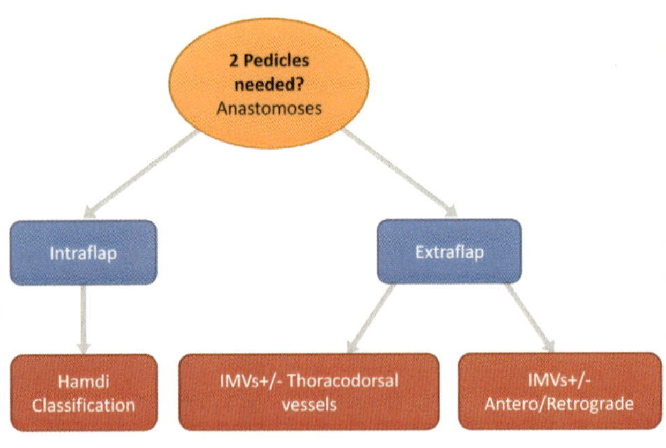


**FIGURE 6 | Flow chart depicting the options in free flap vascular pedicle design for bipedicled microvascular flap anastomoses.**

The next important stage is the evaluation of the superior and inferior "continuities" and branches of the DIE system (**Figure 8**; step 2). We have found that the superior "continuity" of the pedicle can be fragile, especially the venae comitantes, and should be assessed before the pedicle is divided as its vessels collapse post-division and become difficult to evaluate. The critical consideration here is the vein, which tends to be more friable due to its thinner wall. If both the artery and vein of the primary pedicle superior "continuation" have a sufficient caliber and quality, then a superior "continuity" intraflap anastomosis can be made with the secondary pedicle (Hamdi Type IIb or IIIb) (**Figures 5** and **6**). If not, the inferior continuity is considered, which usually supplies the medial row perforators. When basing the flap on lateral row perforators, the ligation of the division leading up to the medial perforators must leave an adequate "stump" for use in Hamdi type IIa and IIIa flap variations (6, 14). Rarely, an artery from the superior "continuity" can be used with a vein from the inferior "continuity" (14, 15) or vice versa. If these "continuities" are not suitable then the second pedicle must be anastomosed in an extraflap arrangement. We avoid the ETS intra-flap anastomoses described by Xu et al. because of the vagaries of this anastomotic type and the concern that it might thrombose due to turbulence at the anastomosis as a consequence of its close proximity to the primary flap anastomosis.

For the recipient vessel selection (**Figure 9**) all the patients in our series had their IMVs exposed using the senior surgeon's total rib-preservation technique (18). In the entire series the primary flap artery was anastomosed to the IMA in an anterograde fashion. The secondary flap artery was anastomosed to the retrograde IMA limb in 64% (16/25) of cases. This reflects the practical ease of a single recipient site and the well-documented adequate retrograde arterial flow (19, 20).

Selecting the appropriate vein for the second pedicle is another crucial step in ensuring pedicled free flap success. Using the same IMV recipients for both pedicles is beneficial because only one recipient site needs to be exposed and the position facilitates the flap inset and shaping. Ideally, two anterograde veins would be used as the recipient vessels to avoid any valves in the retrograde veins (21). We preferentially use the second ICS because of its numerous advantages (18). If the second space is small (<20 mm) we sometimes also expose the third space (**Figure 9**). This serves two purposes:

(a) It may expose the IMV venous confluence and thus provide the easier anterograde venous anastomoses. Often the vein confluence is just under the cranial edge of the third costal cartilage (22, 23).
(b) It lengthens the limbs of the vessels to be used for antero-grade and retrograde anastomoses.

However, care must be taken when dissecting the vessels under the third rib cartilage. This is aided by the observation that there are no side branches of the IMVs directly under the cartilage where visibility would be difficult. The need for meticulous ligation of any tributaries at the superior and inferior aspects of the third costal cartilage is obvious. To facilitate the anastomoses, the third costal cartilage could be sacrificed as in the traditional method of IMV exposure, but we have not found this to be necessary in our series.

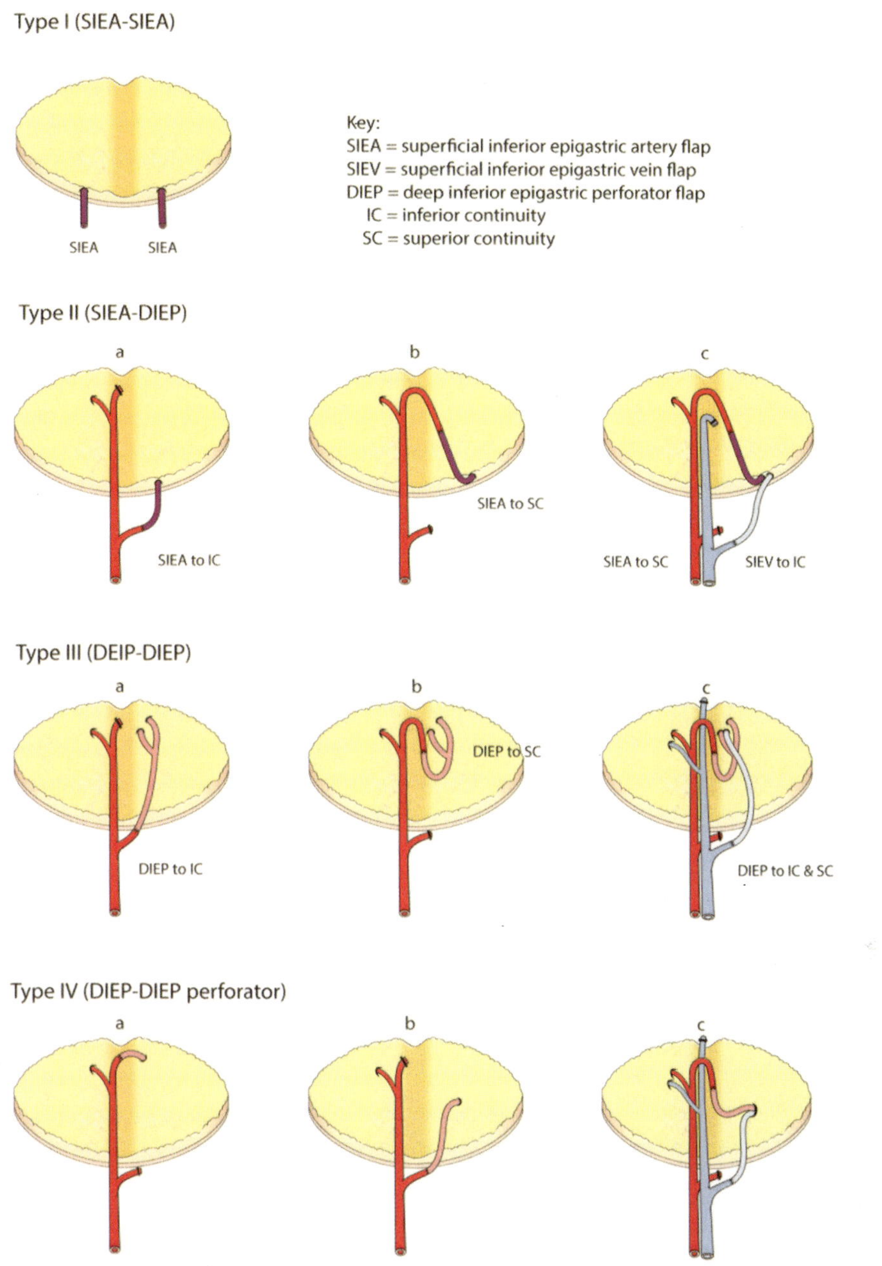


**FIGURE 7 | Comprehensive classification of the variations for intraflap anastomoses in bipedicled abdominal free flaps (modified after Hamdi et al.).**

If two anterograde IM veins are not available we resort to the use of the retrograde limb. In this procedure the vein is clamped with 2 V (venous) Acland clamps at its caudal and cranial ends in the second space and divided at its midpoint (**Figure 9**; step 3). The veins of the primary flap and secondary flaps are anastomosed anterograde and retrograde respectively using venous couplers (**Figure 10**). Some authors have advocated flushing the retrograde vein lumen with heparinized saline to identify any valves or resistance caused by obstruction. We do not believe this to be of any to be of practical significance. If the retrograde limb is not suitable then we consider an *intraflap* vascular arrangement by anastomosing the vein to the superior or inferior continuity.

There may be the rare occurrence in which the veins in both the second and third ICSs are inadequate. In this eventuality ETS anastomosis of the veins may be considered, although none of our cases required this option.

We would only use the TDVs in the axilla as a last resort. Their use would compromise any subsequent use of a salvage latissimus dorsi flap, make the flap inset difficult with anastomoses in two different anatomic locations and lead to lengthened surgical time due to second recipient vessel site exposure. Combined usage of

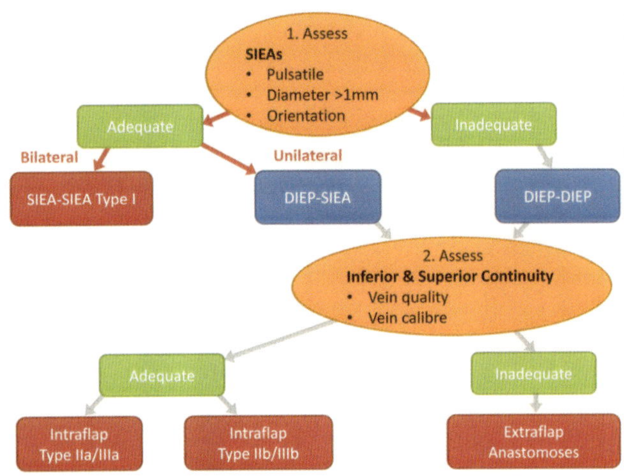


**FIGURE 8 | Flow chart depicting the steps in decision making for the configuration of the flap vessels in abdominal double-pedicled free flap microvascular anastomoses.**

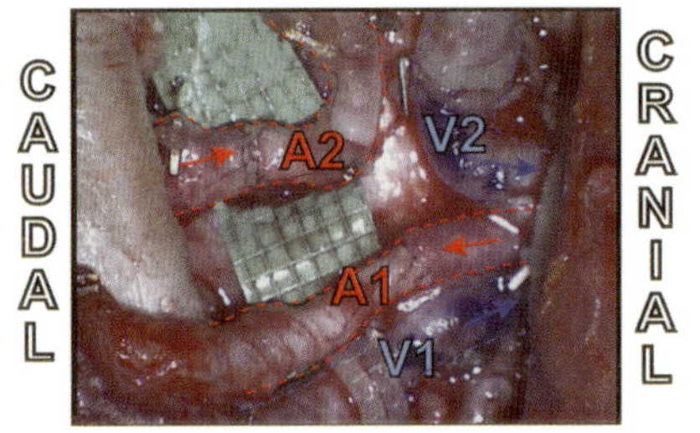


**FIGURE 10 | Intraoperative example of extraflap DIEA–DIEA anastomoses to the internal mammary vessels using two anterograde veins (V1 and V2) both with venous couplers, one antegrade artery (A1) and one retrograde artery (A2).**

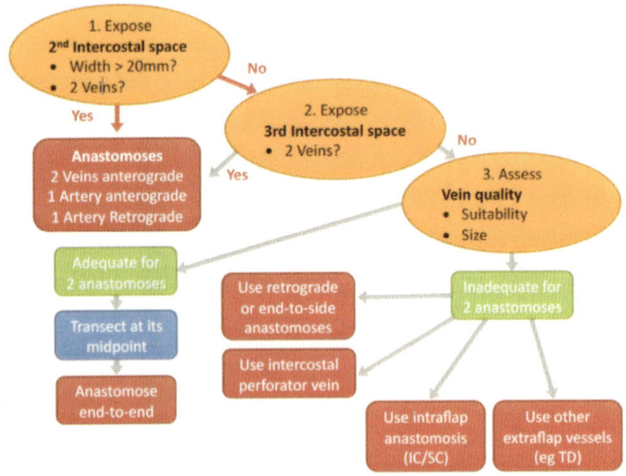


**FIGURE 9 | Flow chart depicting the steps in decision making for determining the configuration of the recipient vessels in abdominal double-pedicled free flap microvascular anastomoses.**

**TABLE 5 | The Malata–Rabey comprehensive classification of double pedicled abdominal free flap anastomoses.**

**A. Intraflap anastomoses**

**Type I** SIEA – SIEA

**Type II** SIEA – DIEP
a. Inferior continuity
b. *Superior continuity*
c. *Combination inferior and superior (vein and artery)*

**Type III** DIEP – DIEP
a. Inferior continuity
b. Superior continuity
c. *Combination of inferior and superior (vein and artery)*

**Type IV** DIEP – DIEP Perforator (left or right)
a. *Inferior continuity (unlikely unless centrally located and long IC)*
b. *Superior continuity*
c. *Combination of inferior and superior (artery and vein): highly unlikely*

**Type V** DIEP – DIEP
a. *End-to-side anastomosis (artery alone) (vein to vena comitans)*
b. *End-to-side anastomosis (artery and vein)*

**B. Extra-flap anastomoses**

**Type I** To a single recipient site: IMVs
a. Flap 1 (both vessels antegrade); Flap 2 (artery retrograde, vein antegrade to second vc)
b. Flap 1 (both vessels antegrade); Flap 2 (both artery and vein retrograde)

**Type II** To a single recipient site: thoracodorsal system
a. Flap 1 (both vessels antegrade); Flap 2 (artery retrograde, vein antegrade to vc)
b. Flap 1 (both vessels antegrade); Flap 2 (both retrograde) – unlikely

**Type III** To two separate recipient sites
a. IMVs and subscapular-thoracodorsal system (preferably above serratus branch)
b. IMVs and pectoral vessels (unlikely)
c. IMVs and other vessels (cephalic vein loop, etc) – when in "trouble"

**C. Combined intraflap and extra-flap anastomoses**

the IMVs and the TDVs for bipedicled anastomoses, however, becomes useful in chest wall reconstruction as the "flattened" flap adequately covers a wide chest defect. It is also easier to use the TDVs if the reconstruction is immediate with an associated axillary lymph node clearance. This exposes the vessels in advance, a key advantage of the subscapular-thoracodorsal system (24, 25).

To ensure good perfusion of the main flap, we perform the primary pedicle anastomosis first after exposing and evaluating the recipient vessels. This also reduces the risk of thrombosis at the secondary anastomoses. In contrast, Xu et al. and the Broomfield group carry out the *intraflap* anastomosis initially (7, 10). We prefer using a coupler for all our venous anastomoses as it is quick, technically easier and helps reduce flap ischemia time. After full flap perfusion, the flap can be inset in a *coned*, *folded*, *stacked*, or *adjacent* arrangement taking great care not to disrupt the anastomoses. When folding the flap we place the flexure inferiorly in order to give the best esthetic appearance, but it can be made superiorly depending on the breast projection desired.

The disadvantages of bipedicled free flaps are their technical complexity, difficulty in flap inset and shaping, tightness of the abdominal closure, prolonged surgical duration and cost. However, we believe that by considering the crucial factors discussed above the surgeon can minimize the donor site morbidity, reduce the duration of flap harvest and vessel anastomosis and optimize the ease of flap inset. From our experience we have proposed a treatment algorithm in **Figures 8** and **9** and a comprehensive classification of bipedicled free flap abdominal reconstructions (**Table 5**; **Figure 7**).

## Conclusion

Bipedicled free flaps can sometimes be necessary in patients undergoing abdominal flap breast reconstruction and can be successfully undertaken in large microvascular surgery centers. They are a reliable and safe option for unilateral autologous breast reconstruction when the volume of tissue required to make a breast mound is larger than that can be transferred on a single flap pedicle. They can greatly benefit the correct patient.

There are numerous techniques for the microsurgical constructs of bipedicled flaps and surgeons intending to perform this surgery should be familiar with them. Our series shows that double-pedicled abdominal free flaps can be safely undertaken with total rib-preservation technique of internal mammary vessel exposure. The algorithm that we have derived from our experience can assist surgeons embarking on this complex microsurgery if they adopt the discussed principles.

## References


1. Hartrampf CR, Scheflan M, Black PW. Breast reconstruction with a transverse abdominal island flap. *Plast Reconstr Surg* (1982) **69**(2):216–25. doi:10.1097/00006534-198202000-00006
2. Holm C, Mayr M, Hofter E, Ninkovic M. Perfusion zones of the DIEP flap revisited: a clinical study. *Plast Reconstr Surg* (2006) **117**(1):37–43. doi:10.1097/01.prs.0000185867.84172.c0
3. Arnez ZM, Scamp T. The bipedicled free TRAM flap. *Br J Plast Surg* (1992) **45**(3):214–8. doi:10.1016/0007-1226(92)90080-H
4. Blondeel PN, Boeckx WD. Refinements in free flap breast reconstruction: the free bilateral deep inferior epigastric perforator flap anastomosed to the internal mammary artery. *Br J Plast Surg* (1994) **47**(7):495–501. doi:10.1016/0007-1226(94)90033-7
5. Agarwal JP, Gottlieb LJ. Double pedicle deep inferior epigastric perforator/muscle-sparing TRAM flaps for unilateral breast reconstruction. *Ann Plast Surg* (2007) **58**(4):359–63. doi:10.1097/01.sap.0000239818.28900.81
6. Hamdi M, Khuthaila DK, Van Landuyt K, Roche N, Monstrey S. Double-pedicle abdominal perforator free flaps for unilateral breast reconstruction: new horizons in microsurgical tissue transfer to the breast. *J Plast Reconstr Aesthet Surg* (2007) **60**(8):904–12;discussion13–4. doi:10.1016/j.bjps.2007.02.016
7. Xu H, Dong J, Wang T. Bipedicle deep inferior epigastric perforator flap for unilateral breast reconstruction: seven years' experience. *Plast Reconstr Surg* (2009) **124**(6):1797–807. doi:10.1097/PRS.0b013e3181bf81cf
8. Beahm EK, Walton RL. The efficacy of bilateral lower abdominal free flaps for unilateral breast reconstruction. *Plast Reconstr Surg* (2007) **120**(1):41–54. doi:10.1097/01.prs.0000263729.26936.31
9. Ali RS, Garrido A, Ramakrishnan V. Stacked free hemi-DIEP flaps: a method of autologous breast reconstruction in a patient with midline abdominal scarring. *Br J Plast Surg* (2002) **55**(4):351–3. doi:10.1054/bjps.2002.3834
10. Figus A, Fioramonti P, Ramakrishnan V. Stacked free SIEA/DIEP flap for unilateral breast reconstruction in a thin patient with an abdominal vertical midline scar. *J Reconstr Microsurg* (2007) **23**(8):523–5. doi:10.1055/s-2007-1022692
11. Schoeller T, Wechselberger G, Roger J, Hussl H, Huemer GM. Management of infraumbilical vertical scars in DIEP-flaps by crossover anastomosis. *J Plast Reconstr Aesthet Surg* (2007) **60**(5):524–8.
12. Chan RK, Przylecki W, Guo L, Caterson SA. Case report. The use of both antegrade and retrograde internal mammary vessels in a folded, stacked deep inferior epigastric artery perforator flap. *Eplasty* (2010) **10**:e32.
13. DellaCroce FJ, Sullivan SK, Trahan C. Stacked deep inferior epigastric perforator flap breast reconstruction: a review of 110 flaps in 55 cases over 3 years. *Plast Reconstr Aesthet Surg* (2011) **127**(3):1093–9.
14. Rabey NG, Erel E, Malata CM. Double-pedicled abdominal free flap using an entirely new microvascular combination of DIEP and SIEA vascular pedicles for unilateral breast reconstruction: a novel addition to the Hamdi classification. *Plast Reconstr Surg* (2012) **130**(5):767e–9e. doi:10.1097/PRS.0b013e318267d995
15. Mohan AT, Patel NG, Malata CM. Combination of the superior and inferior pedicle "continuities" for anastomosis of an SIEA flap to a contralateral DIEP flap in double-pedicled abdominal free flaps: a further modification of the Hamdi classification. *J Plast Reconstr Aesthet Surg* (2014) **67**(10):e237–9. doi:10.1016/j.bjps.2014.06.008
16. Li S, Mu L, Li Y, Xu J, Yang M, Zhao Z, et al. Breast reconstruction with the free bipedicled inferior TRAM flap by anastomosis to the proximal and distal ends of the internal mammary vessels. *J Reconstr Microsurg* (2002) **18**(3):161–8. doi:10.1055/s-2002-28498
17. Ng RL, Youssef A, Kronowitz SJ, Lipa JE, Potochny J, Reece GP. Technical variations of the bipedicled TRAM flap in unilateral breast reconstruction: effects of conventional versus microsurgical techniques of pedicle transfer on complications rates. *Plast Reconstr Surg* (2004) **114**(2):374–84;discussion85–8. doi:10.1097/01.PRS.0000131879.34814.8A
18. Malata CM, Moses M, Mickute Z, Di Candia M. Tips for successful microvascular abdominal flap breast reconstruction utilizing the "total rib preservation" technique for internal mammary vessel exposure. *Ann Plast Surg* (2011) **66**(1):36–42. doi:10.1097/SAP.0b013e3181e19daf
19. Agarwal JP, Ley E, Tieman J. Salvage of SIEA flaps using the retrograde internal mammary system. *Microsurgery* (2010) **30**(7):545–8. doi:10.1002/micr.20791
20. Salgarello M, Visconti G, Barone-Adesi L, Cina A. The retrograde limb of internal mammary vessels as reliable recipient vessels in DIEP flap breast reconstruction: a clinical and radiological study. *Ann Plast Surg* (2013) **74**(4):447–53. doi:10.1097/SAP.0b013e31829fd2e3
21. Mackey SP, Ramsey KW. Exploring the myth of the valveless internal mammary vein – a cadaveric study. *J Plast Reconstr Aesthet Surg* (2011) **64**(9):1174–9. doi:10.1016/j.bjps.2011.03.045
22. Arnez ZM, Valdatta L, Tyler MP, Planinsek F. Anatomy of the internal mammary veins and their use in free TRAM flap breast reconstruction. *Br J Plast Surg* (1995) **48**(8):540–5. doi:10.1016/0007-1226(95)90041-1
23. Clark CP III, Rohrich RJ, Copit S, Pittman CE, Robinson J. An anatomic study of the internal mammary veins: clinical implications for free-tissue-transfer breast reconstruction. *Plast Reconstr Surg* (1997) **99**(2):400–4. doi:10.1097/00006534-199702000-00014
24. Moran SL, Nava G, Behnam AB, Serletti JM. An outcome analysis comparing the thoracodorsal and internal mammary vessels as recipient sites for microvascular breast reconstruction: a prospective study of 100 patients. *Plast Reconstr Surg* (2003) **111**(6):1876–82. doi:10.1097/01.PRS.0000056872.06003.7E
25. Pradas-Irun C, Azzawi K, Malata CM. A plea for recipient vascular pedicle versatility in microvascular breast reconstruction: the conundrum of absent internal mammary veins. *Plast Reconstr Surg* (2012) **129**(2):383e–5e. doi:10.1097/PRS.0b013e31823aeec2

# 15

# Tissue-Engineered Solutions in Plastic and Reconstructive Surgery: Principles and Practice

*Sarah Al-Himdani[1,2†], Zita M. Jessop[1,2†], Ayesha Al-Sabah[1], Emman Combellack[1,2], Amel Ibrahim[1,2,3], Shareen H. Doak[1,4], Andrew M. Hart[5], Charles W. Archer[1,6], Catherine A. Thornton[1,7] and Iain S. Whitaker[1,2*]*

*[1] Reconstructive Surgery and Regenerative Medicine Research Group (ReconRegen), Institute of Life Science, Swansea University Medical School, Swansea, UK, [2] The Welsh Centre for Burns and Plastic Surgery, Morriston Hospital, Swansea, UK, [3] Institute of Child Health, University College London, London, UK, [4] In Vitro Toxicology Group, Institute of Life Science, Swansea University Medical School, Swansea, UK, [5] Canniesburn Plastic Surgery Unit, Centre for Cell Engineering, University of Glasgow, Glasgow, UK, [6] Cartilage Biology Research Group, Institute of Life Science, Swansea University Medical School, Swansea, UK, [7] Human Immunology Group, Institute of Life Science, Swansea University Medical School, Swansea, UK*

**Edited by:**
*Jan A. Plock, University of Zurich, Switzerland*

**Reviewed by:**
*Fatih Zor, Gulhane Military Medical Academy, Turkey*
*Michael P. Chae, Peninsula Health, Australia*

***Correspondence:**
*Iain S. Whitaker*
*i.s.whitaker@swansea.ac.uk*

*[†]Joint first authors.*

**Specialty section:**
*This article was submitted to Reconstructive and Plastic Surgery, a section of the journal Frontiers in Surgery*

Recent advances in microsurgery, imaging, and transplantation have led to significant refinements in autologous reconstructive options; however, the morbidity of donor sites remains. This would be eliminated by successful clinical translation of tissue-engineered solutions into surgical practice. Plastic surgeons are uniquely placed to be intrinsically involved in the research and development of laboratory engineered tissues and their subsequent use. In this article, we present an overview of the field of tissue engineering, with the practicing plastic surgeon in mind. The Medical Research Council states that regenerative medicine and tissue engineering "holds the promise of revolutionizing patient care in the twenty-first century." The UK government highlighted regenerative medicine as one of the key eight great technologies in their industrial strategy worthy of significant investment. The long-term aim of successful biomanufacture to repair composite defects depends on interdisciplinary collaboration between cell biologists, material scientists, engineers, and associated medical specialties; however currently, there is a current lack of coordination in the field as a whole. Barriers to translation are deep rooted at the basic science level, manifested by a lack of consensus on the ideal cell source, scaffold, molecular cues, and environment and manufacturing strategy. There is also insufficient understanding of the long-term safety and durability of tissue-engineered constructs. This review aims to highlight that individualized approaches to the field are not adequate, and research collaboratives will be essential to bring together differing areas of expertise to expedite future clinical translation. The use of tissue engineering in reconstructive surgery would result in a paradigm shift but it is important to maintain realistic expectations. It is generally accepted that it takes 20–30 years from the start of basic science research to clinical utility, demonstrated by contemporary treatments such as bone marrow transplantation. Although great advances have been made in the tissue engineering field, we highlight the barriers that need to be overcome before we see the routine use of tissue-engineered solutions.

**Keywords: tissue engineering, regenerative medicine, stem cells, translation, bioengineering, barriers to translation, translational research, plastic and reconstructive surgery**

# INTRODUCTION

Reconstructive plastic surgery aims to provide living tissue in order to restore both form and function following a wide range of congenital or acquired defects. Operations are complex, often transcending anatomic boundaries. Versatility resulting from surgery on a full range of tissues including skin, fat, nerve, muscle, bone, and cartilage promotes innovation, and with the recent advances in medical imaging (1), microsurgery (2), vascularized composite allotransplantation (3, 4), nanotechnology (5), cell biology, biomaterials (6), and 3D printing (7–10), treatment options for patients are wider than ever before. Even armed with new reconstructive options based on microsurgical principles and transplantation, surgeons have become increasingly cognizant that there is the real potential for a paradigm shift in reconstructive surgery in the medium term via tissue-engineered solutions. The implementation into practice could potentially eliminate the need for donor sites and their morbidity, reduce hospital stay and associated costs (11).

## Relevance of This Article

Contrary to public perception, the diverse workload of reconstructive plastic surgeons comprises a relatively small proportion of purely esthetic procedures (12). The majority of operations undertaken pertain to neoplasia and wound management, with a significant health economic impact (12). Over one million patients are treated per year in NHS England by Plastic Surgeons (13, 14), with evidence suggesting that this workload will continue to increase (15). If you extrapolate these figures worldwide, it is easy to see the clinical need is vast. As a group, reconstructive surgeons are facing more challenging composite defects than ever before coupled with Internet and media savvy patients with increasing expectations (16). Technological innovation in reconstructive surgery in the twentieth century offered the possibility for surgeons to operate on microvascular structures enabling free tissue transfers (2) and extremity replantations. Despite these developments in practice, we are still confronted with shortcomings relating to the availability of donor tissues. In order to overcome this, novel approaches have been investigated. Among these approaches, the most attractive concept is tissue engineering.

Tissue engineering is a modern, interdisciplinary field combining principles of engineering, physics, and the life sciences. It shares a common objective with plastic and reconstructive surgery; "to restore form and function" (17, 18). The long-term aim of tissue engineering is to biomanufacture autologous, vascularized, physiologically relevant solutions to repair and restore complex defects. Successful biomanufacture will depend on the correct blend of cell source, suitable scaffold and ideal microenvironment (19). Answers to these fundamental questions rely on interdisciplinary collaboration between cell biologists, material scientists, biotechnologists, and associated medical specialties (20). Upscaling and widespread use in health services will need close interaction with the cell therapy industry and associated manufacturers.

The surgical community worldwide is becoming increasingly aware of the research landscape. The American Society of Plastic surgeons have highlighted the role of tissue engineering in the future of plastic surgery (21), particularly the need for a focus on translation from bench research to clinical practice. In the United Kingdom, the House of Lords recognized the potential of regenerative medicine to impact on the health service and highlighted the current "lack of coordination" in the field as a whole (22, 23). Recommendations included the development of multidisciplinary working groups (basic scientists, clinicians, investors, manufacturing experts, and regulators), as well as governmental support to drive forward the agenda on regenerative medicine.

There is a need to develop NHS capacity with regional facilities licensed for Good Laboratory Practice (GLP) and current Good Manufacturing Practices (cGMP), which are engaged with a clinical specialty skilled in the manipulation of cells and the viable insertion of tissue-engineered constructs. Skilled in vascularization and in tissue viability/transfer, plastic surgeons already fulfill this role as an interface specialty delivering complex reconstructive techniques to a broad range of other specialties. The regional service structure of plastic surgery within the NHS would further support their capacity to align with regional cGMP facilities and deliver tissue-engineering solutions to a range of medical and surgical specialties.

## Objectives

### Assess the Shortcomings Of

*Traditional Reconstructive Options*

Up till now, restoration of form and function has relied on the use of autologous (rarely allogeneic) tissue, alloplastic implants, or a combination of the two. Although effective, these options have disadvantages that merit highlighting (**Table 1**).

*Tissue-Engineered Solutions*

Although tissue-engineered solutions hold great promise, we must be realistic in that contemporary tissue-engineered constructs implanted into immune-competent animal models have been observed to undergo inflammation, fibrosis, foreign body reaction, and degradation (**Table 1**; **Figure 1**). One of the major problems remains vascularization of larger volume constructs (24), and an issue coming to the fore in modern literature is the potential for tumorigenesis (25).

### Provide an Overview Of

*Fundamental Principles of Tissue Engineering: Cell Source, Scaffold, Assembly Method, and Molecular and Mechanical Signaling*

We discuss the multiple considerations for tissue engineering research in order to highlight the complexity of the field as a whole. This supports the argument for multidisciplinary coordination, which is required to take the field forward. The fundamental principles are summarized in **Figure 2**: cell source, scaffolds, assembly method, subsequent growth (molecular and mechanical signaling), and patient safety. These factors all contribute to the "environment" (19). In simple terms, the cell is required for synthesis of the new tissue matrix, while the scaffold, biomolecules, and the microenvironment provide trophic cues to guide proliferation and differentiation. Growth, induction, and

**TABLE 1 | Advantages and shortcomings of reconstructive solutions for managing tissue defects.**

| Reconstructive solution | Advantages | Disadvantages |
|---|---|---|
| Autologous | • No immunological complications<br>• No ethical constraints<br>• Biologically compatible<br>• Minimal degradation<br>• Fewer legal restrictions<br>• No disease transmission<br>• Challenging harvesting cells in aged or diseased | • Donor site morbidity<br>• Limited quantity of tissue available<br>• Two separate operative sites—greater risk and cost |
| Allogeneic | • No donor site morbidity<br>• Donor cells may have higher viability<br>• Tissue always healthy<br>• Greater quantity of available tissue | • Temporary (i.e., cadaveric skin used in extensive burns)<br>• Tissue typing is required<br>• Immunosuppression may be needed<br>• Risk of disease transmission<br>• Greater legal hurdles<br>• Ethical and psychological challenges |
| Synthetic | • Maintain structural integrity<br>• Predictable and reproducible physical and mechanical properties<br>• Cost effective<br>• Avoids concerns over disease transmission | • Extrusion<br>• Infection<br>• Cannot restore all of specialized tissue/organ functions<br>• Do not respond to biological cues/grow with patient<br>• May provoke an immune/inflammatory/fibrotic reaction<br>• Materials safety testing and manufacturing governance |
| Tissue engineered | • Biocompatible<br>• Good biofunctionality<br>• Good retention of size and shape<br>• No donor site morbidity<br>• Unlimited expansion of cells/tissues<br>• No immunological concerns<br>• Mechanical stability | • Long-term effect unknown<br>• Size often limited by vascularity<br>• Costly<br>• Tumorigenic potential<br>• Difficult to engineer "physiologically relevant/mature tissue" |

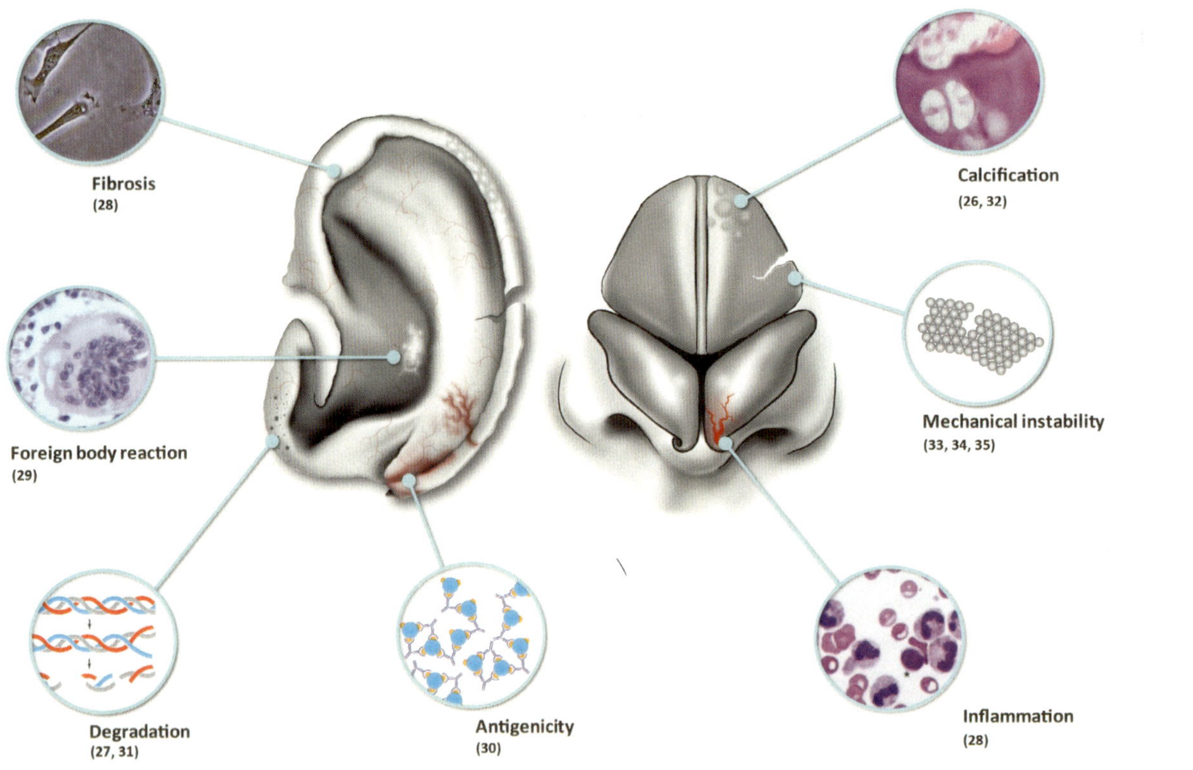


**FIGURE 1** | **Shortcomings of nasal and auricular cartilage tissue engineering.**

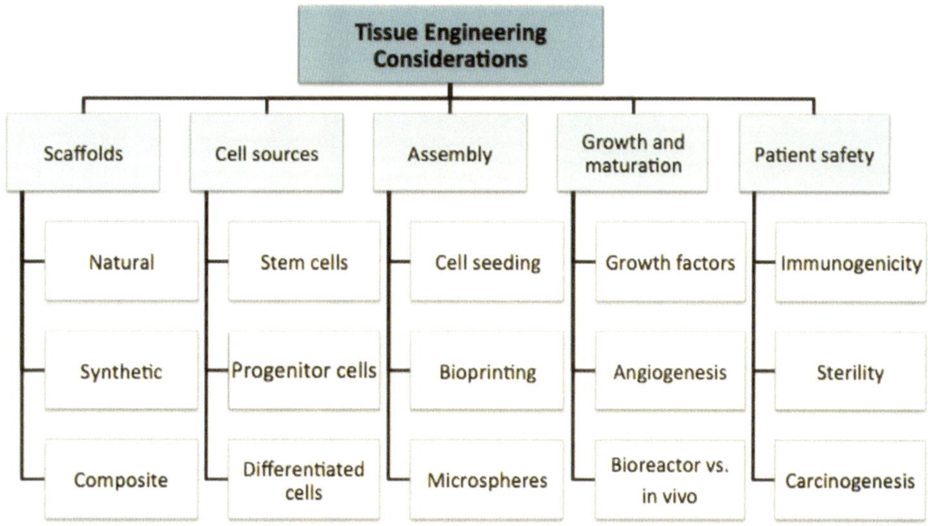


**FIGURE 2** | **Considerations in the field of tissue engineering.**

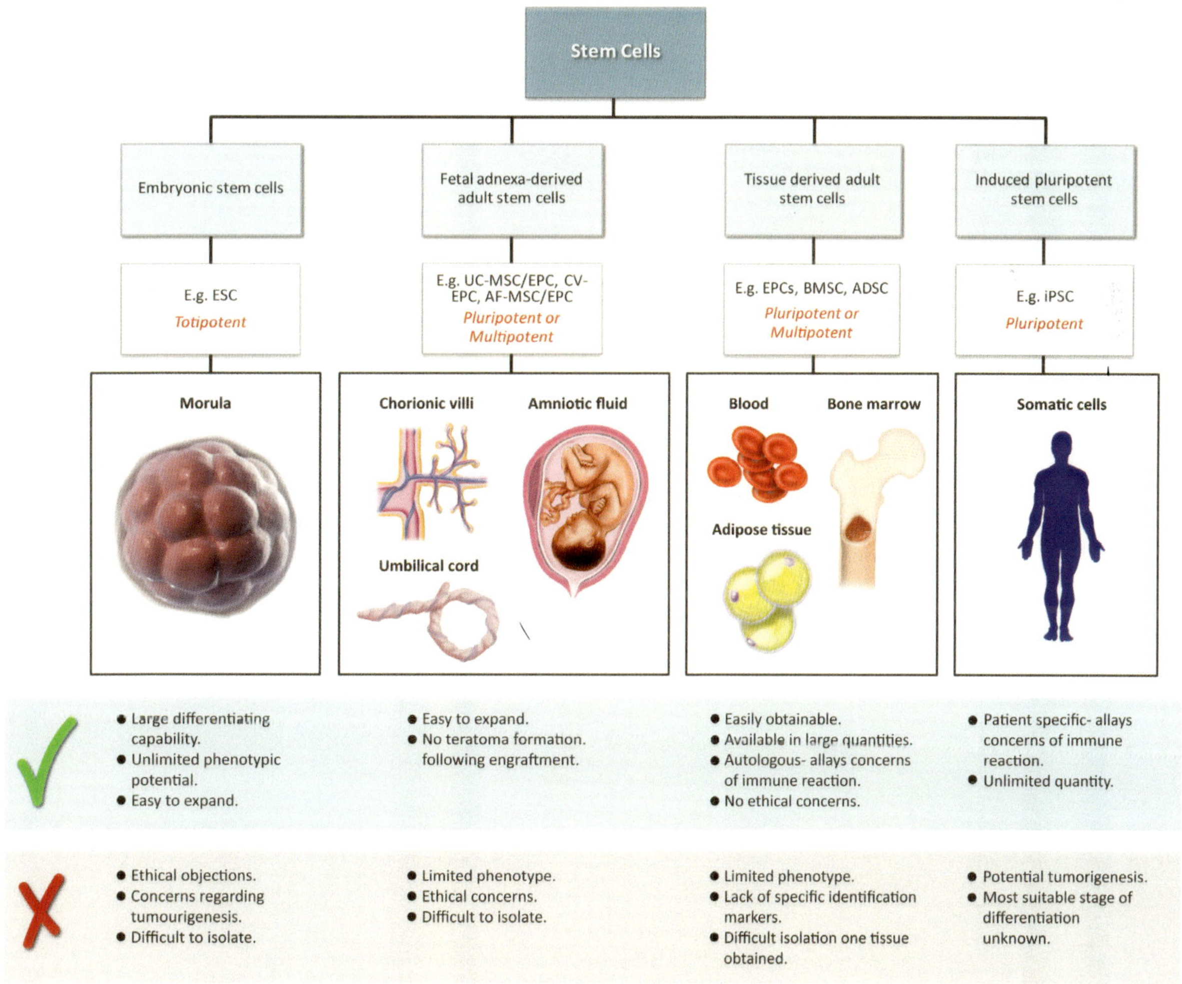


**FIGURE 3** | **Advantages and disadvantages of different cell sources utilized in tissue engineering.**

maintenance of maturation are important for providing durability of the tissue-engineered construct.

### *Cell Sources*

Classical tissue-engineering approaches use *tissue-derived* cells (*not necessarily stem cells*) seeded onto scaffolds (36). These cells may be autologous, allogenic, or xenogenic cells; however, autologous cells are the preferred choice due to the lack of immunogenicity. Cells may be further classified based on differences in their differentiating capabilities (**Figure 3**). Adult somatic cells are fully differentiated, and therefore have restricted future differentiation potential and relatively poor growth, limiting their usefulness for tissue-engineering purposes (37). Progenitor cells are more differentiated than stem cells and are therefore referred to as multipotent rather than pluripotent (38). Stem cells are non-differentiated cells, able to proliferate through multiple generations and differentiate into a variety of cell types (39, 40), and may overcome the limitations of differentiated cells (36) when used for tissue engineering. Pluripotent by definition, stem cells can be derived from embryonic, fetal, or adult (or postnatal somatic) tissue (39). Stem cells are the current preferred cell source for tissue-engineering endeavors and regenerative medicine therapies due to their high potency and capacity for expansion (41). Contemporary research efforts have focused on adult stem cells or progenitor cells for tissue-engineering purposes. The use of embryonic and fetal tissue, although providing pluripotent stem cells with high proliferative potential, raises potential ethical issues as well as safety concerns over tumorigenic potential (42, 43). Adult derived stem cells, which are found among differentiated cells, have been isolated from an increasingly varied number of tissues over the past decade such as bone marrow (i.e., mesenchymal stem cells and hematopoietic stem cells), adipose [adipose-derived stem cells (44)], epithelial (epithelial-derived stem cells), and umbilical cord (cord blood stem cells) tissue (43). Developments made in isolation and culture of adult derived stem cells have improved cell yield during harvest. Subsequent research has focused on manipulating proliferation and differentiation into the desired cell type (45). Adult derived stem cells can only divide a finite number of times and accumulate genetic changes that can limit their supply for tissue-engineering purposes. The discovery of induced pluripotent stem cells (iPSCs) by Takahashi and Yamanaka (46) introduced the idea that a mature differentiated cell could be reverted to a state of pluripotency and multilineage potential (**Figure 4**). While this process, which has been shown to be possible with human cells, creates a potentially limitless source of easily accessible stem cells, it is not without drawbacks (47). Reprograming the cells has raised questions about

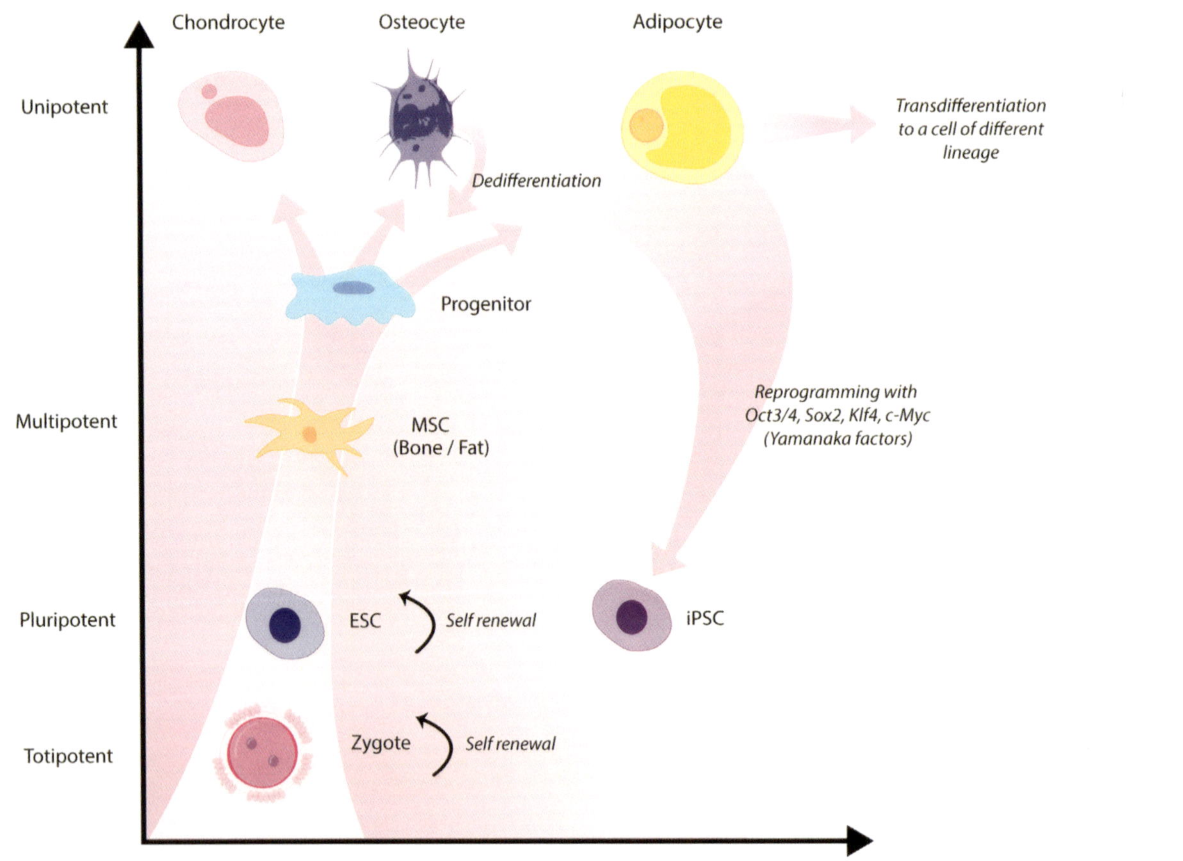


**FIGURE 4 | Hierarchy of stem cells highlighting different degrees of potency**. Yamanaka factors are used to induce differentiated cells to become pluripotent.

epigenetic effects in particular, with a number of papers purporting to show DNA errors that have arisen during the process of inducing pluripotency (47, 48). Questions have also been raised regarding immunogenicity of engineered tissues with iPSCs implanted into a genetically identical mouse able to provoke an unexpected T cell-mediated immune response (49).

To better understand the behavior of specific cell types and their utility for tissue-engineering purposes, there is an increased reliance on advanced technologies (41) to monitor cell phenotype, migration, proliferation, migration, and differentiation both *in vitro* and *in vivo*. Impedance-based systems such as iCELLigence system (ACEA Biosciences) as well as Seahorse XF$^{e}$24 Extracellular Flux Analyzer are allowing real-time monitoring of cellular processes and offer distinct and important advantages over traditional endpoint assays (**Figure 5**). Contemporary imaging modalities such as two photon excited fluorescence microscopy (50) and Raman spectroscopy (51), both with high resolution and depth of penetration (>100 nm, 300 nm and 1 mm, 0.4 mm, respectively) are giving researchers clearer insights into the behavior of different cell types (**Figure 5**).

Further complications arise from the wide donor-to-donor variation in the behavior of cells, particularly stem cell populations, that has become apparent. Human adipose-derived stem cells, an increasingly prevalent source of adult stem cells for studies in tissue engineering, exhibit high donor-to-donor variability with regard to proliferation and differentiation characteristics, and this is not explained simply by donor age (52).

Currently, there is no consensus on the *ideal* cell source for tissue-engineering purposes. A thorough understanding of the advantages and disadvantages of each cell type is crucial to decide on cell selection and the optimal culture conditions in order to engineer specific tissue types.

### *Scaffold Choices*

An appropriate scaffold is crucial to any tissue-engineering strategy. The ideal scaffold provides a framework for cell growth and development, allowing cells to attach, migrate, proliferate, and differentiate while facilitating cellular reorganization into a functional 3D network (**Table 2**).

Desirable characteristics of scaffolds include the following:

- Biomimetic (53)
- Biodegradable (with site specific absorption kinetics) (54–56)
- Appropriate mechanical strength
- Optimal micropores: enabling vascularization and allowing metabolic needs to be met (oxygen and waste product transfer)
- Biocompatible (57)
- Non-immunogenic (58)
- Versatile with regard to manufacturing methods
- Functionalization potential (59)

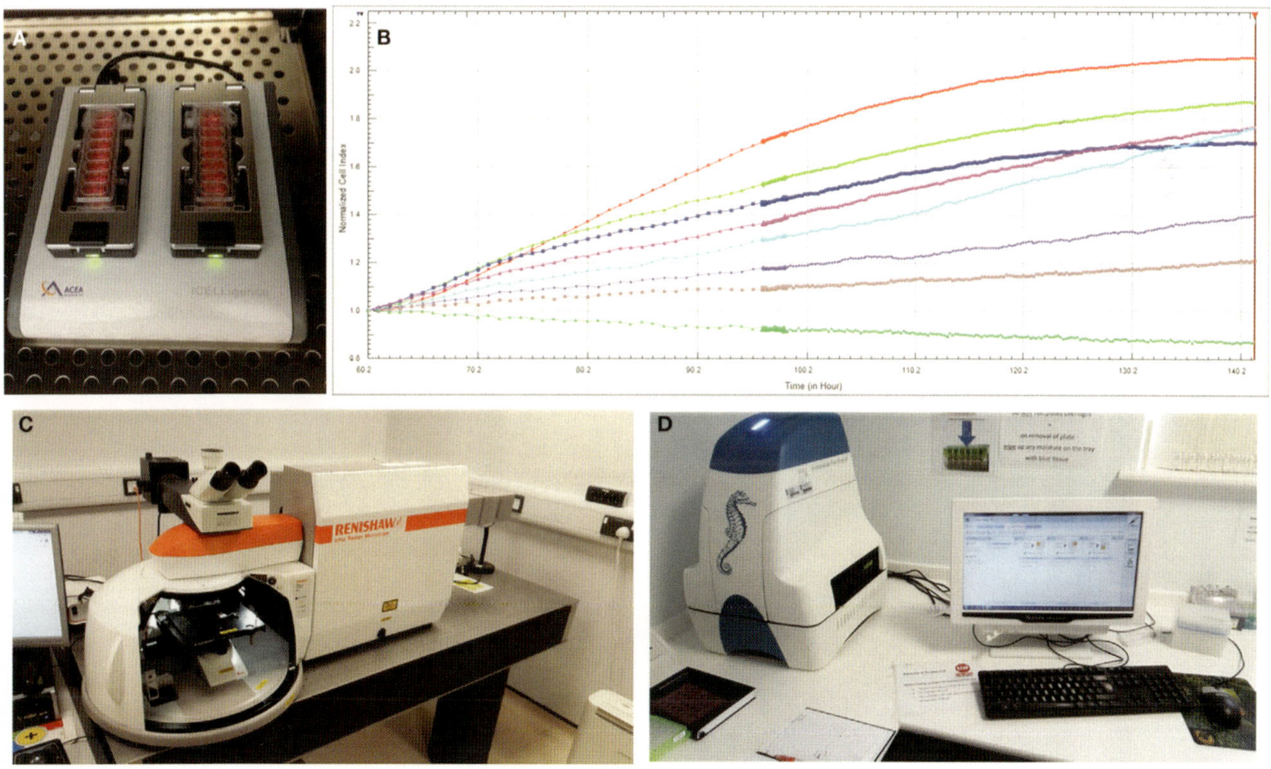


**FIGURE 5 | Advanced technologies for monitoring cell behavior and survival. (A)** ICELLigence impedance based cell assay machine. **(B)** Proliferation curves at different cell seeding densities generated by iCELLigence. **(C)** The Renishaw inVia confocal Raman microscope allows identification of stem cells based on the scattering of photons due to vibrations of molecular bonds. **(D)** Seahorse XF$^{e}$24 Extracellular Flux Analyzer is used for measurement of cellular bioenergetics.

**TABLE 2 | Advantages and disadvantages of biomaterials utilized currently as scaffolds in tissue engineering.**

| Scaffold class | Scaffold subtype | Macrostructure | Microstructure | Chemical composition | Advantages | Disadvantages |
|---|---|---|---|---|---|---|
| Synthetic | Polylactic acid (PLA) | 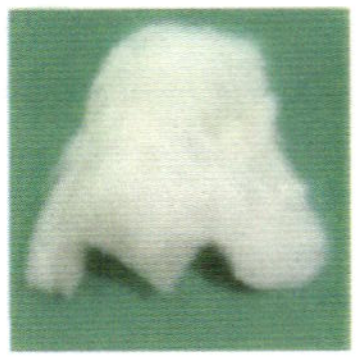 | 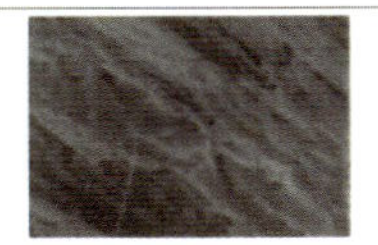 | 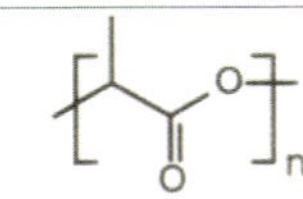 | • More predictable and reproducible mechanical and physical properties<br>• High tensile strength, degradation rate, and elastic modulus (7)<br>• More readily available<br>• Relatively inexpensive | • Immune reaction<br>• Lack biological cues (8)<br>• Toxicity<br>• Infections |
| | Polyglycolic acid (PGA) | 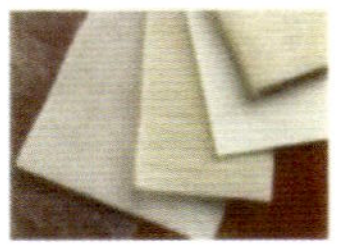 | 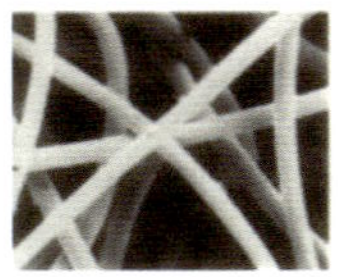 | 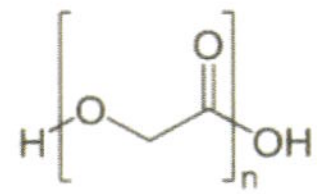 | | |
| | Polyethylene glycol derivatives (PEG) |  | 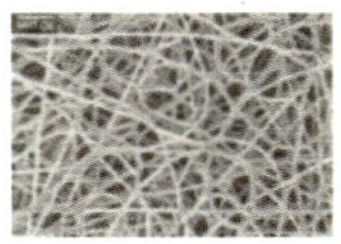 | 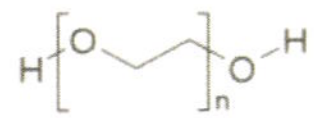 | | |
| Biological | Fibrin | 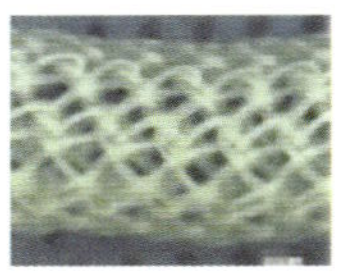 | 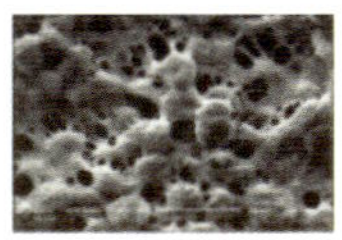 | 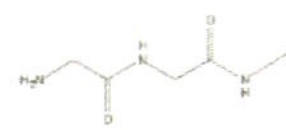 | • Biocompatibility<br>• Cell-controlled degradability<br>• Intrinsic cellular interaction<br>• Hydrated environment<br>• Non-toxic<br>• Mucoadhesive<br>• Cytocompatible (9) | • Batch variations<br>• Limited range of mechanical properties<br>• Less reproducible<br>• Costly<br>• Specific processing conditions (10) |
| | Elastin | 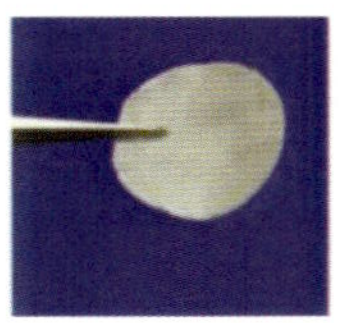 | 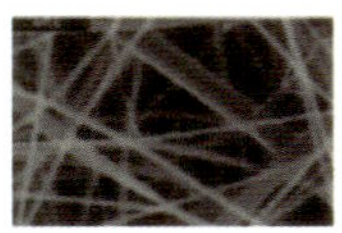 | 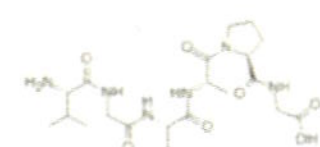 | | |
| | Collagen | 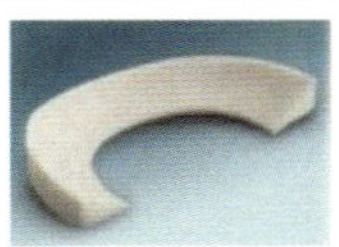 | 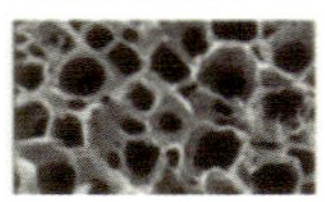 | 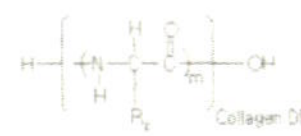 | | |

*(Continued)*

**TABLE 2** | Continued

| Scoffold class | Scaffold subtype | Macrostructure | Microstructure | Chemical composition | Advantages | Disadvantages |
|---|---|---|---|---|---|---|
| | Alginate | 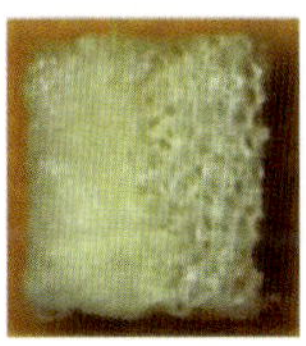 | 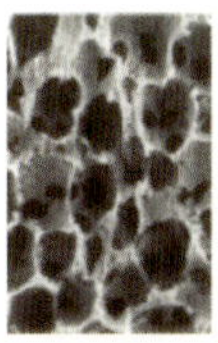 | 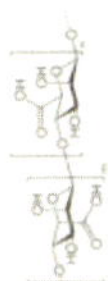 | | |
| | Agarose | 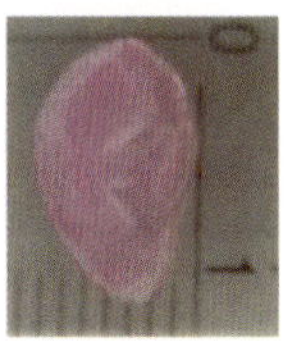 | 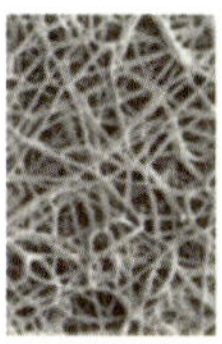 | 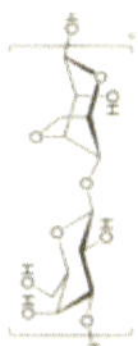 | | |

- 3D control of macroarchitecture
- Various nano- and micro-topographies, stiffnesses, and micro-environments appropriate to the proliferation, migration, and maturation of native or engrafted cells
- Suitable for clinical grade sterilization
- Suitable for industrial production.

Scaffolds are generally classified as biological (organic) or synthetic (inorganic). Engineering of the cell-scaffold construct can be undertaken *in vitro* in a bioreactor or *in vivo* by implanting the construct into the body. Advances in engineering, material science, and biomanufacturing technologies have enabled the design and development of more complex scaffolds using self assembly (60), computer modeling, bioprinting, and nano-technology (60–62). "Functionalized," "decorated," or "smart" biomaterials that incorporate of biomolecular moieties on the surface, aim to orchestrate, and optimize the attachment and growth of cells and the synthesis of new tissue (61, 63). Scaffold size is largely limited by the lack of effective vascularization. Most successful work in the field focuses on understanding native tissue constituents and microarchitecture to allow accurate reproduction of functional tissue (64).

### *Environment*

Consideration of the biophysiochemical 3D environment is crucial for tissue engineering. Cells not only require a scaffold for structural and biological support but also require an environment that provides the correct combination of growth supplements, differentiation signals, perfusion of nutrients, gaseous/waste exchange, pH regulation, and mechanical forces. The metabolic requirements of different tissues are varied and dictate the perfusion, gaseous/waste exchange, pH, and mechanical environment required. There is an increasing awareness that molecular and mechanical signaling is pivotal in the growth and differentiation of tissue-engineered constructs, and in addition to well-known growth factors such as bone morphogenetic proteins, vascular epithelial growth factor, basic fibroblast growth factor FGF-2, and transforming growth factor-β (65), "induction factors," including oxygen tension (66–68), mechanical (69), and electrical stimulation (70), guide subsequent proliferation and differentiation of cells. Cells participate in a web of multidirectional interactions within their niches and tissues of residence [interacting with various nanotopographically sized cues (71)]. This has implications during biomimetic tissue engineering, where the cellular environment (biomolecules), scaffold topography, and other external factors (mechanical and electrical stimulation) require regulation. This is complicated by the fact that cells not only respond to multiple stimuli but also have a direct impact on the environment themselves.

Research in this field is at the interface of cell biologists, engineers, materials scientists, and clinicians and is expanding rapidly. Multidisciplinary teams are working on bioreactor technology, which is vital for *in vitro* tissue engineering. Optimal conditions can to a great extent be applied and controlled through the use of bioreactors to mimic required conditions (72), and specialized bioreactors to help engineer a range of tissues have been developed in recent years (73, 74). Bioreactors are

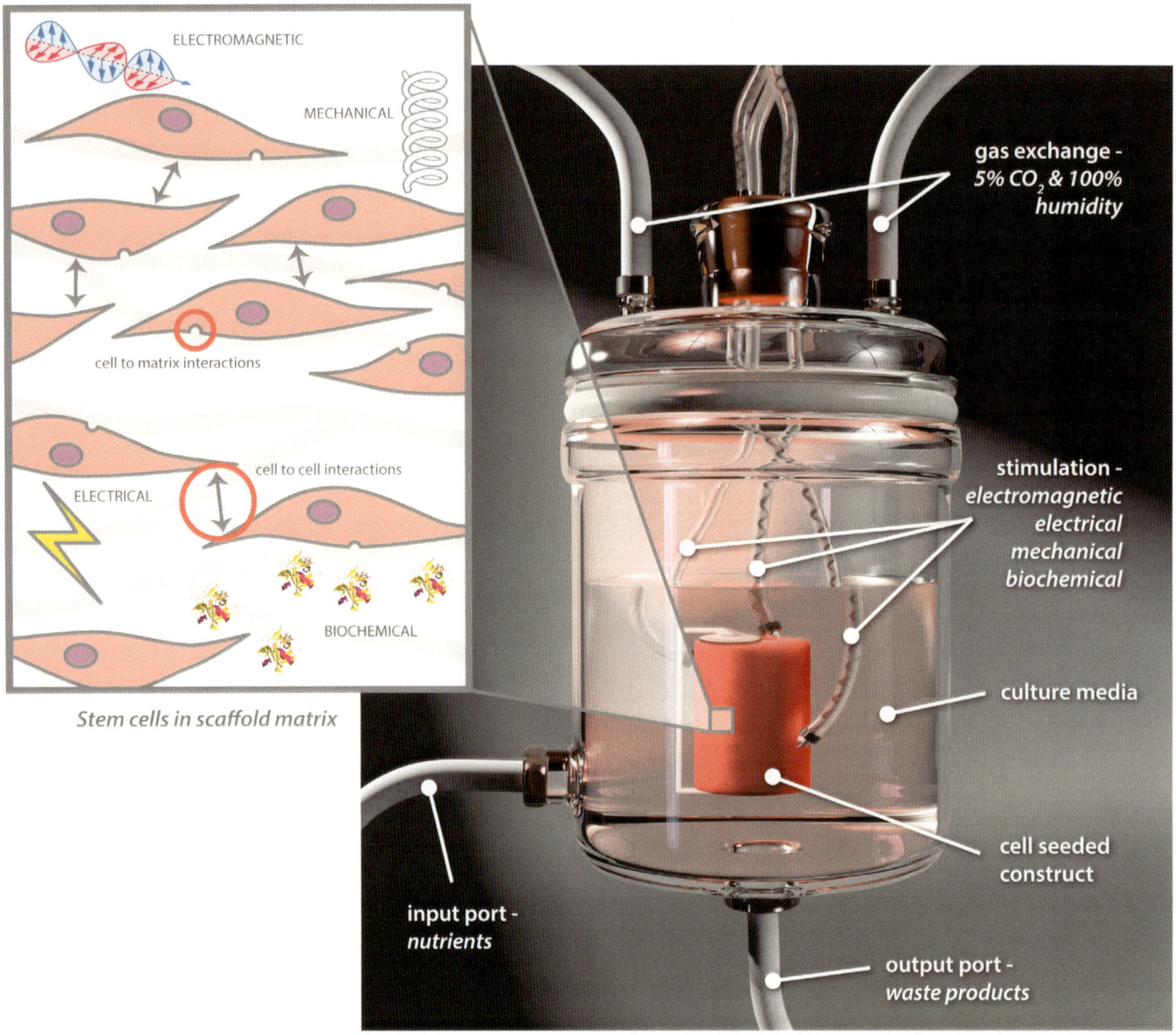


**FIGURE 6 | Different environmental stimuli and the fundamental components of bioreactor technology.**

increasingly being used to provide more complex environments, exposing cells to a range of controllable electrical, electromagnetic, biomolecular, and mechanical cues while varying cell–cell or cell–matrix interactions (**Figure 6**) (73).

## CURRENT BARRIERS TO TRANSLATION

Tissue engineering has the potential for major clinical impact in plastic and reconstructive surgery. Some products using tissue-engineering concepts are already on the market; however, the panacea of functional vascularized composite tissue-engineered constructs is still theoretical. Translation of good basic science research from the laboratory to clinical reality remains a considerable challenge (**Figure 7**). In addition to meeting the scientific challenges of engineering durable and functional tissue for implantation into patients (75), one must also navigate the complex regulatory processes. The regulations controlling the delivery of stem cell therapeutics to the clinic parallel many of those developed for the pharmaceutical industry (76, 77). Guidelines governing the development of cell-based products can be found on websites for the U.S. Food and Drug Administration (FDA),[1] the European Medicines Agency,[2] and related governmental regulatory authorities. The United States Pharmacopeia is an internationally recognized resource defining the currently accepted industry standards for product purity, potency, and quality assurance.[3] These targets are hard to meet outside a large,

[1] http://www.fda.gov/.
[2] http://www.ema.europa.eu/ema.
[3] http://www.usp.org/.

well-equipped commercial enterprise. Many research laboratories attached to clinical facilities do not produce mesenchymal stem cells in accordance with the criteria for either GLP or the more stringent cGMP, both requiring strict operational and certification records relating to all laboratory equipment and reagents used in the cell manufacture process (1, 4, 5).

A clear understanding of the manufacturing workflow is required to allow autologous and allogeneic tissue-engineered product integration into clinical practice (78). Once cells are obtained from a donor, they must be stored in specialized banks and both "scaled-up" (increasing batch size) and "scaled out" (increasing number of batches). There are several challenges in mass production alone including the monitoring of product yield and ensuring purity, potency, and viability throughout the process. Mass production of autologous tissue requires a facility allowing multiple, parallel, patient-specific production lines. Where scaffolds are required, testing and maintenance of quality attributes needs to be undertaken prior to seeding (78). Additional challenges include storage/transportation, contamination, and obtaining regulatory approval.

The long-term safety, efficacy, and functionality of the products also need to be closely assessed (79). Practical considerations that need to be contemplated include the storage environment and shelf life of the manufactured products.

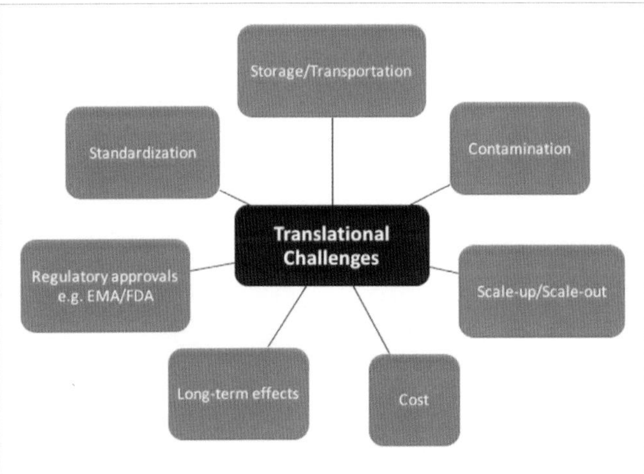


**FIGURE 7 | Barriers to translation in tissue engineering.**

It is also of interest that tissue-engineered products do not easily conform to either of the traditional Food and Drug Administration classification: biologics or devices (80, 81). Combined scaffold and cell-containing devices may be in more than one classification category. For devices, a single confirmatory study is often sufficient for FDA approval. If the product is regulated as a biologic, it must be reviewed and approved by the FDA Center for Biologics Evaluation and Research. If regulated as a drug, several further phases are required prior to FDA approval. Although these regulatory processes above present significant challenges, many countries do have streamlined regulatory processes that might reduce the obstacles faced (82).

## TISSUE ENGINEERING—WHERE ARE WE NOW?

Stable and physiologically relevant (74) tissue replacement with composite engineered tissue remains elusive. Allograft transplantation has been an exciting development for the reconstructive surgeon, but the requirement for long-term immunosuppressive therapy (83), health-care infrastructure, and funding streams means it is not mainstream practice (**Table 3**). Tissue engineering is a promising alternative and has yielded small successes so far. Atala et al. were the first to report tissue-engineered constructs being used in patients (84). This was followed by several reports between 2008 and 2014 in a range of tissues including the trachea (85, 86), urethra (87), and nasal cartilage (88). Results have been varied; tracheal work is currently under investigation due to the deaths of three out of six patients and for nasal cartilage in particular, there was a question mark whether the tissue was replaced by scar or native tissue (89). The current significant barriers to translation for large-volume tissue replacement are the inability to produce "physiologicallty relevant tissue" (74) and difficulties with vascularization (24). Small constructs may succeed based on local angiogenesis (84, 87); however, the metabolic needs of the implanted cells in larger constructs means prevascularisation or the use of vascular pedicles is likely to be necessary (87).

**TABLE 3 | Successful applications of tissue-engineered constructs in humans.**

| Organ/ tissue | No. of patients | Cell source | Outcomes | Reference |
|---|---|---|---|---|
| Bladder | 7 | Bladder urothelial and muscle cells | Improved volume and compliance with no metabolic consequences at mean 46 months follow-up | Atala et al. (84) |
| Trachea | 1 | Recipient MSCs | Functional airway with a normal appearance and mechanical properties at 4 months | Macchiarini et al. (85) |
| Urethra | 5 | Muscle and epithelial cells | Maintenance of wide urethral calibers without strictures, normal architecture on biopsy at 3 months following implantation | Raya-Rivera et al. (87) |
| Nasal cartilage | 5 | Autologous nasal chondrocytes | Good structural stability and respiratory function after 1 year | Fulco et al. (88) |
| Vaginal organs | 4 | Vulval biopsy—epithelial and muscle cells | Tri-layered structure on biopsy with phenotypically normal smooth muscle and epithelia with follow-up up to 8 years | Raya-Rivera et al. (90) |

## CONCLUSION AND FUTURE PERSPECTIVES

Surgical reconstruction using bioengineered tissues has the potential to revolutionize clinical practice. To be successful, one must be able to generate tissue constructs *in vitro* that are morphologically and functionally similar to native tissues. There has been a steady increase in basic science activity in cell therapy and a growing portfolio of cell therapy trials; however, this has not translated to commercial products available for clinical use. To achieve clinical translation, a multidisciplinary approach that successfully integrates engineering and biological methodologies is necessary. Ethical, regulatory, financial, and clinical considerations all present challenges in the translation of tissue-engineered constructs from the laboratory to mainstream clinical practice. Even though The Medical Research Council states that regenerative medicine and tissue engineering "holds the promise of revolutionizing patient care in the 21st century" (91) and that stem cell therapy is viewed as a future "game changer" by the plastic surgery community (92), many are yet to be convinced of this potential within the NHS, with major concerns involving cost-effectiveness, efficacy, reimbursement, and regulation (93). There is little doubt that tissue engineering offers great potential to reduce patient morbidity and mortality, and only co-ordinated and prolonged liaison between clinicians, scientists, and industry will move this from potential to reality.

## GLOSSARY

### Cell Biology

**Differentiation**—The process by which a cell becomes specialized in order to perform a specific function.

**Commitment**—When a cell becomes dedicated to a specific lineage.

**Potency**—The array of commitment opportunities available to a cell.

**Totipotent**—Cells capable of differentiating into any body cell type in addition to extraembryonic or placental cells.

**Multipotent**—Cells capable of differentiating into multiple cell types along one lineage (e.g., hematopoietic stem cells).

**Pluripotent**—Cells that may differentiate into tissues derived from all three germ cell layers.

**Unipotent**—Cells only capable of differentiating into one cell type (e.g., spermatogonial stem cells).

**Clonal**—A population of identical cells derived from the same cell.

**Polyclonal**—A population of cells derived from multiple clones.

**Progenitor**—A cell that has limited potency, but is able to differentiate to another cell type, or differentiate to its target cell lineage.

**Embryonic stem cells**—Embryonically derived pluripotent cells that are obtained from the inner cell mass.

**Induced pluripotent stem cells**—Differentiated cells that are reverted to their pluripotent state via a set of transcription factors.

**Autologous**—Cells or tissues obtained from the same individual.

**Allogeneic**—Cells or tissues obtained from a different individual of the same species.

**Xenogeneic**—Cells or tissues obtained from a different species.

**Extracellular matrix**—Biomolecules synthesized by the cell to provide a suitable environment to support surrounding cells and maintain tissue integrity in response to biochemical and mechanical cues.

### Biomaterials/Scaffolds

**Scaffold**—A 3D biomaterial construct that defines the geometry of the replacement tissue and provides environmental cues that promote tissue regeneration.

**Biomimetic**—Human-made substances, e.g., scaffolds that imitate nature.

**Functionalization**—The modification of scaffolds with bioactive material to enhance the biocompatibility of the scaffold.

**Nanotechnology**—Technology that deals with dimensions and tolerances of less than 100 nm, especially the manipulation of individual atoms and molecules.

**Biomolecular factors**—Biomolecular factors include growth factors, transcription factors, and components of the extracellular matrix.

**Mechanical factors**—External environmental stimuli such as forces generated during everyday movement.

### Manufacturing

**Bioprinting**—the process of generating spatially controlled cell patterns using 3D printing technologies.

**Bioreactor**—System in which conditions are closely controlled to permit or induce certain behavior in living cells or tissues.

**Good Laboratory Practice (GLP)**—System of management controls for laboratories conducting research to ensure consistency, reliability, reproducibility, and high quality of chemical (including pharmaceutical) tests.

**Good Manufacturing Practice (GMP) guidelines**—Regulatory guidelines that outline specific requirements for the handling and processing of human tissue, ensuring safe products of reliable quality.

**Scale-out**—Increasing the number of batches of an engineered product.

**Scale-up**—Increasing batch size on an engineered product.

## AUTHOR CONTRIBUTIONS

SA-H and ZJ completed a literature search and contributed to preparing the manuscript. AA-S, EC, and AI contributed ideas and content to the manuscript. SD, AH, CT, and CA critically revised the manuscript. IW conceived, contributed to the preparation of, and critically revised the manuscript. All the authors read and approved the final manuscript and agreed to be accountable for all aspects of the work.

## ACKNOWLEDGMENTS

The Reconstructive Surgery and Regenerative Medicine Research Group (ReconRegen) is currently supported by funding from the Royal College of Surgeons of England, British Association of Plastic, Reconstructive and Aesthetic Surgeons (BAPRAS), Medical Research Council (MR/N002431/1), ABMU Health Board, and Welsh Assembly Government. The authors thank Mr. Steve Atherton and Ms. Amy Shorter, medical illustrators, ABMU Health Board, for figures.

## REFERENCES


1. Pratt GF, Rozen WM, Chubb D, Ashton MW, Alonso-Burgos A, Whitaker IS. Preoperative imaging for perforator flaps in reconstructive surgery: a systematic review of the evidence for current techniques. *Ann Plast Surg* (2012) 69(1):3–9. doi:10.1097/SPA.0b013e318222b7b7
2. Taylor GI, Daniel RK. The free flap: composite tissue transfer by vascular anastomosis. *Aust N Z J Surg* (1973) 43(1):1–3. doi:10.1111/j.1445-2197.1973.tb05659.x
3. Shores JT, Brandacher G, Lee WPA. Hand and upper extremity transplantation: an update of outcomes in the worldwide experience. *Plast Reconstr Surg* (2015) 135(2):351e–60e. doi:10.1097/PRS.0000000000000892
4. Khalifian S, Brazio PS, Mohan R, Shaffer C, Brandacher G, Barth RN, et al. Facial transplantation: the first 9 years. *Lancet* (2014) 384(9960):2153–63. doi:10.1016/S0140-6736(13)62632-X
5. Nodzo SR, Hohman DW, Chakravarthy K. Nanotechnology: why should we care? *Am J Orthop* (2015) 44(3):E87–8.
6. Naderi H, Matin MM, Bahrami AR. Review paper: critical issues in tissue engineering: biomaterials, cell sources, angiogenesis, and drug delivery systems. *J Biomater Appl* (2011) 26(4):383–417. doi:10.1177/0885328211408946
7. Murphy SV, Atala A. 3D bioprinting of tissues and organs. *Nat Biotechnol* (2014) 32(8):773–85. doi:10.1038/nbt.2958
8. Gerstle TL, Ibrahim AM, Kim PS, Lee BT, Lin SJ. A plastic surgery application in evolution: three-dimensional printing. *Plast Reconstr Surg* (2014) 133(2):446–51. doi:10.1097/01.prs.0000436844.92623.d3
9. Chae MP, Rozen WM, McMenamin PG, Findlay MW, Spychal RT, Hunter-Smith DJ. Emerging applications of bedside 3D printing in plastic surgery. *Front Surg* (2015) 2:25. doi:10.3389/fsurg.2015.00025
10. Kamali P, Dean D, Skoracki R, Koolen PG, Paul MA, Ibrahim AM, et al. The current role of three-dimensional (3D) printing in plastic surgery. *Plast Reconstr Surg* (2016). doi:10.1097/PRS.0000000000003106
11. Golas AR, Hernandez KA, Spector JA. Tissue engineering for plastic surgeons: a primer. *Aesthetic Plast Surg* (2014) 38(1):207–21. doi:10.1007/s00266-013-0255-5
12. Whitaker I, Boyce E. Dismissing the myths: an analysis of 12,483 procedures. All in a years work for a plastic surgical unit. *Internet J World Health Soc Politics* (2009) 6(2).
13. *Hospital Episode Statistics, Admitted Patient Care, England 2012–13.* Health and Social Care Information Centre (2015). Available from: http://www.hscic.gov.uk/catalogue/PUB12566
14. *Hospital Episode Statistics, Outpatient Care.* Health and Social Care Information Centre (2015). Available from: http://www.hscic.gov.uk/searchcatalogue?productid=18356&q=title%3a%22hospital+episode+statistics%22&sort=Relevance&size=10&page=1#top
15. *Recommendation for Plastic Surgery Training 2011.* UK: Centre for Workforce Intelligence a Report from the Royal College of Surgeons of England (2015). Available from: http://www.rcseng.ac.uk/surgeons/surgical-standards/docs/2011-surgical-workforce-census-report
16. Søreide K. Epidemiology of major trauma. *Br J Surg* (2009) 96(7):697–8. doi:10.1002/bjs.6643
17. Sterodimas A, De Faria J, Correa WE, Pitanguy I. Tissue engineering in plastic surgery: an up-to-date review of the current literature. *Ann Plast Surg* (2009) 62(1):97–103. doi.10.1097/SAP.0b013e3181788ec9
18. Skalak R, Fox CF. *Tissue Engineering: Proceeding of a Workshop Held at Granlibakken, Lake Tahoe, California.* New York: Liss (1998).
19. Ikada Y. Challenges in tissue engineering. *J R Soc Interface* (2006) 3(10):589–601. doi:10.1098/rsif.2006.0124
20. Pallua N, Gröger A. Tissue engineering and plastic surgery. In: Klein ME, Neuhann-Lorenz C, editors. *Innovations in Plastic and Aesthetic Surgery.* Berlin, Heidelberg: Springer (2008). p. 17–23.
21. D'Amico RA, Rubin JP. Regenerative medicine and the future of plastic surgery. *Plast Reconstr Surg* (2014) 133(6):1511–2. doi:10.1097/PRS.0000000000000212
22. Committee GBP HOLSAT. *House of Lords – Select Committee on Science and Technology – HL 76.* London: The Stationery Office Limited (2013).
23. O'Dowd A. Peers call for UK to harness "enormous" potential of regenerative medicine. *Br Med J* (2013) 347:f4248. doi:10.1136/bmj.f4248
24. Findlay MW, Dolderer JH, Trost N, Craft RO, Cao Y, Cooper-White J, et al. Tissue-engineered breast reconstruction: bridging the gap toward large-volume tissue engineering in humans. *Plast Reconstr Surg* (2011) 128(6):1206–15. doi:10.1097/PRS.0b013e318230c5b2
25. Freese KE, Kokai L, Edwards RP, Philips BJ, Sheikh MA, Kelley J, et al. Adipose-derived stems cells and their role in human cancer development, growth, progression, and metastasis: a systematic review. *Cancer Res* (2015) 75(7):1161–8. doi:10.1158/0008-5472.CAN-14-2744
26. Bichara DA, O'Sullivan NA, Pomerantseva I, Zhao X, Sundback CA, Vacanti JP, et al. The tissue-engineered auricle: past, present, and future. *Tissue Eng Part B Rev* (2012) 18:51–61. doi:10.1089/ten.TEB.2011.0326
27. Cao Y, Vacanti JP, Paige KT, Upton J, Vacanti CA. Transplantation of chondrocytes utilizing a polymer-cell construct to produce tissue-engineered cartilage in the shape of a human ear. *Plast Reconstr Surg* (1997) 100:297–302. doi:10.1097/00006534-199708000-00001
28. Kamil SH, Vacanti MP, Aminuddin BS, Jackson MJ, Vacanti CA, Eavey RD. Tissue engineering of a human sized and shaped auricle using a mold. *Laryngoscope* (2004) 114:867. doi:10.1097/00005537-200405000-00015
29. Christophel JJ, Chang JS, Park SS. Transplanted tissue-engineered cartilage. *Arch Facial Plast Surg* (2006) 8(2):117–22. doi:10.1001/archfaci.8.2.117
30. Nayyer L, Patel KH, Esmaeili A, Rippel RA, Birchall M, O'Toole G, et al. Tissue engineering: revolution and challenge in auricular cartilage reconstruction. *Plast Reconstr Surg* (2012) 129(5):1123–37. doi:10.1097/PRS.0b013e31824a2c1c
31. Brommer H, Brama PAJ, Laasanen MS, Helminen HJ, van Weeren PR, Jurvelin JS. Functional adaptation of articular cartilage from birth to maturity under the influence of loading: a biomechanical analysis. *Equine Vet J* (2005) 37(2):148–54. doi:10.2746/0425164054223769
32. Kusuhara H, Isogai N, Enjo M, Otani H, Ikada Y, Jacquet R, et al. Tissue engineering a model for the human ear: assessment of size, shape, morphology, and gene expression following seeding of different chondrocytes. *Wound Repair Regen* (2009) 17(1):136–46. doi:10.1111/j.1524-475X.2008.00451.x
33. Nabzdyk C, Pradhan L, Molina J, Perin E, Paniagua D, Rosenstrauch D. Auricular chondrocytes—from benchwork to clinical applications. *In Vivo* (2009) 23(3):369–80.
34. Homicz MR, Schumacher BL, Sah RH, Watson D. Effects of serial expansion of septal chondrocytes on tissue-engineered neocartilage composition. *Otolaryngol Head Neck Surg* (2002) 127:398–408. doi:10.1067/mhn.2002.129730
35. Jian-Wei X, Randolph MA, Peretti GM, Nazzal JA, Roses RE, Morse KR, et al. Producing a flexible tissue-engineered cartilage framework using expanded polytetrafluoroethylene membrane as a pseudoperichondrium. *Plastic Reconstr Surg* (2005) 116(2):577–89. doi:10.1097/01.prs.0000172985.81897.dc
36. Bianco P, Robey PG. Stem cells in tissue engineering. *Nature* (2001) 414(6859):118–21. doi:10.1038/35102181
37. Guillot PV, Cui W, Fisk NM, Polak DJ. Stem cell differentiation and expansion for clinical applications of tissue engineering. *J Cell Mol Med* (2007) 11(5):935–44. doi:10.1111/j.1582-4934.2007.00106.x
38. Shi Q, Rafii S, Wu MH, Wijelath ES, Yu C, Ishida A, et al. Evidence for circulating bone marrow-derived endothelial cells. *Blood* (1998) 92(2):362–7.
39. Thomson JA, Itskovitz-Eldor J, Shapiro SS, Waknitz MA, Swiergiel JJ, Marshall VS, et al. Embryonic stem cell lines derived from human blastocysts. *Science* (1998) 282(5391):1145–7. doi:10.1126/science.282.5391.1145
40. Dominici M, Le Blanc K, Mueller I, Slaper-Cortenbach I, Marini F, Krause D, et al. Minimal criteria for defining multipotent mesenchymal stromal cells. The International Society for Cellular Therapy position statement. *Cytotherapy* (2006) 8(4):315–7. doi:10.1080/14653240600855905
41. Kupfer ME, Ogle BM. Advanced imaging approaches for regenerative medicine: emerging technologies for monitoring stem cell fate in vitro

and in vivo. *Biotechnol J* (2015) 10(10):1515–28. doi:10.1002/biot.201400760
42. Asano T, Sasaki K, Kitano Y, Terao K, Hanazono Y. In vivo tumor formation from primate embryonic stem cells. *Methods Mol Biol* (2006) 329: 459–67.
43. da Silva Meirelles L, Caplan AI, Nardi NB. In search of the in vivo identity of mesenchymal stem cells. *Stem Cells* (2008) 26(9):2287–99. doi:10.1634/stemcells.2007-1122
44. Zuk PA, Zhu M, Mizuno H, Huang J, Futrell JW, Katz AJ, et al. Multilineage cells from human adipose tissue: implications for cell-based therapies. *Tissue Eng* (2001) 7(2):211–28. doi:10.1089/107632701300062859
45. Stock UA, Vacanti JP. Tissue engineering: current state and prospects. *Annu Rev Med* (2001) 52(1):443–51. doi:10.1146/annurev.med.52.1.443
46. Takahashi K, Yamanaka S. Induction of pluripotent stem cells from mouse embryonic and adult fibroblast cultures by defined factors. *Cell* (2006) 126(4):663–76. doi:10.1016/j.cell.2006.07.024
47. Hayden EC. Stem cells: the growing pains of pluripotency. *Nature* (2011) 9:272–4. doi:10.1038/473272a
48. Laurent LC, Ulitsky I, Slavin I, Tran H, Schork A, Morey R, et al. Dynamic changes in the copy number of pluripotency and cell proliferation genes in human ESCs and iPSCs during reprogramming and time in culture. *Cell Stem Cell* (2011) 8(1):106–18. doi:10.1016/j.stem.2010.12.003
49. Zhao T, Zhang Z-N, Rong Z, Xu Y. Immunogenicity of induced pluripotent stem cells. *Nature* (2011) 474(7350):212–5. doi:10.1038/nature10135
50. Chang T, Zimmerley MS, Quinn KP, Lamarre-Jouenne I, Kaplan DL, Beaurepaire E, et al. Non-invasive monitoring of cell metabolism and lipid production in 3D engineered human adipose tissues using label-free multiphoton microscopy. *Biomater* (2013) 34(34):8607–16. doi:10.1016/j.biomaterials.2013.07.066
51. Erlach von TC, Hedegaard MAB, Stevens MM. High resolution Raman spectroscopy mapping of stem cell micropatterns. *Analyst* (2015) 140(6):1798–803. doi:10.1039/c4an02346c
52. Bodle JC, Teeter SD, Hluck BH, Hardin JW, Bernacki SH, Loboa EG. Age-related effects on the potency of human adipose-derived stem cells: creation and evaluation of superlots and implications for musculoskeletal tissue engineering applications. *Tissue Eng Part C Methods* (2014) 20(12):972–83. doi:10.1089/ten.TEC.2013.0683
53. Bhatnagar R, Li S. Biomimetic scaffolds for tissue engineering. *Conf Proc IEEE Eng Med Biol Soc* (2004) 7:5021–3. doi:10.1109/IEMBS.2004.1404387
54. Hollister SJ. Porous scaffold design for tissue engineering. *Nat Mater* (2005) 4(7):518–24. doi:10.1038/nmat1421
55. Hutmacher DW. Scaffolds in tissue engineering bone and cartilage. *Biomaterials* (2000) 21(24):2529–43. doi:10.1016/S0142-9612(00)00121-6
56. Rezwan K, Chen QZ, Blaker JJ, Boccaccini AR. Biodegradable and bioactive porous polymer/inorganic composite scaffolds for bone tissue engineering. *Biomaterials* (2006) 27(18):3413–31. doi:10.1016/j.biomaterials.2006.01.039
57. Kim BS, Mooney DJ. Development of biocompatible synthetic extracellular matrices for tissue engineering. *Trends Biotechnol* (1998) 16(5):224–30. doi:10.1016/S0167-7799(98)01191-3
58. Lutolf MP, Hubbell JA. Synthetic biomaterials as instructive extracellular microenvironments for morphogenesis in tissue engineering. *Nat Biotechnol* (2005) 23(1):47–55. doi:10.1038/nbt1055
59. Sanghvi AB, Miller KP-H, Belcher AM, Schmidt CE. Biomaterials functionalization using a novel peptide that selectively binds to a conducting polymer. *Nat Mater* (2005) 4(6):496–502. doi:10.1038/nmat1397
60. Barnes CP, Sell SA, Boland ED, Simpson DG, Bowlin GL. Nanofiber technology: designing the next generation of tissue engineering scaffolds. *Adv Drug Deliv Rev* (2007) 59(14):1413–33. doi:10.1016/j.addr.2007.04.022
61. Furth ME, Atala A, Van Dyke ME. Smart biomaterials design for tissue engineering and regenerative medicine. *Biomaterials* (2007) 28(34):5068–73. doi:10.1016/j.biomaterials.2007.07.042
62. Wong YS, Tay CY, Wen F. Engineered polymeric biomaterials for tissue engineering. *Curr Tissue Eng* (2012) 1:41–53.
63. Anderson DG, Burdick JA, Langer R. Materials science. Smart biomaterials. *Science* (2004) 305(5692):1923–4. doi:10.1126/science.1099987
64. Lanza R, Langer R, Vacanti JP. *Principles of Tissue Engineering*. 4th ed. Academic Press (2013). 1 p.
65. Chen F-M, Zhang M, Wu Z-F. Toward delivery of multiple growth factors in tissue engineering. *Biomaterials* (2010) 31(24):6279–308. doi:10.1016/j.biomaterials.2010.04.053
66. Leijten J, Georgi N, Moreira Teixeira L, van Blitterswijk CA, Post JN, Karperien M. Metabolic programming of mesenchymal stromal cells by oxygen tension directs chondrogenic cell fate. *Proc Natl Acad Sci U S A* (2014) 111(38):13954–9. doi:10.1073/pnas.1410977111
67. Fotia C, Massa A, Boriani F, Baldini N, Granchi D. Prolonged exposure to hypoxic milieu improves the osteogenic potential of adipose derived stem cells. *J Cell Biochem* (2015) 116(7):1442–53. doi:10.1002/jcb.25106
68. De Miguel MP, Alcaina Y, la Maza de DS, Lopez-Iglesias P. Cell metabolism under microenvironmental low oxygen tension levels in stemness, proliferation and pluripotency. *Curr Mol Med* (2015) 15(4):343–59. doi:10.2174/1566524015666150505160406
69. Correia V, Panadero JA, Ribeiro C, Sencadas V, Rocha JG, Gomez Ribelles JL, et al. Design and validation of a biomechanical bioreactor for cartilage tissue culture. *Biomech Model Mechanobiol* (2016) 15(2):471–8. doi:10.1007/s10237-015-0698-5
70. Hernández-Bule ML, Paíno CL, Trillo MÁ, Úbeda A. Electric stimulation at 448 kHz promotes proliferation of human mesenchymal stem cells. *Cell Physiol Biochem* (2014) 34(5):1741–55. doi:10.1159/000366375
71. Griffin MF, Butler PE, Seifalian AM, Kalaskar DM. Control of stem cell fate by engineering their micro and nanoenvironment. *World J Stem Cells* (2015) 7(1):37–50. doi:10.4252/wjsc.v7.i1.37
72. Pörtner R, Nagel-Heyer S, Goepfert C, Adamietz P, Meenen NM. Bioreactor design for tissue engineering. *J Biosci Bioeng* (2005) 100(3):235–45. doi:10.1263/jbb.100.235
73. Hansmann J, Groeber F, Kahlig A, Kleinhans C, Walles H. Bioreactors in tissue engineering – principles, applications and commercial constraints. *Biotechnol J* (2013) 8(3):298–307. doi:10.1002/biot.201200162
74. Abbott RD, Kaplan DL. Strategies for improving the physiological relevance of human engineered tissues. *Trends Biotechnol* (2015) 33(7):401–7. doi:10.1016/j.tibtech.2015.04.003
75. Hunziker E, Spector M, Libera J, Gertzman A, Woo SL-Y, Ratcliffe A, et al. Translation from research to applications. *Tissue Eng* (2006) 12(12):3341–64. doi:10.1089/ten.2006.12.3341
76. Halme DG, Kessler DA. FDA regulation of stem-cell-based therapies. *N Engl J Med* (2006) 355(16):1730–5. doi:10.1056/NEJMhpr063086
77. Fink DW. FDA regulation of stem cell-based products. *Science* (2009) 324(5935):1662–3. doi:10.1126/science.1173712
78. Hunsberger J, Harrysson O, Shirwaiker R, Starly B, Wysk R, Cohen P, et al. Manufacturing road map for tissue engineering and regenerative medicine technologies. *Stem Cells Transl Med* (2015) 4(2):130–5. doi:10.5966/sctm.2014-0254
79. Berry MG, Stanek JJ. The PIP mammary prosthesis: a product recall study. *J Plast Reconstr Aesthet Surg* (2012) 65(6):697–704. doi:10.1016/j.bjps.2012.02.019
80. Lu L, Arbit HM, Herrick JL, Segovis SG, Maran A, Yaszemski MJ. Tissue engineered constructs: perspectives on clinical translation. *Ann Biomed Eng* (2015) 43(3):796–804. doi:10.1007/s10439-015-1280-0
81. Uppal RS, Sabbagh W, Chana J, Gault DT. Donor-site morbidity after autologous costal cartilage harvest in ear reconstruction and approaches to reducing donor-site contour deformity. *Plast Reconstr Surg* (2008) 121(6):1949–55. doi:10.1097/PRS.0b013e318170709e
82. Birchall MA, Seifalian AM. Tissue engineering's green shoots of disruptive innovation. *Lancet* (2014) 384(9940):288–90. doi:10.1016/S0140-6736(14)60533-X
83. Whitaker IS, Duggan EM, Alloway RR, Brown C, McGuire S, Woodle ES, et al. Composite tissue allotransplantation: a review of relevant immunological issues for plastic surgeons. *J Plast Reconstr Aesthet Surg* (2008) 61(5):481–92. doi:10.1016/j.bjps.2007.11.019
84. Atala A, Bauer SB, Soker S, Yoo JJ, Retik AB. Tissue-engineered autologous bladders for patients needing cystoplasty. *Lancet* (2006) 367(9518):1241–6. doi:10.1016/S0140-6736(06)68438-9
85. Macchiarini P, Jungebluth P, Go T, Asnaghi MA, Rees LE, Cogan TA, et al. Clinical transplantation of a tissue-engineered airway. *Lancet* (2008) 372(9655):2023–30. doi:10.1016/S0140-6736(08)61598-6

86. Baiguera S, Birchall MA, Macchiarini P. Tissue-engineered tracheal transplantation. *Transplantation* (2010) 89(5):485–91. doi:10.1097/TP.0b013e3181cd4ad3
87. Raya-Rivera A, Esquiliano DR, Yoo JJ, Lopez-Bayghen E, Soker S, Atala A. Tissue-engineered autologous urethras for patients who need reconstruction: an observational study. *Lancet* (2011) 377(9772):1175–82. doi:10.1016/S0140-6736(10)62354-9
88. Fulco I, Miot S, Haug MD, Barbero A, Wixmerten A, Feliciano S, et al. Engineered autologous cartilage tissue for nasal reconstruction after tumour resection: an observational first-in-human trial. *Lancet* (2014) 384(9940):337–46. doi:10.1016/S0140-6736(14)60544-4
89. Russell AJ. The end of the beginning for tissue engineering. *Lancet* (2014) 383(9913):193–5. doi:10.1016/S0140-6736(13)62110-8
90. Raya-Rivera AM, Esquiliano D, Fierro-Pastrana R, López-Bayghen E, Valencia P, Ordorica-Flores R, et al. Tissue-engineered autologous vaginal organs in patients: a pilot cohort study. *Lancet* (2014) 384(9940):329–36. doi:10.1016/S0140-6736(14)60542-0
91. Medical Research Council. *Regenerative Medicine and Stem Cells*. Available from: http://www.mrc.ac.uk/research/initiatives/regenerative-medicine-stem-cells/ (accessed January 26, 2017).
92. Ozturk S, Karagoz H, Zor F. The future of plastic surgery: surgeon's perspective. *J Craniofac Surg* (2015) 26(8):e708–13. doi:10.1097/SCS.0000000000002204
93. Davies BM, Rikabi S, French A, Pinedo-Villanueva R, Morrey ME, Wartolowska K, et al. Quantitative assessment of barriers to the clinical development and adoption of cellular therapies: a pilot study. *J Tissue Eng* (2014) 5(0):2041731414551764. doi:10.1177/2041731414551764

# 16

# The challenge for reconstructive surgeons in the twenty-first century: manufacturing tissue-engineered solutions

*Zita M. Jessop[1,2*†], Sarah Al-Himdani[1,2†], Marc Clement[3,4] and Iain Stuart Whitaker[1,2]*

*[1] Reconstructive Surgery and Regenerative Medicine Research Group (ReconRegen), Institute of Life Science, Swansea University Medical School, Swansea, UK, [2] The Welsh Centre for Burns and Plastic Surgery, Morriston Hospital, Swansea, UK, [3] School of Management, Swansea University, Swansea, UK, [4] Institute of Life Science, Swansea University Medical School, Swansea, UK*

**Keywords: tissue engineering, regenerative medicine, plastic and reconstructive surgery, translational research, biomanufacturing, barriers to translation**

***Edited and reviewed by:***
*Ramin Shayan, O'Brien Institute, Australia; St Vincent's Hospital Melbourne, Australia*

****Correspondence:***
*Zita M. Jessop*
*zitajessop@gmail.com*

*†Zita M. Jessop and Sarah Al-Himdani are joint first authors*

***Specialty section:***
*This article was submitted to Reconstructive and Plastic Surgery, a section of the journal Frontiers in Surgery*

## BACKGROUND

These are exciting times in the field of plastic and reconstructive surgery. Meaningful advances in a wide range of basic science and clinical spheres have been made in the field in recent years, with direct translation to patient care. As a community, we are fortunate to be involved in such a vast, complex, increasingly interdisciplinary, rapidly expanding, and intellectually challenging field of surgery. Plastic surgery aims to restore "form and function" following a wide range of congenital or acquired defects, with procedures often transcending anatomic boundaries. This versatility promotes innovation, and with the recent advances in medical imaging (1), microsurgery (2), composite tissue allotransplantation (3, 4), nanotechnology (5), cell biology and biomaterials (6), and 3D printing (7), treatment options for patients are wider than ever before. For centuries, the "reconstructive ladder" was restricted to local flaps and skin grafts. Although these autologous options are reliable, plastic surgeons, with their constant wish to refine techniques, have become increasingly cognizant that there is the real potential for a paradigm shift in reconstructive surgery in the medium term. Tissue-engineered solutions (**Figure 1A**) offer the potential to alleviate the need for donor sites and their associated morbidity and to reduce hospital stay and associated costs (8).

## EXTENT OF THE PROBLEM

Reconstructive plastic surgeons have a diverse workload and contrary to the perceptions of the media, it comprises a relatively small proportion of purely aesthetic procedures (9). The majority of operations relate to wound management and neoplasia, with a significant health economic impact (9). In the year 2013–2014 alone, over one million patients were treated in NHS England by plastic surgeons (10, 11). Evidence suggests that this workload will continue to increase (12). With a continual supply of major trauma and neoplasia, plastic surgeons are facing more challenging composite defects than ever before coupled with internet and media savvy patients with increasing expectations (13).

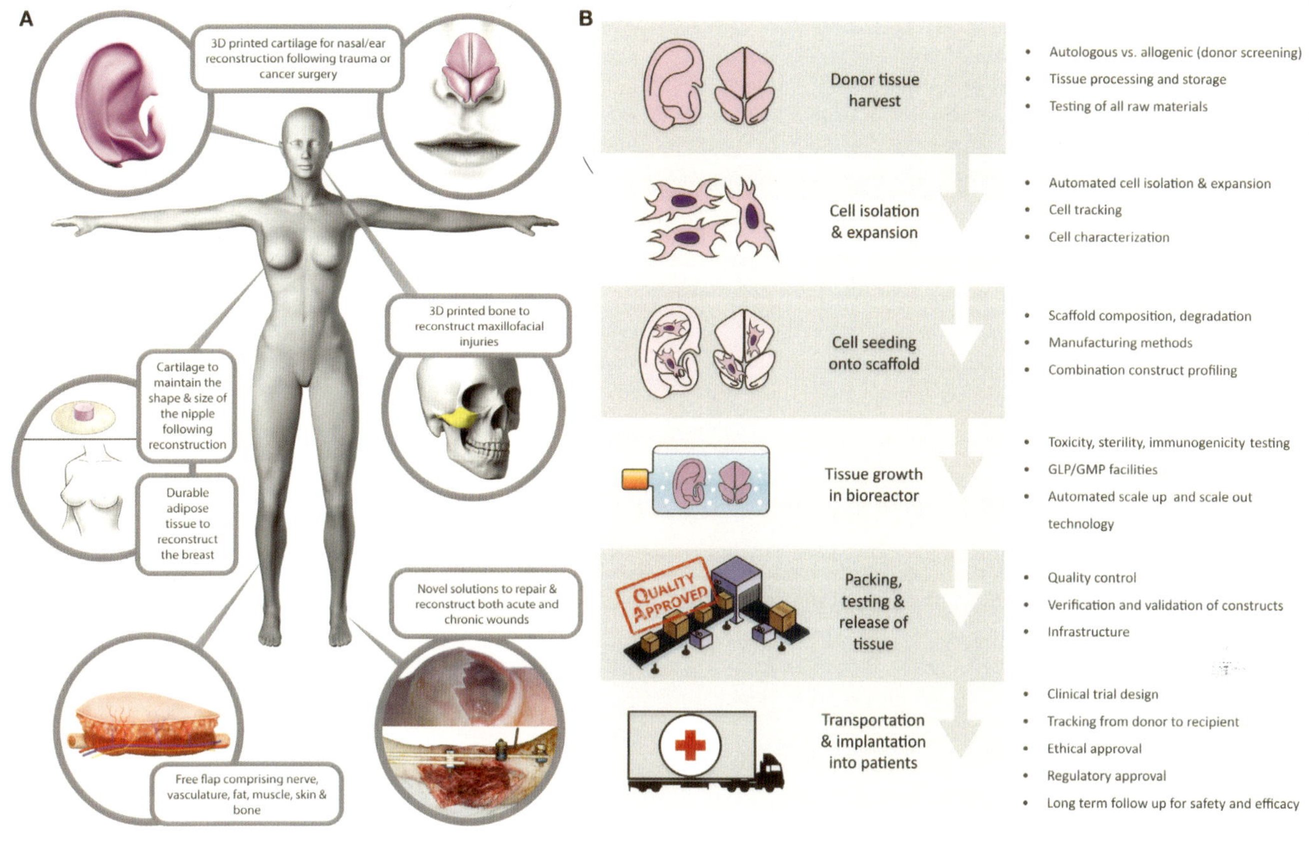


**FIGURE 1 | (A)** Tissue-engineered reconstructive solutions. **(B)** Potential barriers to translation at each level of the tissue-engineering supply chain.

## INNOVATIONS IN RECONSTRUCTIVE SURGERY

Technological innovation in plastic and reconstructive surgery in the twentieth century revolutionized the specialty, opening up the possibility for surgeons to operate on microvascular structures using specialized microscopes and instruments, enabling them to undertake free tissue transfers (2) and extremity replantations. Despite these developments in practice, we are still confronted with shortcomings relating to the availability of donor tissues. In order to overcome this, novel approaches have been investigated. Transplantation of organs and tissues, first performed by a plastic surgeon and Nobel laureate (Dr. Joseph Murray) in 1954 (14, 15), has rapidly expanded over the twentieth century from traditional solid organ transplant to a range of vascularized composite tissue allografts including the upper extremity (3) and face (4). Although excellent medium-term outcomes have been reported, there have been ongoing debates surrounding ethical (16, 17), psychological, and medical issues in the long term, especially relating to the effects of immunosuppression (18). The more attractive concept, obviating the need for long-term immunosuppression, is tissue engineering. The Medical Research Council states that regenerative medicine and tissue engineering "holds the promise of revolutionizing patient care in the twenty-first century" and the UK government highlighted regenerative medicine as one of the key areas, which could provide a global competitive advantage for the UK (19, 20). In 2014, it was highlighted as one of the eight great technologies in the industrial strategy government manifesto worthy of significant investment.

## THE CHALLENGES

Tissue engineering is a modern, interdisciplinary field combining principles of engineering, physics, and life sciences. It shares a common objective with plastic and reconstructive surgery: "to restore form and function" (21, 22). The surgical community worldwide is becoming increasingly aware of the research landscape. The American Society of Plastic surgeons have highlighted the role of tissue engineering in the future of plastic surgery (23), particularly the need for a focus on translation from bench research to clinical practice, which would provide clarity on avenues for upscaling and tissue engineering supply chains (**Figure 1B**).

Although the UK government and others have recognized the potential of regenerative medicine and tissue engineering to impact on the health service, they also highlighted the current "lack of coordination" in the field as a whole (24). Despite recent *in vitro* and *in vivo* studies attesting to the feasibility of tissue engineering for use in a range of clinical scenarios (25–30), barriers have been identified that are inhibiting clinical translation (**Figure 1B**). These barriers to translation are deep rooted at the basic science level, manifesting in insufficient understanding of the safety and durability of tissue-engineered constructs (31, 32). Understandably, before these hurdles are overcome, investors are unwilling to shoulder the financial, ethical, and regulatory burden of translational research that may not be commercially viable, which then impacts on funding and further progress in the field (33).

## Scientific Unknowns

The term "tissue engineering" was first coined almost 30 years ago, with skin being one of the first to be used clinically (34). Despite numerous successes in this exciting field, there have been very few reports of successful clinical translation. This is due to a combination of factors, including lack of clarity regarding ideal cell sources and scaffolds (35), methods of vascularizing larger constructs (36), reliable cell and construct characterization pre-implantation and evidence of safety (37), and durability in large animal models (35). This is not surprising given the complexity of research in this field that cross cuts cell biology, material science, biochemistry, and engineering. As cells are complex, dynamic, and interactive, it is crucial to have a solid scientific foundation regarding their stability, functional capacity, and response to host environment (38). It is generally accepted that it takes 20–30 years from the start of basic science research to clinical utility, demonstrated by contemporary treatments such as bone marrow transplantation (39).

## Ethical and Regulatory Milestones

There is a lack of international standards for the use of stem cell and tissue engineering therapies in human patients, which has led to the use of unproven treatments in unregulated international clinics which damages the research in this field (40, 41). Stem cell hype has also generated unrealistic patient hopes, which raises ethical concerns when initiating clinical trials of cell-based therapies (42). Tissue-engineered constructs do not easily fit into the U.S. Food and Drug Administration (FDA) and the European Medicines Agency (EMA) classifications for medical products (43). Since many of these constructs are complex and consist of more than one component, i.e., biomolecule, cell, and biomaterial, they are classed as combination products that fall under the advanced therapy medicinal products (ATMPs) category (44, 45). The review of any regulated product is therefore undertaken on a case-by-case basis but generally considers four aspects: product manufacture, preclinical testing (laboratory and animal models), clinical performance, and product labeling according to claim of intended use. These processes are time, labor, and money intensive and have often been criticized for lack of clarity and inconsistencies between different regulatory agencies (46, 47), which have in turn hindered the availability of products in some areas. The tissue-engineering field is still in early development and hence regulatory requirements are also continuing to evolve with it. There is now increasing dialog between the international TERMIS committees and regulatory bodies in order to work toward a consensus on regulatory requirements in order to foster innovation while continuing to ensure the safety and efficacy of tissue-engineered solutions (46).

## Lack of Funding

Despite investment in the tissue-engineering sector from a number of companies, the high production costs, unrealistic promises from the scientific community, and regulatory hurdles have limited successful clinical translation and commercial success of these early products (48–50). It has been suggested that alliances between companies or collaboration between industry and government funding agencies, who can share expertise as well as the financial burden, will be the key to driving translation from bench to bedside through clinical trials (33, 49). Partnerships within and across different sectors, such as the CASMI Translational Stem Cell Consortium (CTSCC) (51) (an academic-industry consortium), are already emerging and aim to identify key hurdles in commercialization. There is also an increasing focus on developing "translation centers" such as Harvard Stem Cell Institute (HSCI), Centre for Commercialisation of Regenerative Medicine (CCRM), and the Cell Therapy Catapult (51).

## Infrastructure for Scale Up and Scale Out

Biomanufacturing is an often overlooked but vital process of clinical translation (52). Once a successful tissue-engineered construct has been developed and tested in the laboratory, there are a number of considerations when driving the product toward clinical trials and widespread commercial use. Many methods of cell isolation, expansion, differentiation, and seeding onto scaffolds continue to be variable bench processes. These processes need to be refined by using batch-tested reagents, defined culture and bioreactor conditions, and automated techniques to ensure the process is quality controlled and able to be verified and validated according to regulatory requirements (38). A key component is the transition from manual laboratory based techniques to certified good manufacturing practice (cGMP) processes, which require a sound business model, significant infrastructure, personnel and automated scale-up and scale-out strategies. In order to set up these processes for widespread use in health services, there needs to be synergized communication between basic researchers, clinicians, industry experts, and regulators. There are initiatives to set up translational hubs for ATMPs, such as the European Advanced Translational Research Infrastructure in Medicine (EATRIS), in order to fill the gap between basic science and clinical practice and overcome the bottlenecks for translation (45).

# CONCLUSION

There is a clear and unmet clinical need for an adequate solution to reconstruct tissue defects following tumor resections, severe trauma, or deep burns, which removes the morbidity and mortality associated with donor sites. Tissue engineering, with its potential to biomanufacture constructs to repair and restore complex defects, holds great promise (53). The innovative and complex nature of these constructs results in a number of scientific, ethical, regulatory, financial, and infrastructural challenges, which currently hinder clinical translation. Answers to the fundamental scientific questions as well as our ability to overcome the translational challenges rely on multidisciplinary working groups (academia, clinicians, patient representatives, investors, manufacturing experts, and regulators) as well as governmental support (54) before we will see widespread use of tissue-engineered constructs in reconstructive surgery.

## AUTHOR CONTRIBUTIONS

ZJ and SA-H undertook the literature review and drafted the manuscript. MC revised the manuscript. IW conceived the study and revised the manuscript. All authors read and approved the final manuscript.

## ACKNOWLEDGMENTS

Mr. Steve Atherton RMIP MIMI, Medical Illustrator, ABMU Health Board for **Figure 1**. Mr. Luke Whitmore for his help in literature retrieval and bibliographic secondary linkage.

## FUNDING

Medical Research Council UK, Royal College of Surgeons of England, ABMU Health Board Research & Development

## REFERENCES

1. Pratt GF, Rozen WM, Chubb D, Ashton MW, Alonso-Burgos A, Whitaker IS. Preoperative imaging for perforator flaps in reconstructive surgery: a systematic review of the evidence for current techniques. *Ann Plast Surg* (2012) **69**:3–9. doi:10.1097/SPA.0b013e318222b7b7
2. Taylor GI, Daniel RK. The free flap: composite tissue transfer by vascular anastomosis. *Aust N Z J Surg* (1973) **43**:1–3. doi:10.1111/j.1445-2197.1973.tb05659.x
3. Shores JT, Brandacher G, Lee WP. Hand and upper extremity transplantation: an update of outcomes in the worldwide experience. *Plast Reconstr Surg* (2015) **135**:351e–60e. doi:10.1097/PRS.0000000000000892
4. Khalifian S, Brazio PS, Mohan R, Shaffer C, Brandacher G, Barth RN, et al. Facial transplantation: the first 9 years. *Lancet* (2014) **384**:2153–63. doi:10.1016/S0140-6736(13)62632-X
5. Nodzo SR, Hohman DW, Chakravarthy K. Nanotechnology: why should we care? *Am J Orthop* (2015) **44**:E87–8.
6. Naderi H, Matin MM, Bahrami AR. Review paper: critical issues in tissue engineering: biomaterials, cell sources, angiogenesis, and drug delivery systems. *J Biomater Appl* (2011) **26**:383–417. doi:10.1177/0885328211408946
7. Murphy SV, Atala A. 3D bioprinting of tissues and organs. *Nat Biotechnol* (2014) **32**:773–85. doi:10.1038/nbt.2958
8. Golas AR, Hernandez KA, Spector JA. Tissue engineering for plastic surgeons: a primer. *Aesthetic Plast Surg* (2014) **38**:207–21. doi:10.1007/s00266-013-0255-5
9. Mason L, Whitaker L, Boyce D. Dismissing the myths: an analysis of 12,483 procedures. All in a years work for a plastic surgical unit. *The Internet Journal of World Health and Societal Politics* (2008) **6**(2).
10. Hospital Episode Statistics, Admitted Patient Care, England 2012–13. Health and Social Care Information Centre. [Cited 2015 Oct 7]. Available from: http://www.hscic.gov.uk/catalogue/PUB12566
11. Hospital Episode Statistics, Outpatient care, April 2015. Health and Social Care Information Centre. [Cited 2015 Oct 7]. Available from: http://www.hscic.gov.uk/searchcatalogue?productid=18356&q=title%3a%22hospital+episode+statistics%22&sort=Relevance&size=10&page=1#top
12. Recommendation for Plastic Surgery Training 2011. UK: Centre for Workforce Intelligence a Report from the Royal College of Surgeons of England. [Cited 2015 Oct 7]. Available from: http://www.rcseng.ac.uk/surgeons/surgical-standards/docs/2011-surgical-workforce-census-report
13. Søreide K. (2009). Epidemiology of major trauma. *Br J Surg* 96: 697–8. doi:10.1002/bjs.6643
14. Harrison JH, Merrill JP, Murray JE. Renal homotransplantation in identical twins. *Surg Forum* (1956) **6**:432–6.
15. Cannon B, Murray JE. Plastic surgery: tissue and organ homotransplantation. *N Engl J Med* (1956) **255**:900–4. doi:10.1056/NEJM195611082551906
16. Wiggins OP, Barker JH, Martinez S, Vossen M, Maldonado C, Grossi F, et al. On the ethics of facial transplantation research. *Am J Bioeth* (2004) **4**(3):1–12.
17. McDowell N. Surgeons struggle with ethical nightmare of face transplants. *Nature* (2002) **420**:449. doi:10.1038/420449a
18. Whitaker IS, Duggan EM, Alloway RR, Brown C, McGuire S, Woodle ES, et al. Composite tissue allotransplantation: a review of relevant immunological issues for plastic surgeons. *J Plast Reconstr Aesthet Surg* (2008) **61**:481–92. doi:10.1016/j.bjps.2007.11.019
19. Committee GBP HOLSAT. *House of Lords – Select Committee on Science and Technology – HL 76*. London: The Stationery Office Limited (2013).
20. O'Dowd A. Peers call for UK to harness "enormous" potential of regenerative medicine. *BMJ* (2013) **347**:f4248. doi:10.1136/bmj.f4248
21. Sterodimas A, De Faria J, Correa WE, Pitanguy I. Tissue engineering in plastic surgery: an up-to-date review of the current literature. *Ann Plast Surg* (2009) **62**:97–103. doi:10.1097/SAP.0b013e3181788ec9
22. Skalak R, Fox CF. *Tissue Engineering*. Alan R. Liss, New York (1988).
23. D'mico RA, Rubin JP. Regenerative medicine and the future of plastic surgery. *Plast Reconstr Surg* (2014) **133**:1511–2. doi:10.1097/PRS.0000000000000212
24. House of Lords Science and Technology Committee. 28 Jun 2013. [Cited 2015 Oct 7]. Available from: http://www.parliament.uk/hlscience
25. Kim YS, Choi YJ, Lee SW, Kwon OR, Suh DS, Heo DB, et al. Assessment of clinical and MRI outcomes after mesenchymal stem cell implantation in patients with knee osteoarthritis: a prospective study. *Osteoarthritis Cartilage* (2015): S1063–4584. doi:10.1016/j.joca.2015.08.009
26. Findlay MW, Dolderer JH, Trost N, Craft RO, Cao Y, Cooper-White J, et al. Tissue-engineered breast reconstruction: bridging the gap toward large-volume tissue engineering in humans. *Plast Reconstr Surg* (2011) **128**:1206–15. doi:10.1097/PRS.0b013e318230c5b2
27. Georgiou M, Golding JP, Loughlin AJ, Kingham PJ, Phillips JB. Engineered neural tissue with aligned, differentiated adipose-derived stem cells promotes peripheral nerve regeneration across a critical sized defect in rat sciatic nerve. *Biomaterials* (2015) **37**:242–51. doi:10.1016/j.biomaterials.2014.10.009
28. Patrick CW. Breast tissue engineering. *Annu Rev Biomed Eng* (2004) **6**:109–30. doi:10.1146/annurev.bioeng.6.040803.140032
29. Bichara DA, O'Sullivan N-A, Pomerantseva I, Zhao X, Sundback CA, Vacanti JP, et al. The tissue-engineered auricle: past, present, and future. *Tissue Eng Part B Rev* (2012) **18**:51–61. doi:10.1089/ten.TEB.2011.0326
30. Reichert JC, Hutmacher DW. Bone tissue engineering. In: Pallua N, Suscheck CV, editors. *Tissue Engineering*. Berlin, Heidelberg: Springer (2010). p. 431–56.
31. Gad SC, McCord MG. *Safety Evaluation in the Development of Medical Devices and Combination Products*. 3rd ed. Cary: CRC Press (2008).
32. Derksen M-H. *Engineering Flesh; Towards Professional Responsibility for "Lived Bodies" in Tissue Engineering*. Eindhoven: 3TU Ethics (2008).
33. Hewson SM, Fehlings LN, Messih M, Fehlings MG. The challenges of translating stem cells for spinal cord injury and related disorders: what are the barriers and opportunities? *Expert Rev Neurother* (2013) **13**:143–50. doi:10.1586/ern.12.157
34. Keck M, Lumenta DB, Kamolz L-P. Skin tissue engineering. In: Kamolz LP, Lumenta DP, editors. *Dermal Replacements in General, Burn, and Plastic Surgery*. Vienna: Springer (2013). p. 13–25.
35. Ikada Y. Challenges in tissue engineering. *J R Soc Interface* (2006) **3**:589–601. doi:10.1098/rsif.2006.0124
36. Novosel EC, Kleinhans C, Kluger PJ. Vascularization is the key challenge in tissue engineering. *Adv Drug Deliv Rev* (2011) **63**:300–11. doi:10.1016/j.addr.2011.03.004
37. Klinger RY, Blum JL, Hearn B, Lebow B, Niklason LE. Relevance and safety of telomerase for human tissue engineering. *Proc Natl Acad Sci U S A* (2006) **103**:2500–5. doi:10.1073/pnas.0508184103

38. Parenteau NL. Commercial development of cell-based therapeutics: strategic considerations along the drug to tissue spectrum. *Regen Med* (2009) **4**:601–11. doi:10.2217/rme.09.29
39. Nakano T, Era T, Kodama H, Honjo T. Development of blood cells from mouse embryonic stem cells in culture. In: Ikehara S, Takaku F, Good RA, editors. *Bone Marrow Transplantation*. Tokyo: Springer Science & Business Media (2012). p. 9–19.
40. Cohen CB, Cohen PJ. International stem cell tourism and the need for effective regulation. Part I: Stem cell tourism in Russia and India: clinical research, innovative treatment, or unproven hype? *Kennedy Inst Ethics J* (2010) **20**:27–49. doi:10.1353/ken.0.0305
41. Lau D, Ogbogu U, Taylor B, Stafinski T, Menon D, Caulfield T. Stem cell clinics online: the direct-to-consumer portrayal of stem cell medicine. *Cell Stem Cell* (2008) **3**:591–4. doi:10.1016/j.stem.2008.11.001
42. The darker side of stem cells. *Nature* (2012) **483**:5. doi:10.1038/483005a
43. Panetta NJ, Gupta DM, Longaker MT. Bench to bedside: navigating industry, the FDA and Venture Capital. In: Chang J, Gupta G, editors. *Tissue Engineering for the Hand*. World Scientific Publishing Co. (2010). p. 253–69.
44. Hellman KB. Engineered tissues: the regulatory path from concept to market. In: Fisher JP, editor. *Tissue Engineering Advances in Experimental Medicine and Biology*. Boston, MA: Springer. p. 363–76.
45. Belardelli F, Rizza P, Moretti F, Carella C, Galli MC, Migliaccio G. Translational research on advanced therapies. *Ann Ist Super Sanita* (2011) **47**:72–8. doi:10.4415/ANN_11_01_15
46. Bertram T, Hellman KB, Bayon Y, Ellison S, Wilburn SRS. The regulatory imperative: international perspective. *Tissue Eng Part B Rev* (2013) **19**:191–3. doi:10.1089/ten.teb.2012.0654
47. Bertram TA, Tentoff E, Johnson PC, Tawil B, Van Dyke M, Hellman KB. Hurdles in tissue engineering/regenerative medicine product commercialization: a pilot survey of governmental funding agencies and the financial industry. *Tissue Eng Part A* (2012) **18**:2187–94. doi:10.1089/ten.TEA.2012.0186
48. Wilan KH, Scott CT, Herrera S. Chasing a cellular fountain of youth. *Nat Biotechnol* (2005) **23**:807–15. doi:10.1038/nbt1005-1315c
49. Pangarkar N, Hutmacher DW. Invention and business performance in the tissue-engineering industry. *Tissue Eng* (2004) **9**:1313–22. doi:10.1089/10763270360728224
50. Trounson A. Integration and translation: driving stem cell therapies toward the clinic. *Regen Med* (2008) **3**:269–73. doi:10.2217/17460751.3.3.269
51. French A, Bure K, Brindley DA. CASMI TSCC launch event, Paris, France, July 2013: an assessment of the key barriers to the commercialization and clinical adoption of pluripotent stem cell therapies. *Rejuvenation Res* (2014) **17**(1):84–8. doi:10.1089/rej.2014.1545
52. French A, Buckler RL, Brindley DA. Commercialization of regenerative medicine: learning from spin-outs. *Rejuvenation Res* (2013) **16**(2):164–70. doi:10.1089/rej.2013.1423
53. Pallua N, Suschek CV. *Tissue Engineering: From Lab to Clinic*. Berlin, Heidelberg: Springer (2010).
54. Pallua N, Gröger A. Tissue engineering and plastic surgery. In: Eisenmann-Klein M, Nuehann-Lorenz C, editors. *Innovations in Plastic and Aesthetic Surgery*. Berlin, Heidelberg: Springer (2010). p. 17–23.

# 17

# Superior Vena Cava (SVC) Endovascular Reconstruction with Implanted Central Venous Catheter Repositioning for Treatment of Malignant SVC Obstruction

*Stephanie Volpi, Francesco Doenz and Salah D. Qanadli**

*Cardio-Thoracic and Vascular Unit, Department of Radiology, Centre Hospitalier Universitaire Vaudois (CHUV), Lausanne, Switzerland*

**Edited by:**
*Christos V. Ioannou, University of Crete, Greece*

**Reviewed by:**
*Rosa María Moreno Carriles, Hospital Universitario de La Princesa, Spain*
*Nikolaos Kontopodis, University Hospital of Heraklion, Greece*
*Joseph J. Naoum, Lebanese American University, Lebanon*
*Elias Kehayas, University Hospital of Heraklion, Greece*

***Correspondence:**
*Salah D. Qanadli*
*salah.qanadli@chuv.ch*

**Specialty section:**
*This article was submitted to Vascular Surgery, a section of the journal Frontiers in Surgery*

Superior vena cava (SVC) syndrome is a group of clinical signs caused by the obstruction or compression of SVC and characterized by edema of the head, neck, and upper extremities, shortness of breath, and headaches. The syndrome may be caused by benign causes but most of the cases are caused by lung or mediastinal malignant tumors. Stenting of SVC has become widely accepted as the palliative treatment for this condition in malignant diseases, as it offers rapid relief of symptoms and improves the quality of life. Preserving previously placed central venous catheters (CVCs) is a major issue in this population. We report the case of a patient with SVC syndrome caused by tumoral obstruction due to central small-cell lung cancer who had right subclavian implanted CVC and a preferential head and neck venous drainage through the left internal jugular and brachiocephalic vein (BCV). We describe a complex procedure of SVC reconstruction with two different objectives: left recanalization and stent placement to ensure head and neck venous drainage and right BCV stenting for CVC repositioning and subsequent replacement. We also review published cases of SVC obstructions stenting with catheter repositioning. The patient experienced quick relief of symptoms after treatment. Chemotherapy was rapidly delivered through the preserved implanted CVC access. A 3-month follow-up computed tomography showed stents patency.

**Keywords: superior vena cava syndrome, endovascular stenting, lung cancer, central venous catheter protection, vena cava obstruction**

## INTRODUCTION

Endovascular stent-based revascularization is used as a therapeutic measure in patients with superior vena cava (SVC) obstructions (1). It does not interfere with subsequent antitumor treatments and provides urgent relief of symptoms (2, 3). Additionally, stenting greatly improves the quality of life of patients (4–7) with a good long-term patency, especially in patients with benign causes (1). Revascularization in patients with malignant causes of obstructions aims of course to ensure venous drainage but also in several cases where the patient had or need the central venous catheters (CVCs) to preserve the CVC function and/or route for insertion. We report the history of a patient who developed SVC syndrome due to extensive extravascular tumor-related obstruction and who previously received implanted CVC for the purpose of chemotherapy. The endovascular approach consisted on treating venous obstructions while preserving the CVC function using bilateral asymmetric stenting and endovascular CVC-repositioning maneuvers.

## CASE PRESENTATION

### Patient

A 60-year-old male patient with central small-cell lung cancer having brain, adrenal gland, and bones metastasis (stage IV) underwent right-sided subclavian CVC implantation 3 months ago for a first-line chemotherapy (cisplatin and etoposide).

He was admitted to the emergency department with symptoms suggestive of SVC syndrome, including distended collateral neck veins, plethora of the face, and dyspnea.

Computed tomography (CT) chest venography evidenced central tumor growth with the obstruction of the SVC and the encirclement of both brachiocephalic veins (BCVs). Neither endoluminal component nor thrombus formation was identified. The left internal jugular vein (IJV) was larger than the right, corresponding to a major left venous return from the head and neck.

The diagnosis of subacute SVC syndrome related to tumor progression was established. To provide rapid relief of severe venous congestion and its associated morbidity, endovascular management was decided.

The CVC was still functional on radiographic evaluation. In an attempt to preserve the CVC for any subsequent chemotherapy, we opted to deploy two kissing stents in order to cover the SVC downstream and both BCVs. The CVC tip had to be moved into the ipsilateral BCV before stent placement. A written consent was obtained from the patient.

### Procedure

We performed the procedure in the radiology vascular-operating room using X-ray guidance under local anesthesia (10 mL of 1% lidocaine) with conscious sedation (intravenous administration of 1 mg midazolam). Standard physiological monitoring (pulse, blood pressure, oxygen saturation, and electrocardiogram) was carried out during the procedure. Antibiotic prophylaxis administrated parentally was 2 g cefazolin. Both the right and left femoral veins were cannulated with 80-cm long 10 French sheaths to facilitate the passage of large-diameter balloons and stents.

The tight stenosis of the SVC and left BCV was crossed with a 5-Fr vertebral curve catheter (Terumo, Tokyo, Japan) and a 0.035-inch-angled hydrophilic guidewire (Terumo) *via* a femoral approach, and an SVC angiogram was carried out. Results showed a large filling defect of the SVC and left BCV stenosis with the presence of collateral veins (**Figure 1A**).

As it was not possible to cross the SVC and right BCV from the right femoral approach, the right basilic vein was punctured with a 20-G needle. A 45-cm long six-French introducer sheath was inserted and a phlebography was performed, revealing a subtotal stenosis of the right BCV in its central two-thirds with multiple collateral channels (**Figure 1B**). Mechanical recanalization of the right BCV and SVC occlusion was achieved with a 0.035-inch-angled hydrophilic guidewire from access through the basilic vein (Terumo) supported by a vertebral curve 5-French catheter (Terumo). When the guidewire had traversed the occluded segment, it was grasped with a one-loop snare on the opposite side from the femoral approach and retrieved through the hemostatic valve sheath in a "teleferic" mode. This allowed future insertion of a balloon or a stent over the guidewire. Once both BCVs have been recanalized, the tip of the CVC was snared and withdrawn into the right subclavian vein using a trifoil EN-snare (Merit Medical, South Jordan, USA) through a right basilic vein access (**Figure 2A**). Conventional percutaneous balloon angioplasty of the left BCV and SVC with a 4-mm diameter balloon was performed first (Passeo™ 35, Biotronik, Berlin, Germany). Bilateral kissing self-expandable Sinus-XL Flex stents (Optimed, Ettlingen, Germany) were deployed from the left BCV vein to the SVC (a 14-mm nominal diameter and 150 mm in length) and from the right BCV to the SVC (a 14-mm nominal diameter and 100 mm in length) (**Figure 2B**). The choice of stent diameters was guided by pretherapeutic data from CT with oversizing stents by up to 2-mm reference vessel diameter, in a non-involved BCV segment to help

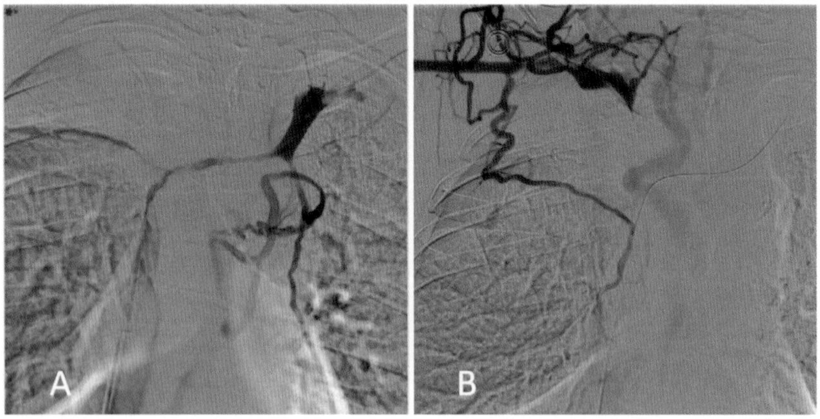


**FIGURE 1** | Digital subtraction phlebography from the left **(A)** and right **(B)** subclavian veins showed superior vena cava and both the right and left brachiocephalic vein stenosis with collateral channels.

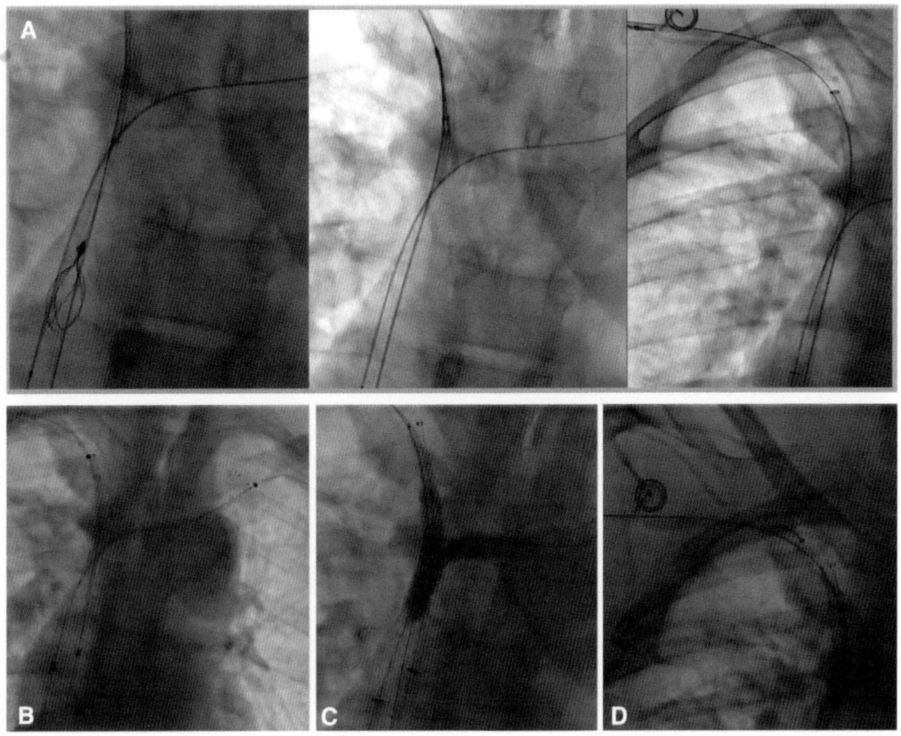

**FIGURE 2** | **(A)** In an attempt to preserve the central venous catheter (CVC) for further chemotherapy, the CVC tip was removed before stenting from the superior vena cava into the right subclavian vein using a trifoil EN-snare from access through the basilic vein. **(B)** Bilateral kissing stents deployment (a 14-mm nominal diameter and 150- and 100-mm nominal lengths, Sinus-XL Flex, Optimed) and **(C)** balloon angioplasty (an 8-mm diameter balloon within the right stent, a 10-mm diameter balloon within the left stent) of superior vena cava (SVC) and the bilateral caudal portion of the brachiocephalic veins were performed. **(D)** Using a snare-loop technique, the CVC tip was removed in the SVC within the stent to facilitate subsequent chemotherapy.

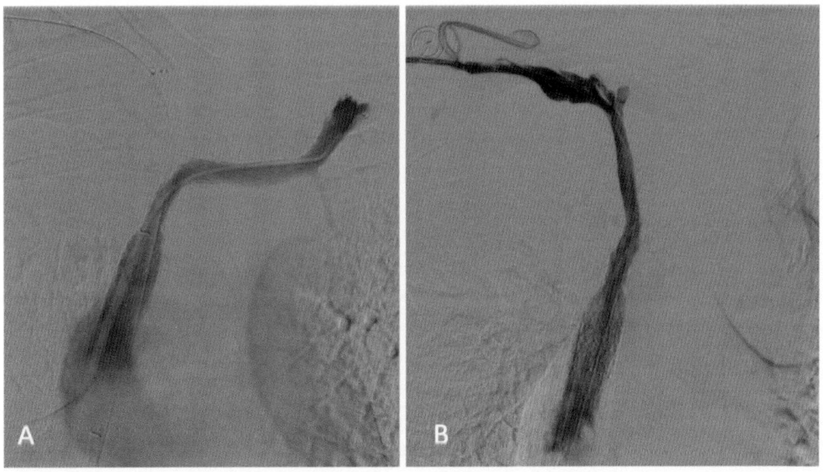

**FIGURE 3** | Left **(A)** and right **(B)** subclavian venograms obtained after stents placement showed restoration of superior vena cava and both brachiocephalic veins patency without collateral channels. No significant residual stenosis was observed within the stents.

reduce delayed stent migration (8, 9). Kissing balloon angioplasty was then performed within the stents using a 10-mm diameter balloon (Armada™ 35, Abbott Vascular, Chicago, USA) into the left-sided stent and an 8-mm diameter balloon (Armada™ 35, Abbott Vascular) into the right-sided stent (**Figure 2C**).

Finally, the CVC was carefully replaced in the SVC within the stent (**Figure 2D**) using the same "snare-loop" technique.

A final cavogram showed improvement in the luminal diameter of the SVC and both BCVs with a free flow of contrast material into the right atrium and no collateral veins (**Figure 3**).

Intravenous 7,000-IU heparin (5,000-IU heparin bolus at the beginning of the procedure followed by an administration of 2,000 IU after balloon angioplasty) was given *via* femoral venous sheath during the procedure. The procedure was successfully completed within 2 h.

## Follow-up

The patient experienced quick relief of symptoms and was discharged home 48 h later, with a prescription of 60 mg enoxaparin and 100 mg/day acetylsalicylic acid for 3 months. No procedure-related complications occurred. The sixth round of chemotherapy (carboplatine and etoposide) was administrated a week after recanalization.

At a 3-month follow-up, the patient was asymptomatic without recurrence of his previous symptoms, and no mechanical problem of the CVC was observed. CT venography showed stents expansion and patency with no collateral drainage (**Figure 4**).

The patient died 4 months following the stenting procedure. The leading cause of death was neurologic complications related to brain metastasis.

# DISCUSSION

The treatment of SVC syndrome using percutaneous transluminal stenting is a well-accepted technique with usually rapid symptom relief in these patients (10–12). The complications of this procedure including rupture of the SVC or stent migration are rare (12–14).

In our institution as in many centers, self-expanding bare-metal stents are the most common types of stents usually deployed in SVC obstructions (9, 12, 15, 16). Balloon-expandable stents are not recommended because of vein diameter differences between the distal- and proximal-landing zones and the short length of stents. Even if the use of covered stents versus bare-metal stents has suggested superior patency rates with covered stents after 12 months in malignant SVC obstruction (17), covered stents should be used with caution due to concerns of stent migration and covering venous collaterals, particularly if placing a covered stent across the brachiocephalic confluence. Slow-balloon pre-dilatation is required if the occlusive lesion precludes the passage of the stent delivery system. We also routinely perform post-stent dilatation if there is a >30% residual stenosis. This appears to be required in most of the patients (7, 15).

Data on the performance of bilateral stenting are limited. Dyet et al. stated that they had discontinued bilateral stent placement in SVC syndrome, having seen that unilateral placement was also clinically effective (16). Two studies found equally good initial clinical success in both groups, but a higher proportion of obstructive complications were seen in the bilateral group (18, 19). The bilateral technique is technically more demanding, and it is also more expensive and time-consuming.

When both BCVs are invaded by the tumor, unilateral BCV revascularization is sufficient and provides higher flow through the stent than when both BCVs are revascularized (20). The choice of recanalization side is based on the preferential head and neck venous drainage side or the inability to access both sides (1, 20, 21). CT phlebography is usually the modality of choice to determine the location of SVC obstruction and the involvement of BCV, and to provide an evaluation of head and neck venous drainage *via* internal jugular vein size (21). In our case, the left IJV vein was the major venous return from the head and neck, whereas the right IJV was thin. Therefore, the SVC downstream and the left BCV had to be recanalized to relieve symptoms.

Three options were considered. The first one was an SVC stenting with repositioning of the CVC just before and after stenting (1, 22, 23). CVCs are usually removed before stenting to prevent catheter fixation between the stent and the vessel wall with the associated risk of catheter dysfunction or catheter loss (24). To avoid catheter removal and the associated strain and risks of a new CVC insertion for the patient, a technique of repositioning before and after stenting was proposed, as previously described by Qanadli et al. (25). This option may have been considered in case of focal SVC stenosis without BCV veins involvement.

The second option would have been the SVC and left BCV stenting to assure head and neck venous drainage without preserving the CVC. This option may have led to catheter dysfunction or catheter loss. However, chemotherapy is also the standard form of treatment of malignant SVC syndrome. After rapid relief of

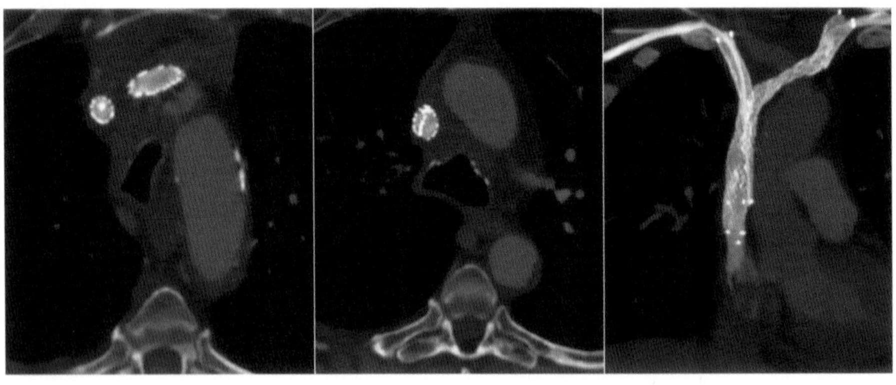

**FIGURE 4** | A 3-month follow-up computed tomography (axial sections and coronal section in maximum intensity projection) demonstrated bilateral stents patency without collateral veins. The left-sided stent, which ensures head and neck venous drainage, had a larger expansion than the right-sided one.

**TABLE 1** | Literature review of reported cases on technical differences of catheter repositioning during the treatment of SVC obstruction.

| Patient sex/age (years) | CVC type | CVC position/ tip | SVC obstruction stenosis/ occlusion | BCV obstruction stenosis/ occlusion | CVC-repositioning approach | Stenting SVC | Stenting RBCV/ LBCV | SVC reconstruction |
|---|---|---|---|---|---|---|---|---|
| F/61 (22) | Hickmann | R SCV/NS | 0/0 | 1/0 | Ipsilateral IVJ | 0 | 1/0 | 0 |
| M/61 (22) | Hickmann | R SCV/NS | 1/0 | 1/0 | Ipsilateral IVJ | 0 | 1/0 | 0 |
| F/76 (22) | Hickmann | L IJV/NS | 0/0 | 1/0 | Ipsilateral CV | 0 | 0/1 | 0 |
| M/61 (22) | Hickmann | L IJV/NS | 1/0 | 1/0 | Ipsilateral CV | 0 | 0/1 | 0 |
| M/63 (22) | Hickmann | L IJV/NS | 0/0 | 1/0 | Ipsilateral CV | 0 | 1/0 | 0 |
| F/77 (22) | Hickmann | R IJV/NS | 0/0 | 1/0 | Ipsilateral CV | 0 | 1/0 | 0 |
| F/24 (22) | ICVC | L BCV/NS | 1/0 | 0/1 | Contralateral CV | 1 | 0/0 | 0 |
| M/51 (22) | ICVC | L BCV/NS | 1/0 | 0/1 | Contralateral CV | 1 | 0/0 | 0 |
| M/48 (24) | ICVC | L SCV/SVC | 0/1 | 0/0 | Ipsilateral BV | 1 | 0/0 | 0 |
| F/49 (25) | ICVC | R SCV/SVC | 0/1 | 0/0 | Ipsilateral BV | 1 | 0/0 | 0 |
| F/44 (28) | ICVC | L SCV/SVC | 1/0 | 0/0 | R femoral vein | 1 | 0/0 | 0 |
| M/54 (29) | ICVC | L SCV/SVC | 1/0 | 0/1 | R IJV + L IJV | 1 | 0/1 | 0 |
| M/60[a] | ICVC | R SCV/SVC | 0/1 | 1/1 | Ipsilateral BV + R femoral vein | 2 | 1/1 | 1 |

*BCV, brachiocephalic vein; BV, basilica vein; CVC, central venous catheters; CV, cubital vein; ICVC, implanted central venous catheter; IJV, internal jugular vein; L, left; NS, not specified; R, right; SVC, superior vena cava.*
*[a]Refers to our article.*

symptoms after stenting, there is a need to continue the scheduled coadjuvant treatments (chemotherapy, radiotherapy, or both) (26). In this situation, unilateral stenting while preserving CVC access by leaving a peripherally inserted central catheter or an arm port CVC over the basilica vein access guidewire would have been another possibility.

A bilateral kissing stent deployment in order to cover the SVC downstream and both BCVs with CVC repositioning was the third and preferred option. This SVC reconstruction had two different objectives for each side. Left recanalization assured head and neck venous drainage, whereas right recanalization permitted CVC repositioning and subsequent in-stent replacement.

A last possibility is to deploy two different self-expandable stents, with a larger one in the SVC and left BCV. A larger stent would provide higher flow through it, reducing the risk of obstructive complications (27). In our case, the priority was to keep the left-sided flow patency to ensure head and neck drainage. We have oversized balloon angioplasty within the left-sided stent (a 10-mm diameter) comparatively to balloon angioplasty within the right-sided stent (an 8-mm diameter). Follow-up CT confirmed a larger expansion of the left-sided stent.

We reviewed published case reports of SVC stenting with catheter repositioning (**Table 1**). All previous cases reported CVC repositioning through the stent used in the treatment of SVC syndrome (22, 24, 25, 28, 29). Only two patients had SVC occlusion.

Our case reports for the first time SVC and BCV reconstruction, for the purpose of not only treating venous obstruction but also preserving CVC function. Because of the bilateral involvement of BCV, one axis (one stent) was used to treat venous obstruction and the second one (one stent) was implanted to create a venous access and save CVC function.

## CONCLUDING REMARKS

In conclusion, even if unilateral stent placement is preferable in most patients with SVC syndrome because it is as clinically efficient as bilateral placement while offering lower cost, easier procedure, and lower rates of complications, bilateral stenting has to be considered in selected patients to avoid catheter loss or to facilitate subsequent catheter insertion. The procedure is safe and improves patients' quality of life without the need of a second intervention for CVC placement.

## AUTHOR CONTRIBUTIONS

All authors listed have made a substantial, direct, and intellectual contribution to this work and approved it for publication.

## REFERENCES

1. Breault S, Doenz F, Jouannic AM, Qanadli SD. Percutaneous endovascular management of chronic superior vena cava syndrome of benign causes: long-term follow-up. *Eur Radiol* (2017) 27(1):97–104. doi:10.1007/s00330-016-4354-y
2. Nicholson AA, Ettles DF, Arnold A, Greenston M, Dyet JF. Treatment of malignant vena cava obstruction: metal stents or radiation therapy. *J Vasc Interv Radiol* (1997) 8:781–8. doi:10.1016/S1051-0443(97)70660-2
3. Niu S, Xu YS, Cheng L, Cao C. Stent insertion for malignant superior vena cava syndrome: effectiveness and long-term outcome. *Radiol Med* (2017) 122(8):633–8. doi:10.1007/s11547-017-0767-1
4. Kuo TT, Chen PL, Shih CC, Chen IM. Endovascular stenting for end-stage lung cancer patients with superior vena cava syndrome post first-line treatments – a single-center experience and literature review. *J Chin Med Assoc* (2017) 80(8):482–6. doi:10.1016/j.jcma.2017.04.005
5. Lanciego C, Pangua C, Chacon JI, Velasco J, Boy RC, Viana A, et al. Endovascular stenting as the first step in the overall management of malignant

superior vena cava syndrome. *AJR Am J Roentgenol* (2009) 193(2):549–58. doi:10.2214/AJR.08.1904

6. Lacombe P, Qanadli SD, Mignon F, Sissakian JF, Barré O, El Hajjam M, et al. Superior vena cava endoprosthesis. *Rev Mal Respir* (1999) 16(Suppl 3): S157–61.
7. Nagata T, Makutani S, Uchida H, Kichikawa K, Maeda M, Yoshioka T, et al. Follow-up results of 71 patients undergoing metallic stent placement for the treatment of a malignant obstruction of the superior vena cava. *Cardiovasc Intervent Radiol* (2007) 30(5):959–67. doi:10.1007/s00270-007-9088-4
8. Taylor JD, Lehmann ED, Belli AM, Nicholson AA, Kessel D, Robertson IR, et al. Strategies for the management of SVC stent migration into the right atrium. *Cardiovasc Intervent Radiol* (2007) 30(5):1003–9. doi:10.1007/s00270-007-9109-3
9. Mokry T, Bellemann N, Sommer CM, Heussel CP, Bozorgmehr F, Gnutzmann D, et al. Retrospective study in 23 patients of the self-expanding sinus-XL stent for treatment of malignant superior vena cava obstruction caused by non-small cell lung cancer. *J Vasc Interv Radiol* (2015) 26(3):357–65. doi:10.1016/j.jvir.2014.11.019
10. Rizvi AZ, Kalra M, Bjarnason H, Bower TC, Schleck C, Gloviczki P. Benign superior vena cava syndrome: stenting is now the first line of treatment. *J Vasc Surg* (2008) 47:372–80. doi:10.1016/j.jvs.2007.09.071
11. Qanadli SD, El Hajjam M, Mignon F, de Kerviler E, Rocha P, Barré O. Subacute and chronic benign superior vena cava obstructions: endovascular management by self-expanding metallic stents. *AJR Am J Roentgenol* (1999) 173(1):159–64. doi:10.2214/ajr.173.1.10397119
12. Ganeshan A, Hon LQ, Warakaulle DR, Morgan R, Uberoi R. Superior vena caval stenting for SVC obstruction: current status. *Eur J Radiol* (2009) 71(2):343–9. doi:10.1016/j.ejrad.2008.04.014
13. Devcic Z, Techasith T, Banerjee A, Rosenberg JK, Sze DY. Technical and anatomic factors influencing the success of inferior vena caval stent placement for malignant obstruction. *J Vasc Interv Radiol* (2016) 27(9):1350–60. doi:10.1016/j.jvir.2016.02.030
14. Smayra T, Otal P, Chabbert V, Chemla P, Romero M, Joffre F, et al. Long-term results of endovascular stent placement in the superior caval venous system. *Cardiovasc Intervent Radiol* (2001) 24(6):388–94. doi:10.1007/s00270-001-0055-1
15. Fagedet D, Thony F, Timsit JF, Rodiere M, Monnin-Bares V, Ferretti GR, et al. Endovascular treatment of malignant superior vena cava syndrome: results and predictive factors of clinical efficacy. *Cardiovasc Intervent Radiol* (2013) 36(1):140–9. doi:10.1007/s00270-011-0310-z
16. Dyet JF, Nicholson AA, Cook AM. The use of the wallstent endovascular prosthesis in the treatment of malignant obstruction of the superior vena cava. *Clin Radiol* (1993) 48:381–5. doi:10.1016/S0009-9260(05)81105-5
17. Gwon DI, Ko GY, Kim JH, Shin JH, Yoon HK, Sung KB. Malignant superior vena cava syndrome: a comparative cohort study of treatment with covered stents versus uncovered stents. *Radiology* (2013) 266(3):979–87. doi:10.1148/radiol.12120517
18. Dinkel HP, Mettke B, Schmid F, Baumgartner I, Triller J, Do DD. Endovascular treatment of malignant superior vena cava syndrome: is bilateral wallstent placement superior to unilateral placement? *J Endovasc Ther* (2003) 10:788–97. doi:10.1583/1545-1550(2003)010<0158:PTOPPU>2.0.CO;2
19. Lanciego C, Chacón JL, Julián A, Andrade J, López L, Martinez B, et al. Stenting as first option for endovascular treatment of malignant superior vena cava syndrome. *AJR Am J Roentgenol* (2001) 177:585–93. doi:10.2214/ajr.177.3.1770585
20. Uberoi R. Quality assurance guidelines for superior vena cava stenting in malignant disease. *Cardiovasc Intervent Radiol* (2006) 29(3):319–22. doi:10.1007/s00270-005-0284-9
21. Qanadli SD, El Hajjam M, Bruckert F, Judet O, Barré O, Chagnon S, et al. Helical CT phlebography of the superior vena cava: diagnosis and evaluation of venous obstruction. *AJR Am J Roentgenol* (1999) 172(5):1327–33. doi:10.2214/ajr.172.5.10227511
22. Stockx L, Raat H, Donck J, Wilms G, Marchal G. Repositioning and leaving in situ the central venous catheter during percutaneous treatment of associated superior vena cava syndrome: a report of eight cases. *Cardiovasc Intervent Radiol* (1999) 22(3):224–6. doi:10.1007/s002709900371
23. Clark K, Chick JF, Reddy SN, Shin BJ, Nadolski GJ, Clark TW, et al. Concurrent central venous stent and central venous access device placement does not compromise stent patency or catheter function in patients with malignant central venous obstruction. *J Vasc Interv Radiol* (2017) 28(4):602–7. doi:10.1016/j.jvir.2016.12.1222
24. Bovenschulte H, Bangard C, Lackner KJ. Superior vena cava stent implantation: preserving an indwelling port catheter by temporary shift of the brachiocephalic vein. *Rofo* (2010) 182(3):274–5. doi:10.1055/s-0028-1109993
25. Qanadli SD, Mesurolle B, Sissakian JF, Chagnon S, Lacombe P. Implanted central venous catheter-related acute superior vena cava syndrome: management by metallic stent and endovascular repositioning of the catheter tip. *Eur Radiol* (2000) 10(8):1329–31. doi:10.1007/s003300000361
26. Pérez CA, Presant CA, Van Amburg AL. Management of superior vena cava syndrome. *Semin Oncol* (1978) 5:123–35.
27. Yim CD, Sane SS, Bjarnason H. Superior vena cava stenting. *Radiol Clin North Am* (2000) 38(2):409–24. doi:10.1016/S0033-8389(05)70171-8
28. Perno J, Putnam SG, Cohen GS, Ball D. Endovascular treatment of superior vena cava syndrome without removing a central venous catheter. *J Vasc Interv Radiol* (1999) 10(7):917–8. doi:10.1016/S1051-0443(99)70137-5
29. Isfort P, Penzkofer T, Goerg F, Mahnken AH. Stenting of the superior vena cava and left brachiocephalic vein with preserving the central venous catheter in situ. *Korean J Radiol* (2011) 12(5):629–33. doi:10.3348/kjr.2011.12.5.629

# 18

# Impact on Patient Care of a Multidisciplinary Center Specializing in Colorectal and Pelvic Reconstruction

*Alejandra Vilanova-Sánchez[1,2], Carlos Albert Reck[3], Richard J. Wood[2], Cristina Garcia Mauriño[4], Alessandra C. Gasior[2], Robert E. Dyckes[2], Katherine McCracken[2], Laura Weaver[2], Devin R. Halleran[2], Karen Diefenbach[2], Dennis Minzler[4], Rebecca M. Rentea[2], Christina B. Ching[2], Venkata Rama Jayanthi[4], Molly Fuchs[2], Daniel Dajusta[2], Geri D. Hewitt[2] and Marc A. Levitt[2]**

[1] Pediatric Surgery, Colorectal and Pelvic Surgery Division, Hospital Universitario La Paz, Madrid, Spain, [2] Center for Colorectal and Pelvic Reconstruction (CCPR), Nationwide Children's Hospital, Columbus, OH, United States, [3] Vienna General Hospital, Vienna, Austria, [4] Nationwide Children's Hospital, Columbus, OH, United States

**Edited by:**
Pietro Bagolan,
Bambino Gesù Ospedale Pediatrico (IRCCS), Italy

**Reviewed by:**
Peter F. Nichol,
University of Wisconsin-Madison, United States
Elke Ruttenstock,
Hospital for Sick Children, Canada

***Correspondence:**
Marc A. Levitt
marc.levitt@nationwidechildrens.org

**Specialty section:**
This article was submitted to Pediatric Surgery, a section of the journal Frontiers in Surgery

**Aim of the study:** Many patients with an anorectal malformation (ARM) or pelvic anomaly have associated urologic or gynecologic problems. We hypothesized that our multidisciplinary center, which integrates pediatric colorectal, urologic, gynecologic and GI motility services, could impact a patient's anesthetic exposures and hospital visits.

**Methods:** We tabulated during 2015 anesthetic/surgical events, endotracheal intubations, and clinic/hospital visits for all patients having a combined procedure.

**Main results:** Eighty two patients underwent 132 combined procedures (**Table 1**). The median age at intervention was 3 years [0.2-17], and length of follow up was 25 months [7-31]. The number of procedures in patients who underwent combined surgery was lower as compared to if they had been done independently [1(1-5) vs. 3(2-7) ($p < 0.001$)]. Intubations were also lower [1[1-3] vs. 2[1-6]; $p < 0.001$]. Hospital length of stay was significantly lower for the combined procedures vs. the theoretical individual procedures [8 days [3-20] vs. 10 days [4-16]] $p < 0.05$. Post-operative clinic visits were fewer when combined visits were coordinated as compared to the theoretical individual clinic visits (urology, gynecology, and colorectal) [1[1-4] vs. 2[1-6]; $p = < 0.001$].

**Conclusions:** Patients with anorectal and pelvic malformations are likely to have many medical or surgical interventions during their lifetime. A multidisciplinary approach can reduce surgical interventions, anesthetic procedures, endotracheal intubations, and hospital/outpatient visits.

**Keywords: anorectal malformation (ARM), hirschsprung disease, multidiscipinary collaboration, combined procedure, colorectal surgery, impact on patient care**

## INTRODUCTION

Anorectal malformations (ARM), and a variety of complex pelvic anomalies have a high prevalence of urologic and gynecologic malformations with future consequences in urologic and fecal continence as well as sexual and reproductive health (1–4). Also, patients with spinal anomalies such as myelomeningocele have a high prevalence of neurogenic bladder and bowel leading to incontinence (5). Due to the complexity of these malformations these patients require multiple clinic visits, hospital admissions, and surgical procedures during their lifetime. Moreover, due to the broad scope of these malformations, numerous specialists in different surgical areas such as pediatric colorectal surgery, urology, and gynecology need to be involved in their care.

Good outcomes have been well described with surgical and medical multidisciplinary teams, reducing morbidity as well as cost and hospital stays when treating complex medical conditions, in both adult and pediatric populations (6–8). However, to our best knowledge, there is no reference showing the impact of a multidisciplinary approach in a Pediatric Colorectal Center.

In 2014, we developed a Center devoted to complex colorectal and pelvic care, with the primary goal to reduce the social and familial impact, the surgical and medical burden of care in this particular population. We aimed to describe our experience in a multidisciplinary center that treats patients with complex pelvic malformation and assess the impact of the collaborative approach to their care regarding surgical procedures, anesthetics events, and hospital and clinic visits.

## METHODS

### Data Collection

A retrospective review of patients having multidisciplinary treatment, with the involvement of more than one surgical team was performed from 1/2015 to 1/2016. The type of malformation, teams involved, type of anesthesia, procedures performed, length of hospital stay, number of clinic visits, complications, and duration of follow up were recorded.

We compared our results with the data we would have obtained if the procedures would have been done without the collaboration between services, meaning that a patient would have had individually procedures with individual anesthetic events, endotracheal intubation (if required), and single hospital admission and post-operative clinic visits.

To calculate the theoretical length hospital stay for individual procedures, the mean stay for the individual surgeries performed in our service during the same period for the same group of surgeons (year 2015) was recovered from the hospital database. For example: Mean of Hospital stay of Bilateral reimplant: 2 days. Mean of Colostomy closure: 4 days.

If they would had the procedures separately, they would have needed 6 days in 2 different hospital admission, 2 different anesthetics events and endotracheal intubations, 2 separate postoperative clinic visits and therefore hospital visits. If with the collaborative approach we found a patient having a colostomy closure and bilateral reimplant in the same anesthetic event with the same endotracheal intubation who needed 5 days of hospital admission we calculated: 1 surgical/anesthetic event, 1 endotracheal intubation, and only 1 post-operative clinic visit. That patient would have saved 1 anesthesia, 1 endotracheal intubation and 1 day of hospital admission.

### Statistical Analysis

Age of patients at time of combined surgical intervention, combined procedures per patient, anesthetic events, number of endotracheal intubation, hospital stay and clinic visits with and without collaboration were compared using Mann—Whitney test for continuous variables and chi-square test for categorical variables, and data presented as median (range) or frequencies (percentages) accordingly. Analyses were conducted GraphPad Prism v.6 (GraphPad Software; La Jolla, CA), with a two-sided $p$-value of $< 0.05$ considered statistically significant.

## SELECTION OF PATIENTS FOR COMBINED PROCEDURES

All patients able to have a combined procedure were discussed in a collaborative meeting. In that weekly team meeting, all the care providers in our Center are present: pediatric colorectal surgeons, pediatric urologists, pediatric and adolescent gynecologists, nurses and nurse practitioners, anesthesiologists, operating room staff, and social workers. We discuss the type of intervention needed, anesthetics risk, and modality of postoperative treatment and pain control. We also discussed the post-operative follow up plan for all of the disciplines involved in their care.

## LIMITATION OF THE STUDY

The theoretical number of independent procedures, independent anesthetic procedures, endotracheal intubations, and independent hospital admissions days are data that were telescope and attributed to our population. Due to the variables that we are comparing we could not compare the same procedures done combined and separately for the same population of patients during the same period. The most objective way to compare both approaches was to compare medians assuming the patients have the same characteristics and demographic characteristics in both groups. Regarding complications, we could not compare the rates of complications for the procedures done separately and combined as we did not have the data for the independent procedures available. Starting in 2016, the data has been collected prospectively (for both groups), and we will be able to report complications rate comparing both groups in the future.

## RESULTS

During the 1 year study period, a total of 285 patients underwent 469 surgical procedures in our Center. Of these, 82 patients underwent 132 combined procedures including: urology, gynecology plus colorectal (87), urology plus colorectal (34), or gynecology plus colorectal (11). Of the 82 patients, 56 (68%)

**TABLE 1** | Description of the services involved in the combined procedures.

| | | |
|---|---|---|
| Malformation | Complex ARM | 75 |
| | Spinal Anomaly | 5 |
| | Sacrococcygeal Teratoma | 2 |
| Combined procedures | Colorectal + Urology + Gynecology | 87 |
| | Colorectal + Urology | 34 |
| | Colorectal + Gynecology | 11 |
| Reason for collaboration | Practical Advantage | 115 |
| | Tissue sharing | 9 |
| | Single Pelvic Exploration | 8 |

were previously operated elsewhere and attended our clinic for definitive pelvic reconstruction or evaluation for a reoperation. Twenty six patients (32%) had not undergone prior definitive surgery before evaluation or treatment at our Center. The median age at the time of the combined procedures was 3 years [0.2–21]. The most frequent type of malformation was complex ARM, followed by cloaca and spinal anomalies (**Table 1**).

We divided the combined procedures into 3 categories based on the main reason for the collaboration (**Table 2**).

The first group of procedures were those we decided to be combined in order to save an anesthetic, visits to the hospital, and/or for a practical advantage (115). Seventy five of these procedures (57%) were minor procedures such an examination of the perineum under anesthesia combined with vaginoscopy and cystoscopy, with the three teams present at the procedure. This simple combination of procedures saved 150 anesthesia inductions, 150 hospital visits and allowed operative planning for future reconstruction if needed.

The second group of combined procedures were those which could not have been done without collaboration due to sharing of tissues (9) (**Table 2**). These include 3 appendices used for both Malone and Mitrofanoff, 5 sigmoid colons used for both bladder augment and sigmoid resection (in patients with colonic dysmotility needing a colonic resection) and 1 redo PSARP and rectal patch used for urethral repair of urethral stricture after primary PSARP.

The third group of patients was selected for a combined procedure to enter the pelvis only once in complex pelvic malformations, including the 3 combined teams working together performing complex urologic, gynecologic and colorectal reconstruction (8).

The median number anesthetic events per patient and therefore hospital visits were significantly lower in those who underwent combined procedures vs. if the procedures would have been done independently [combined 1 [1-5], individual 3[2-7]].

The number of patients who required endotracheal intubation in any of their combined procedures was 36, with a total of 42 endotracheal intubations performed. The median number of intubations per patient was significantly lower when combined procedures were performed vs. theoretical individually performed surgeries. [combined; 1[1-3], individual 2[1-6]; $p < 0.001$] (**Table 3**).

A total of 43 procedures required hospital admission. The median number of hospital stay in days was significantly lower for the combined procedures vs. theoretical individual procedures (8 days [3-20] vs. 10 days [4-16]; $p < 0.001$).

A total of 46 patients had a total of 67 multidisciplinary clinic visits. The median number of clinic visits and therefore visits to the hospital during the study period per patient was significantly lower when combined clinic visits were coordinated vs. theoretical individually visits (urology,gynecology, and colorectal) [combined; 1[1-4], individual 2[1-6]; $P = < 0.001$].

The median length of follow up has been 25 months [7-31].

In the post-operative period, 6 patients had complications that required a conservative treatment (5 wound infections, 1 scrotal hematoma). Three patients needed reintervention in the same hospital admission (2 pelvic abscesses with IR drainage placement, 1 rectovaginal fistula with colostomy creation). In the long term follow up, 1 patient needed a Mitrofanoff revision, and 1 malone revision, both for a skin level stricture.

## DISCUSSION

Patients with congenital anorectal and pelvic malformations as well as other many chronic health impairments require regular episodes of hospital visits or anesthetic exposures. These children are medically fragile and need frequent hospitalizations, emergency department visits, and surgical procedures. The presence of a chronic condition, such as complex pelvic malformation, may also limit or alter social interactions, due to fecal or urinary incontinence, and distinguish children from their peers, which can increase their anxiety and depression in early ages (9). It has been well documented in many medical fields, in both adults and children, that a multidisciplinary approach can improve healthcare in complex illnesses. With a multi-specialist work team approach, health care burden, patient self-perception of illness and family responsibilities can be minimized as well as a reduction of surgical procedures and therefore exposure to anesthetics (10–14). Although, this has been proven in other conditions, this is the first study to our knowledge reporting on the impact on medical care associated with an interdisciplinary approach for children with complex congenital pelvic/anorectal malformations.

In this study, we analyzed the burden of care in patients presenting to our multidisciplinary Colorectal and Pelvic Reconstruction Center who underwent a surgical procedure from January 2015 and January 2016. We provided combined procedures with more than one service involved to 82 patients, performing 132 combined procedures. The majority of combined procedures 75 (57%) were done with the primary objective of minimizing the hospital visits, or to shorten anesthetics exposure or minor procedures. This first group of combined procedures saved 150 anesthesia inductions and 150 hospital visits.

Our goal was to minimize multiple anesthetic exposures in children, which have been related to an increased risk for later development of ADHD and mental disabilities (15, 16). In studies demonstrating an association of anesthesia with disability, only children with multiple anesthetic exposures have

**TABLE 2 |** Description of the combined porcedures and reason for combined surgery.

| Type of collaboration | Number of procedures | Combined procedures |
|---|---|---|
| Practical advantage | 115 | 75 Cystoscopy + Examination under anesthesia + vaginoscopy<br>8 Colostomy closure + assessment Mullerian structures<br>6 Colostomy closure + orchidopexy<br>5 Colostomy closure + circumcision<br>4 Colostomy closure + hypospadias repair<br>3 Colostomy closure + ureteral reimplantation<br>2 Colostomy closure + scrotoplasty<br>1 Colostomy closure + malone + ureteral reimplant + vesicostomy closure<br>1 Colostomy closure + nephrectomy<br>1 Colostomy closure + orchiectomy + scrotoplasty + utricule resection<br>1 Redo PSARP + introitoplasty + vaginal septum removal<br>1 Redo PSARP + lap Malone + resection remnant of the original fístula (ROOF) + penoscrotal web release<br>1 Redo PSARP + lap Malone + circumcision + penoscrotal transposition<br>1 Redo PSARP + Malone + orchidopexy + scrotoplasty<br>1 Redo PSARP + ROOF excision + ureteral reimplant<br>1 Sigmoid resection + Malone + Mitrofanoff revision +Inspection mullerian structures + vaginoscopy<br>1 Neo-Malone + Mitrofanoff revision + cystoscopy |
| Tissue sharing | 9 | 5 Sigmoid colon used for bladder augment +BN sling + sigmoid resection in dysfunctional colon + Mitrofanoff<br>3 Split Appendix used for Malone + Mitrofanoff<br>1 Redo PSARP + rectal patch used for urethral stricture repair |
| Single pelvic exploration | 8 | 2 Colonic pull through + bladder augment + BN sling + Mitrofanoff + vaginal replacement + ileostomy creation<br>1 Redo Cloaca repair + vaginal replacement + bladder augment<br>1 Redo Cloaca repair + ileostomy creation + left ureteral reimplant + vaginal replacement<br>1 Redo Cloaca repair + Neo-Malone + ileostomy creation + bilateral ureteral reimplant + mitrofanoff + vaginal Replacement<br>1 Redo PSARP + Bladder augmen t+ Monti + Introitoplasty +inspection mullerian structures<br>1 Cloaca repair + Bladder augment + vesicostomy + nephrectomy + vaginal replacement |
| Total | 132 | |

*PSARP, Posterior sagittal anorectoplasty; ROOF, Remamnt of the origianl fistula; BN, Bladder neck.*

**TABLE 3 |** Comparison of the number of anesthetic inductions, clinic vistis, and endotracheal intubations perfomed per patient with and without a multidisciplinary approach.

| Intervention | With multidisciplinary team | Without multidisciplinary team | Total interventions saved | Intervention saved per patient | *p*-value |
|---|---|---|---|---|---|
| Anesthetic inductions | 132 | 346 | 214 | 2.6 (1–6) | $p < 0.001$ |
| Endotracheal intubations | 50 | 101 | 51 | 0.6 (0–3) | $p < 0.001$ |
| Clinic visits | 67 | 156 | 89 | 11.17 (1–2) | $p < 0.001$ |

been associated with deficits, but an effect with a single exposure has not been identified (17, 18). Environmental factors though may be important in the development of mental issues after anesthesia (19).

We also reduced the number of endotracheal intubations by 50% (from 101 to 50) with a mean saved per patient ratio of 0.6 (range 0–3) ($p < 0.0001$). This reduction directly minimized the risk of developing congenital subglottic stenosis in children due in part to multiple endotracheal intubations or long period of intubations (20–22).

The second groups of procedures were scheduled as combined cases for tissue sharing advantages. We used the appendix for both Malone and Mitrofanoff in children with neurogenic bowel and bladder (23). This way we avoided the risk of a new intervention or the risk of the creation of either a neo-Malone or a small bowel Monti procedure with a bowel anastomosis. We also shared the sigmoid in 5 children needing colonic resection for colonic dysmotility and needing a bladder augmentation. In a patient with an anal and urethral stricture after a primary PSARP, we used a rectal patch for repair of a post-operative urethral stricture done at the time of the redo PSARP. These procedures could not have been done without a collaborative approach.

The third groups of patients are those with very complex urologic, gynecologic, and colorectal diseases requiring repair of all three organ systems. We had several reasons to combine their operations in addition to saving hospital visits, anesthetic exposure and the number of endotracheal intubations namely the ability to avoid entering the pelvis multiple times. The distinct advantages to this approach include: Colorectal surgery involving colonic pull through and pelvic anastomosis have been directly related with infertility (24–26), and multiple pelvic and abdominal surgeries are directly associated with a higher risk of bowel obstruction and the need for emergent surgery. Adhesiolysis in repeat abdominal surgery may increase the incidence of inadvertent bowel injury and increases the operating time and as well as future chronic abdominal and pelvic pain (27, 28).

The total hospital days saved was 103 and the mean saved per patient was 1.25 (range 0–5) ($p < 0.0001$). By reducing the number of days of hospital admission, we reduced the burden of medication, antibiotics, the risk of nosocomial infection and psychologic and economic impact on the patient and the family. By lowering the post-operative clinic visits, we also reduced the cost of travel to the clinic for the family as well as the number of unattended work/school days. Post-operative combined clinic visits were reduced by 42%, and every patient saved at least 1–2 clinic visits.

In summary, we can conclude that patients with anorectal and pelvic malformations are likely to have many medical or surgical interventions during their lifetime. Our data shows that if they are treated using a multidisciplinary approach, hospital length of stay, clinic visits and surgical and anesthetic procedures can be minimized. This reduces both the burden of care as well as the financial impact of medical care. We believe that this model of care could be reproducible in other parts of the health care system.

## AUTHOR'S NOTE

This study was reviewed and approved by Institutional Review Board at Nationwide Children's Hospital, Columbus Ohio, with the study registry number IRB14-00232 being part of the Colorectal registry at the Center for colorectal and pelvic reconstruction, Nationwide Children'sHospital.

## AUTHOR CONTRIBUTIONS

AV-S: Main author. CR, AG, KM, RD, DM, KD, CC, and DD: Data collection. RW, VJ, GH, DRH, and MF: Editor of manuscript. CG, RR, and LW: Data analysis. ML: Senior author. All authors of this research paper have directly participated in the planning, execution, or analysis of this study. All authors of this paper have read and approved the final version submitted.

## REFERENCES


1. Levitt MA, Stein DM, Peña A. Gynecologic concerns in the treatment of teenagers with cloaca. *J Pediatr Surg.* (1998) 33:188–93.
2. Goossens WJ, de Blaauw I, Wijnen MH, de Gier RP, Kortmann B, Feitz WF. Urological anomalies in anorectal malformations in The Netherlands: effects of screening all patients on long-term outcome. *Pediatr Surg Int.* (2011) 27:1091–7. doi: 10.1007/s00383-011-2959-4
3. Rigueros Springford L, Connor MJ, Jones K, Kapetanakis VV, Giuliani S. Prevalence of active long-term problems in patients with anorectal malformations: a systematic review. *Dis Colon Rectum.* (2016) 59:570–80. doi: 10.1097/DCR.0000000000000576
4. Skerritt C, Sánchez AV, Lane VA, Wood RJ, Hewitt GD, Breech LL, et al. Menstrual, sexual, and obstetrical outcomes after vaginal replacement for vaginal atresia associated with anorectal malformation. *Eur J Pediatr Surg.* (2016) 27:495–502. doi: 10.1055/s-0036-1593610
5. Chan YY, Sandlin SK, Kurzrock EA. Urological outcomes of myelomeningocele and lipomeningocele. *Curr Urol Rep.* (2017) 18.35. doi: 10.1007/s11934-017-0684-9
6. Alizo G, Sciarretta JD, Gibson S, Muertos K, Holmes S, Denittis F, et al. Multidisciplinary team approach to traumatic spinal cord injuries: a single institution's quality improvement project. *Eur J Trauma Emerg Surg.* (2017) 44:245–250. doi: 10.1007/s00068-017-0776-8
7. Stephens MR, Lewis WG, Brewster AE, Lord I, Blackshaw GR, Hodzovic I, et al. Multidisciplinary team management is associated with improved outcomes after surgery for esophageal cancer. *Dis Esophagus* (2006) 19:164–71. doi: 10.1111/j.1442-2050.2006.00559.x
8. Bratton DL, Price M, Gavin L, Glenn K, Brenner M, Gelfand EW, et al. Impact of a multidisciplinary day program on disease and healthcare costs in children and adolescents with severe asthma: a two-year follow-up study. *Pediatr Pulmonol.* (2001) 31:177–89. doi: 10.1002/ppul.1027
9. Gortmaker SL, Walker DK, Weitzman M, Sobol AM. Chronic conditions, socioeconomic risks, and behavioral problems in children and adolescents. *Pediatrics* (1990) 85:267–76.
10. Berman S, Rannie M, Moore L, Elias E, Dryer LJ, Jones MD Jr. Utilization and costs for children who have special health care needs and are enrolled in a hospital-based comprehensive primary care clinic. *Pediatrics* (2005) 115:e637–42. doi: 10.1542/peds.2004-2084
11. Junor EJ, Hole DJ, Gillis CR. Management of ovarian cancer: referral to a multidisciplinary team matters. *Br J Cancer* (1994) 70:363–70.
12. Collaco JM, Aherrera AD, Au Yeung KJ, Lefton-Greif MA, Hoch J, Skinner ML. Interdisciplinary pediatric aerodigestive care and reduction in health care costs and burden. *JAMA Otolaryngol Head Neck Surg.* (2015) 141:101–5. doi: 10.1001/jamaoto.2014.3057
13. Bocca G, Corpeleijn E, van den Heuvel ER, Stolk RP, Sauer PJ. Three-year follow-up of 3-year-old to 5-year-old children after participation in a multidisciplinary or a usual-care obesity treatment program. *Clin Nutr.* (2014) 33:1095–100. doi: 10.1016/j.clnu.2013.12.002
14. von Kodolitsch Y, Rybczynski M, Vogler M, Mir TS, Schüler H, Kutsche K, et al. The role of the multidisciplinary health care team in the management of patients with Marfan syndrome. *J Multidiscip Healthc.* (2016) 9:587–614. doi: 10.2147/JMDH.S93680
15. Sprung J, Flick RP, Katusic SK, Colligan RC, Barbaresi WJ, Bojanić K, et al. Attention-deficit/hyperactivity disorder after early exposure to procedures requiring general anesthesia. *Mayo Clin Proc.* (2012) 87:120–9. doi: 10.1016/j.mayocp.2011.11.008
16. Wilder RT, Flick RP, Sprung J, Katusic SK, Barbaresi WJ, Mickelson C, et al. Early exposure to anesthesia and learning disabilities in a

population-based birth cohort. *Anesthesiology* (2009) 110:796–804. doi: 10.1097/01.anes.0000344728.34332.5d
17. DiMaggio C, Sun LS, Li G. Early childhood exposure to anesthesia and risk of developmental and behavioral disorders in a sibling birth cohort. *Anesth Analg.* (2011) 113:1143–51. doi: 10.1213/ANE.0b013e3182147f42
18. Flick RP, Katusic SK, Colligan RC, Wilder RT, Voigt RG, Olson MD, et al. Cognitive and behavioral outcomes after early exposure to anesthesia and surgery. *Pediatrics* (2011) 128:e1053–61. doi: 10.1542/peds.2011-0351
19. Ing C, DiMaggio C, Whitehouse A, Hegarty MK, Brady J, von Ungern-Sternberg BS, et al. Long-term differences in language and cognitive function after childhood exposure to anesthesia. *Pediatrics* (2012) 130: e476–85. doi: 10.1542/peds.2011-3822
20. Jefferson ND, Cohen AP, Rutter MJ. Subglottic stenosis. *Semin Pediatr Surg.* (2016) 25:138–43. doi: 10.1053/j.sempedsurg.2016.02.006
21. Ortiz R, Dominguez E, De La Torre C, Hernandez F, Encinas JL, Lopez-Fernandez S, et al. Early endoscopic dilation and mitomycin application in the treatment of acquired tracheal stenosis. *Eur J Pediatr Surg.* (2014) 24:39–45. doi: 10.1055/s-0033-1357754
22. Kruse KE, Purohit PJ, Cadman CR, Su F, Aghaeepour N, Hammer GB. Subglottic stenosis following cardiac surgery with cardiopulmonary bypass in infants and children. *Pediatr Crit Care Med.* (2017) 18:429–33. doi: 10.1097/PCC.0000000000001125
23. VanderBrink BA, Levitt MA, Defoor WR, Alam S. Creation of an appendicovesicostomy Mitrofanoff from a preexisting appendicocecostomy utilizing the spilt appendix technique. *J Pediatr Surg.* (2014) 49:656–9. doi: 10.1016/j.jpedsurg.2013.12.021
24. The Cochrane Collaboration. Barrier agents for adhesion prevention after gynaecological surgery. In: *Cochrane Database of Systematic Reviews.* Chichester: John Wiley & Sons, Ltd (1996). p. 135. (Abstract from 7th Congress of the European Society for Gynaecological Endoscopy; vol. 177).
25. Rajaratnam SG, Eglinton TW, Hider P, Fearnhead NS. Impact of ileal pouch-anal anastomosis on female fertility: meta-analysis and systematic review. *Int J Colorectal Dis.* (2011) 26:1365–74. doi: 10.1007/s00384-011-1274-9
26. Mavros MN, Velmahos GC, Lee J, Kaafarani HM. Adhesiolysis-related morbidity in abdominal surgery: an analysis of 5940 cases from the ACS-NSQIP database. *J Surg Res.* (2014) 186:675. doi: 10.1016/j.jss.2013.11.822
27. ten Broek RP, Issa Y, van Santbrink EJ, Bouvy ND, Kruitwagen RF, Jeekel J, et al. Burden of adhesions in abdominal and pelvic surgery: systematic review and met-analysis. *BMJ.* (2013) 347:f5588. doi: 10.1136/bmj.f5588
28. Hindocha A, Beere L, Dias S, Watson A, Ahmad G. Adhesion prevention agents for gynaecological surgery: an overview of Cochrane reviews. *Cochrane Database Syst Rev.* (2015) 1:CD011254. doi: 10.1002/14651858.CD011254

# 19

# Current Limitations of Surgical Robotics in Reconstructive Plastic Microsurgery

*Youri P. A. Tan* [1]*, *Philippe Liverneaux* [2] *and Jason K. F. Wong* [1,3]

[1] *The Manchester Centre for Plastic Surgery and Burns, Manchester University NHS Foundation Trust, Manchester, United Kingdom,* [2] *Department of Hand Surgery, University Hospital of Strasbourg, FMTS, University of Strasbourg, Icube CNRS, Illkirch, France,* [3] *Blond McIndoe Laboratories, Division of Cell Matrix Biology and Regenerative Medicine, University of Manchester, Manchester, United Kingdom*

Surgical robots have the potential to provide surgeons with increased capabilities, such as removing physiologic tremor, scaling motion and increasing manual dexterity. Several surgical specialties have subsequently integrated robotic surgery into common clinical practice. Plastic and reconstructive microsurgical procedures have not yet benefitted significantly from technical developments observed over the last two decades. Several studies have successfully demonstrated the feasibility of utilising surgical robots in plastic surgery procedures, yet limited work has been done to identify and analyse current barriers that have prevented wide-scale adaptation of surgical robots for microsurgery. Therefore, a systematic review using PubMed, MEDLINE, Embase and Web of Science databases was performed, in order to evaluate current state of surgical robotics within the field of reconstructive microsurgery and their limitations. Despite the theoretical potential of surgical robots, current commercially available robotic systems are suboptimal for plastic or reconstructive microsurgery. Absence of bespoke microsurgical instruments, increases in operating time, and high costs associated with robotic-assisted provide a barrier to using such systems effectively for reconstructive microsurgery. Consequently, surgical robots provide currently little overall advantage over conventional microsurgery. Nevertheless, if current barriers can be addressed and systems are specifically designed for microsurgery, surgical robots may have the potential of meaningful impact on clinical outcomes within this surgical subspeciality.

**Keywords: reconstructive surgery, plastic surgery, microsurgery, surgical robotics, robotic surgery**

**Edited by:**
*Vijay S. Gorantla, University of Pittsburgh Medical Center, United States*

**Reviewed by:**
*Fatih Zor, Wake Forest Institute for Regenerative Medicine, United States*
*Oren Lapid, Academic Medical Center (AMC), Netherlands*

***Correspondence:**
*Youri P. A. Tan*
*youri.tan@nhs.net*

**Specialty section:**
*This article was submitted to Reconstructive and Plastic Surgery, a section of the journal Frontiers in Surgery*

## 1. INTRODUCTION

Progressive changes in robotic and computer-guided systems have significantly altered operating practice across different medical and surgical specialties. Surgical robots can extend the capabilities of surgeons by reducing fine tremors, increasing manual dexterity and offering real-time 3D visualisation during endoscopic surgery (1, 2). This allows for highly precise movement in narrow and difficult-to-access spaces, and subsequently opens the door for minimally invasive surgery (**Figure 1**). In addition to enhancing surgical skills and improving ergonomics during surgery, minimally invasive surgery is associated with shorter hospitalisation and reduced risk of adverse complications (3, 4). Recent success of surgical robots, particularly the da Vinci Surgical System® (Intuitive Surgical™, Sunnyvale, CA), has created a thriving multibillion-dollar industry. Numerous companies are now focusing on

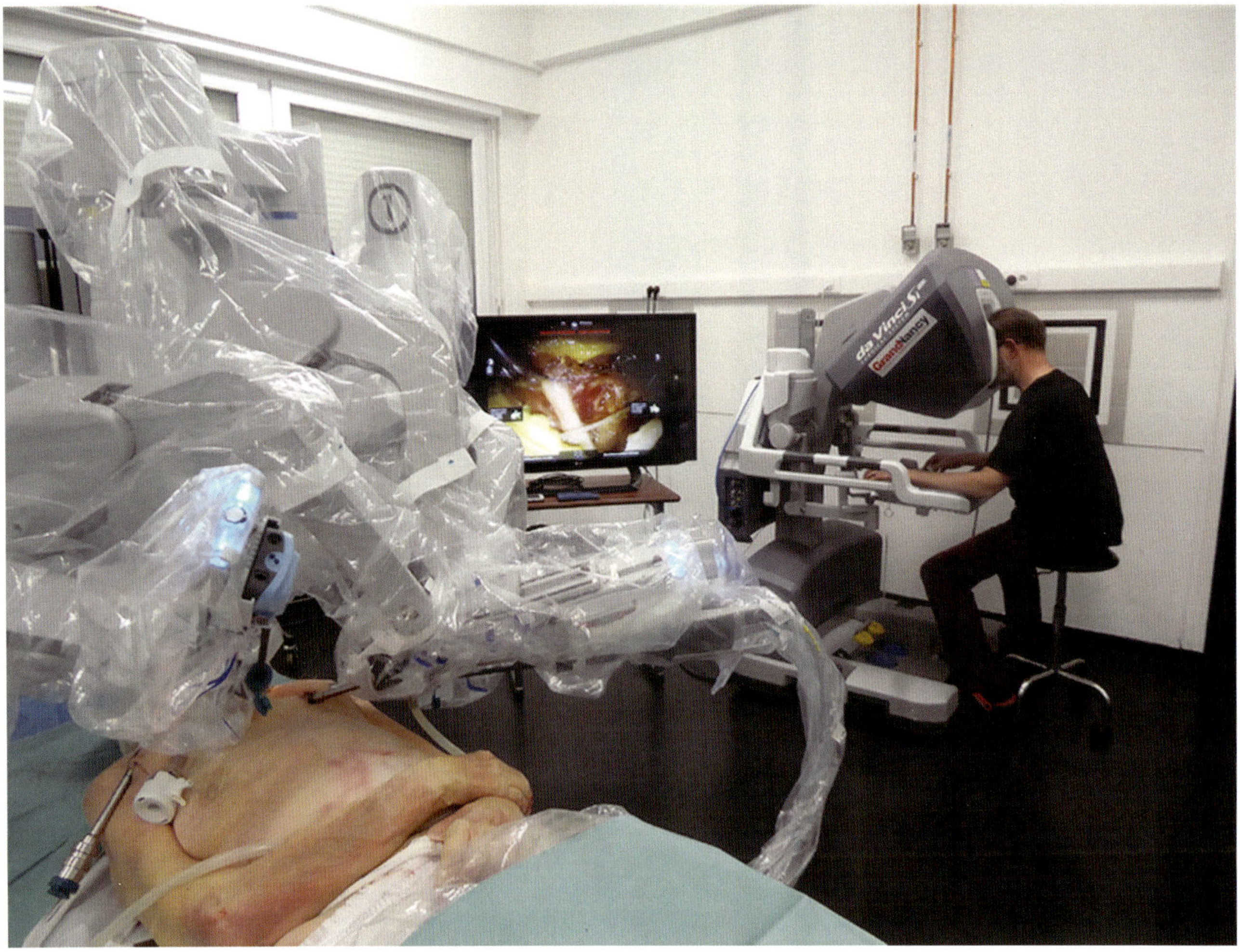

**FIGURE 1 |** Endoscopic robot-assisted C7 nerve root retrophalangeal transfer from the contralateral healthy side: a cadaver feasibility study. Installation of a da Vinci SI® robot (Intuitive Surgical™, Sunnyvale, CA). In the first plane, the cadaver is in a supine position and the robot is installed at the head to dissect the left brachial plexus. In the second plane, a 2D monitor shows the suture of the two current C7 roots. In the third plane, the operator, installed at the surgical console, telemanipulates the robot's arms. The working space is kept open by blowing CO2 at 10 mmHg.

this market in order to gain a stake in this valuable industry. Verily Life Sciences™ (formerly Google Life Sciences™) and Johnson & Johnson™ are collaborating on the development of a surgical robotic system through Verb Surgical™. Medtronic™ has made sizeable investments in Mazor Robotics™ that focusses on the development of surgical robots for spine and brain surgery. Furthermore, other less-known companies, such as Auris Surgical Robotics™, Cambridge Medical Robotics™ and TransEnterix Surgical™, have each announced their own surgical robotics platform. While several novel teleoperated surgical robotic systems are expected to become available within the foreseeable future, the next generation of partial autonomous surgical robots, capable of suturing skin and creating soft-tissue anastomosis without direct input from surgeons, is already being tested in research laboratories (5).

## 1.1. Surgical Robotics in Plastic Surgery

Despite numerous technical advancements in surgical robotics in recent years, only a small proportion of surgical specialties have benefited notably from these innovations. Within the United States, approximately 85% of radical prostatectomies were done robotically in 2013. Radical prostatectomies are now more commonly performed using a robot-assisted technique compared to laparoscopic surgery (6, 7). Similarly, uptake of robotic-assisted surgery has been increasing rapidly among gynaecology within a relatively short time frame. A survey among gynaecologist oncology training centres revealed that 24% of US gynaecologist oncologists perform robotic-assisted surgery, whereas 95% of US gynaecological oncology fellows are trained to use the da Vinci Surgical System® (8).

Contrary to the developments within urological and gynaecological surgery, the field of plastic and reconstructive surgery has seen little utilisation of surgical robotics and computer-assisted systems in the operating theatre. Despite plastic surgery's limited use of endoscopic surgery, specific advantages of currently available robotic systems, such as removal of physiologic tremor and improved dexterity, can theoretically provide significant aid during microsurgical procedures.

Motivated by the possibility of enhancing the practical skills required during surgery and combining this with imaging modalities, plastic surgeons have studied the feasibility of integrating robots into clinical practice. Several clinical studies have shown that robotic microsurgery for plastic and reconstructive procedures is feasible. Early studies in rats highlighted that robotic-assisted surgery can aid during microsurgery. In 2000, Li et al. successfully demonstrated 1 mm femoral artery anastomosis in Sprague-Dawley rats using a four-degrees-of-freedom telemanipulator system (SRI International, Menlo Park, CA) with equal anastomotic patency rates compared to conventional microsurgical anastomosis (9). A larger comparison in 2005 between conventional microsurgery and microsurgery using the Zeus Robotic Surgical System® (Computer Motion™, Goleta, CA) to perform end-to-end anastomoses of 1 mm femoral arteries in Sprague-Dawley rats with interrupted 10–0 suture achieved similar results (10). Later studies in pigs also revealed positive results in more complex scenarios, such as free-flap surgery and limb replantation (11, 12). Success in a variety of animal studies, subsequently translated into the first human trials of robotic-assisted surgery to harvest the internal mammary vessels to provide the recipient pedicle for free-flap breast reconstruction. Granting a relatively high complication rate in 20 patients (6 take-backs, and loss of 2 muscle flaps), Boyd et al. highlighted that robotic harvest of the internal mammary vessels was feasible (13). As surgical robots became more available in hospitals, they were applied to a wider range of plastic surgical procedures, such as free-flap reconstruction (14, 15), brachial plexus (16, 17) and peripheral nerve surgery (18). Yet, despite the theoretical benefits positive results, plastic surgery did not follow the trend to incorporate surgical robots on a larger scale. Adaptation of surgical robots within plastic surgery is currently limited to very few reconstructive microsurgical procedures. Sole subspecialty within plastic surgery that has utilised robotic-assisted surgery is oropharyngeal surgery, on the grounds that the da Vinci Surgical System® is FDA approved for transoral robotic head and neck surgery. Nevertheless, using surgical robots during plastic surgery procedures remains a rare occurrence.

In order to maximise the potential of surgical robots in plastic and reconstructive surgery, barriers and shortcomings of surgical robots have to be addressed. In this paper, we examine previous studies and identify limitations of surgical robots and indirect barriers that have prevented widespread utilisation. This will help us determine what are the requirements for future robotic systems to address the needs in reconstructive microsurgery. The aim of our systematic review is to increase awareness of the imperfections of the current generation of surgical robots and prevent these from occurring in future robotic systems.

## 2. METHODOLOGY

A literature search was performed using MEDLINE, PubMed, Embase and Web of Science. The search term "robot* microsurgery" was used for all four databases: MEDLINE, Embase, PubMed and Web of Science. Our search was limited to full-text articles written in English and published between January 2000 and July 2017. Only papers that directly utilised surgical robots in either a laboratory or clinical settings were included. Emphasis was put on feasibility studies, case reports, case series and so on, whereas literature reviews were excluded. Both human and animal studies were included in our search. For each paper, abstracts were assessed based on relevance to robotics within plastic reconstructive microsurgery. Publications purely related to other surgical specialties, such as urology and neurosurgery were excluded. In addition, engineering or technical papers proposing novel robotic systems were also omitted. Articles that passed initial screening were subsequently reviewed full text and data regarding limitations, disadvantages and barriers of surgical robotics in plastic and reconstructive microsurgery was extracted.

## 3. RESULTS

Our search yielded a total of 1,848 articles, and after removal of duplicates we obtained 962 unique articles. Eight hundred and forty articles were subsequently excluded after screening of abstracts based on our inclusion criteria as described in our methodology. Hundred and twenty-two full-text papers were assessed for further analysis, which resulted in exclusion of 84 articles and inclusion of 38 papers (**Figure 2**). Analysis of all papers in our review revealed that the 53% ($n$ = 20) of papers that utilised surgical robotic systems during microsurgical procedures are feasibility studies. The remainder of papers were case series ($n$ = 10), case reports ($n$ = 4) and cohort studies ($n$ = 2). The da Vinci Surgical System® was the most common surgical robotic system that was used ($n$ = 31). Other papers either used the Zeus Robotic Surgical System®, Automated Endoscopic System for Optical Positioning® (Computer Motion™, Goleta, CA) or a custom surgical robot (**Table 1**).

Fourteen papers examined the use of surgical robotics in live humans patients (13–26), five studies exclusively focussed on human cadaver specimens (27–31), while two papers described the use of surgical robots in both human cadavers and live patients (32, 33). Fourteen papers evaluated the use of surgical robotics exclusively in animal models (9–12, 34–43), and one paper used both animal models and human cadaver material (44). A relatively small proportion of papers ($n$ = 2) that were included in our review used artificial material to investigate the use of surgical robotic systems in reconstructive microsurgery (45, 46). Nearly all studies, 93% ($n$ = 13) that described the use of surgical robots in live human patients utilised the da Vinci Surgical System®. The exact versions of the da Vinci Surgical System® used across the different studies, for example, da Vinci S®, da Vinci Si®, da Vinci Xi®, could not be determined due to this specific data being omitted from a number of papers that were included in our review. Only one single study did not use the da Vinci Surgical System® in patients, instead the Automated Endoscopic System for Optical Positioning® was used. A total of 114 patients were operated on with the assistance of surgical robotics. Despite accounting for only 35% of studies (14, 15, 20, 22, 23, 25, 32), head and neck surgery accounted for 51% ($n$ = 58) of patients that were operated on with the aid of

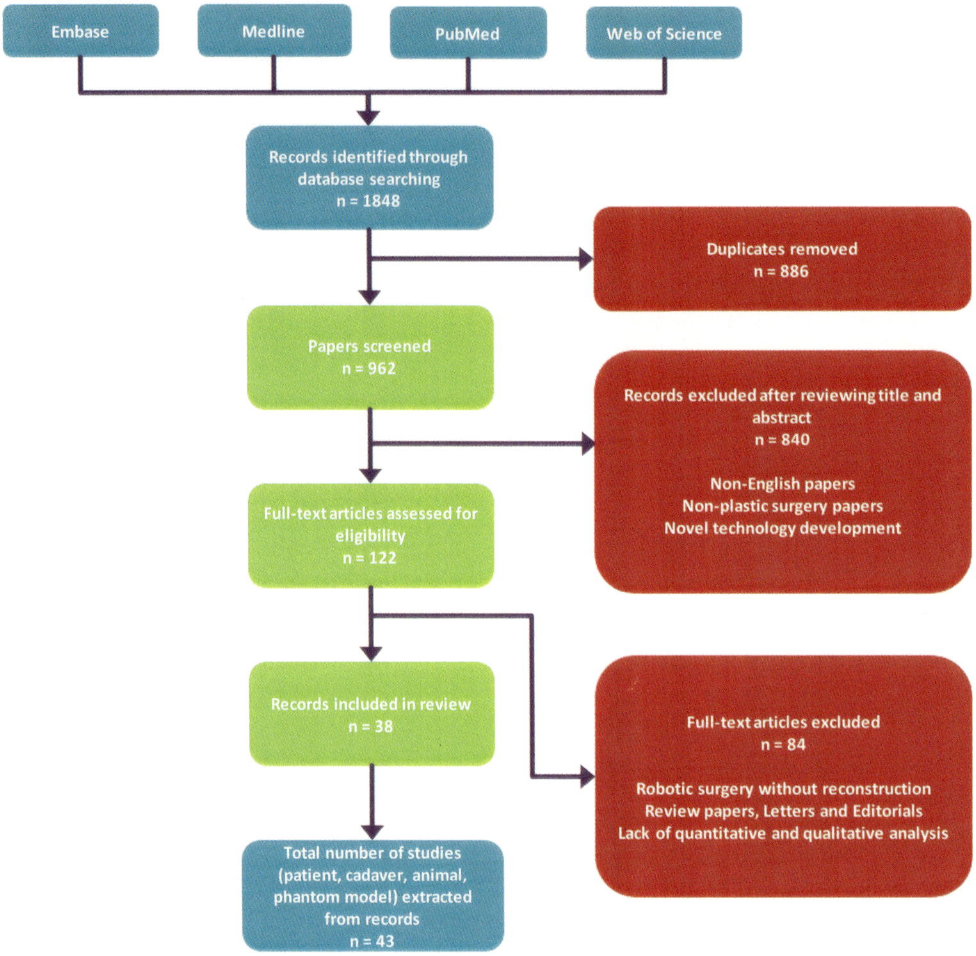


**FIGURE 2** | Flowchart of the database search strategy used in this review.

surgical robotics. Reconstruction of the oropharynx following malignancy was the most common indication for transoral robotic-assisted surgery. Among this cohort, 40 patients underwent oropharyngeal reconstruction using a free radial forearm fasciocutaneous flap (14, 15, 20, 23, 25, 32), 4 patients were reconstructed using an anterolateral thigh flap (14, 20, 23), 1 patient benefitted from a facial artery myomucosal flap (23) and 1 patient had their defect repaired via primary closure (23). Apart from oropharyngeal malignancy, 10 patients underwent transoral robotic-assisted surgery for cleft palate repair (22) and 2 patients had scalp defects repaired using a free latissimus dorsi muscle flap (32). Breast surgery was the second most common surgical procedure during which surgical robotic systems were used ($n = 26$) (13, 32). Twenty patients had internal mammary vessels harvested using the Automated Endoscopic System for Optical Positioning® for breast reconstruction (13). Six patients underwent robotic harvest of the latissimus dorsi muscle for free muscle transfer reconstruction of the breast (32). Furthermore, 12 patients underwent robot-assisted reconstructive upper-limb surgery during (18, 19, 21, 24), 7 patients received surgery for lower limb defects (24, 26, 33), 6 patients were operated on for pelvic reconstruction (26) and 5 patients had brachial plexus surgery (16, 17, 24) (**Table 2**).

**TABLE 1** | Limitations of surgical robotics.

| | Number of papers | Percentage |
|---|---|---|
| Total number of papers | 38 | 100 |
| **SURGICAL ROBOT** | | |
| da Vinci Surgical System® | 31 | 81.6 |
| Zeus Robotic Surgical System® | 3 | 7.9 |
| Automated Endoscopic System for Optical Positioning® | 1 | 2.6 |
| Other | 3 | 7.9 |
| **DISADVANTAGES** | | |
| Inadequate instrumentation | 17 | 44.7 |
| Increase in operating time | 17 | 44.7 |
| Absence of tactile feedback | 16 | 42.1 |
| High cost | 13 | 34.2 |
| Space requirements | 10 | 26.3 |

Analysis of any disadvantages or drawbacks of using surgical robotics for plastic reconstructive microsurgery, revealed five

**TABLE 2 |** Surgical robotics and interventions in patients.

| | Number of patients | Percentage |
|---|---|---|
| Total number of patients | 114 | 100 |
| **SURGICAL ROBOT** | | |
| da Vinci Surgical System® | 94 | 82.5 |
| Automated Endoscopic System for Optical Positioning® | 20 | 17.5 |
| **SURGICAL TREATMENT** | | |
| Head and neck surgery | | |
| Oropharynx repair radial forearm fasciocutaneous flap | 40 | 35.1 |
| Oropharynx repair anterolateral thigh flap | 4 | 3.5 |
| Oropharynx repair facial artery myomucosal flap | 1 | 0.9 |
| Oropharyngeal repair primary closure | 1 | 0.9 |
| Cleft palate reconstruction | 10 | 8.8 |
| Latissimus dorsi harvest | 2 | 1.8 |
| Breast surgery | | |
| Internal mammary vessel harvest | 20 | 17.5 |
| Latissimus dorsi harvest | 6 | 5.3 |
| Upper limb surgery | | |
| Peripheral nerve translocation | 7 | 6.1 |
| Peripheral nerve repair | 4 | 3.5 |
| Ulnar artery reconstruction | 1 | 0.9 |
| Lower limb surgery | | |
| Rectus muscle harvest | 5 | 4.4 |
| Peripheral nerve repair | 2 | 1.8 |
| Pelvic surgery | | |
| Rectus muscle harvest | 6 | 5.3 |
| Brachial plexus surgery | | |
| Brachial plexus reconstruction | 5 | 4.4 |

common obstacles (**Table 1**). Seventeen papers highlighted that the use of surgical robotics was associated with an increase in operating room time. Factors contributing to the increase in time were additional time necessary for setting up the surgical robot before a procedure (12, 15, 16, 36) and the additional time required to perform then actual procedure. Li et al. noted that total completion time was 2.6 times longer using a robotic-assisted technique compared to conventional microsurgery (9). Similarly, cleft palate repair by Nguyen et al., showed that the mean surgical duration for transoral robotic-assisted surgery was 122 ± 8 min, compared to 87 ± 6 min for the control group (22). An increase in operating time can partially be accounted to difficulties with surgical tools. Seventeenpapers mentioned that the current tools available in current robotic systems are inadequate for reconstructive microsurgical procedures. The lack of true microsurgical instruments creates a barrier for surgeons to handle delicate equipment and tissue. Consequently, needle tearing and difficulties in manipulating tissue has been observed. Interestingly, 16 papers mention that the lack of haptic feedback during surgery can be considered as a deficit. Simultaneously, several authors state that visual feedback can compensate for the lack of tactile feedback when operating on fragile tissue. While surgical robots are nowadays a common occurrence many hospitals across the world, the cost of acquiring and maintaining a surgical robot has been a frequent point of concern. Subsequently, 13 papers argue the cost of surgical robots prohibit their use. Especially in plastic surgery, limited data exists on the clinical benefits of surgical robots over conventional surgical intervention that would justify the adaptation of surgical robotics in common practice. Only one study assessed long-term outcome between robotic-assisted surgery compared to conventional reconstructive surgery. They discovered that functional post-operative outcomes 3 months following robotic-assisted oropharyngeal reconstruction is superior to conventional surgery ($p = 0.005$) (25). Finally, 10 papers highlighted that the size of surgical robotics can proof problematic in smaller operating theatres. Most operating rooms are not designed to facilitate large robots, therefore surgical workflow can be impeded.

## 4. DISCUSSION

Following a variety of proof of concept studies in animal models and human cadavers, significant success has been documented in utilising surgical robots in patients within plastic surgery. There is a wide range of surgical procedures in which robotic surgery is feasible, including head and neck reconstruction, free-flap harvest and nerve reconstruction (**Table 2**). Improved visualisation of the operating field, enhanced dexterity and elimination of tremor are valuable aids when performing complex procedures on microscopic level. Consequently, the potential of surgical robotics is promising. Despite positive results from feasibility studies, uptake of surgical robotics within plastic surgery has been limited. The use of surgical robotics in day-to-day practice is restricted to a small subset of procedures, which is congruent with currently available literature. The majority of studies considered in this review are case reports or small case series with less than five patients. These provide valuable insight into important aspects of plastic surgery, such as microvascular anastomosis and nerve repair that form the basis of complex reconstruction. Although this may act as a stepping stone to conduct further research into surgical robotics in reconstructive microsurgery on a larger scale, this has not yielded in publication of larger studies. Yet, one area within the field of plastic surgery is currently leading the game when it comes to utilising surgical robots in common practice. Robotic head and neck reconstruction has seen remarkable progress over the last few years. Transoral robotic surgery is currently gaining popularity and is providing new approaches to oropharyngeal access in resection of cancers and cleft palate reconstruction. To date, results from transoral surgery have been promising, and importantly, data indicating this has been derived from comparative cohort studies (15, 25). Biron et al. compared transoral robotic surgery ($n = 18$) to the lip-splitting mandibulotomy approach ($n = 29$) for primary resection of oropharyngeal carcinomas with radial forearm free-flap reconstruction. Patients who underwent robotic resection and reconstruction were discharged from hospital approximately 5.3 days earlier, and estimated overall cost of admission was lower (\$18,522.18 vs \$24,932.16) compared to conventional surgery (15). Analysis of functional outcome by Tsai et al.

between robotic-assisted free-flap oropharyngeal reconstruction ($n$ = 14) and conventional free-flap reconstruction ($n$ = 33) revealed that Functional Intraoral Glasgow Scale (47) was significantly better 3 months post-operatively in patients who underwent robotic reconstruction ($p$ = 0.005) (25). As the indications for surgical robots are gradually increasing, the demand for adequate training and obtaining hands-on experience is rising. As such, the level of interest in this field is emerging and driven the creation of professional bodies, such as the Robotic-Assisted Microsurgical & Endoscopic Society (RAMES), to provide surgeons with training opportunities with robotic technology. Nevertheless, while increasing awareness of surgical robots through educational events encourages adaption of such systems on a larger scale, the future of surgical robots mainly will rely on the outcome of larger clinical studies. The availability of strong evidence from large studies is essential in order to determine if there is an overall benefit of surgical robotics over conventional microsurgery. A lack of meaningful evidence is currently the main barrier in order to assess whether surgical robots should be incorporated within plastic surgery on a larger scale.

## 4.1. Limitations of Surgical Robotics

### 4.1.1. Instrumentation

A significant proportion of studies that were assessed in this review state that the absence of adequate instrumentation specifically designed for microsurgery poses a major limitation of current robotic surgical systems. The majority of published articles relied on the da Vinci surgical robot for assessing the feasibility of robotic microsurgery. While this particular system is licensed for minimally invasive surgery in seven surgical specialties, it is neither indicated nor designed for open plastic reconstructive microsurgery. The majority of instruments compatible with the da Vinci are considered to be too large for fine manipulation of delicate tissue normally seen during microsurgery. Success has been observed by utilising the da Vinci's Black Diamond Micro Forceps for operating on small vessels and nerves (14, 20, 25, 36). Yet, lack of a comprehensive set of appropriate microsurgical instruments means that handling submillimetre tissue and equipment is challenging and time-consuming process. Common elements of a microsurgical procedure, such as dissecting blood vessels, applying vessel clamps and handling fine sutures, become more difficult when using a surgical robot compared to conventional microsurgery. In addition to oversized instruments, the variety of instruments of surgical tools does not cover the full scope of tissue encountered during microsurgery. Numerous operations involving upper or lower limbs involve manipulating a variety of tissue with different characteristics, such as skin, vessels and bones. To date, no robotic system exists that provides the tools necessary to perform procedures in which all different types of tissue are involved. As a result, performing procedures that involve both soft and hard tissues cannot be achieved purely using surgical robotics (12). In addition, the extent of macroscopic and microscopic techniques used during reconstructive surgery make robotic use inefficient. Consequently, it requires continuous switching between conventional and robotic-assisted microsurgery, which is labourious and a time-consuming process.

Besides adequate surgical tools to operate on delicate tissue, appropriate optical aids to magnify and improve visualisation of the surgical field are essential during microsurgery. The da Vinci surgical robot provides endoscopic 3D imaging system capable of up to 10× magnification through digital zoom. Unfortunately, the image magnification and quality of da Vinci surgical robot is below standards compared to that of surgical microscopes (23). As microsurgical procedures occasionally may require magnification beyond what is currently offered with the da Vinci, this system is limited in its use. Integration of surgical microscopes or other imaging systems capable of delivering adequate optical magnification while maintaining high image quality is desirable. Overall, the scarcity of adequate microsurgical instruments and robotic systems tailored to the requirements of plastic and reconstructive microsurgery prohibits using the theoretical potential of surgical robots.

### 4.1.2. Tactile Feedback

A recurring aspect of surgical robotics which some clinicians have argued as a disadvantage is the lack of tactile feedback when operating. A substantial proportion of papers reviewed, mention the absence of haptic feedback in current surgical robots as a drawback ($n$ = 17). However, whether this is a disadvantage is controversial. Despite criticising the lack of haptic feedback, several go on to mention that tactile feedback is non-essential and can be compensated for by other means (11, 12, 28). While being able to sense the amount of forces exerted on delicate tissue may at first glance seem essential, it has been shown that visual feedback during microsurgery can reliably compensate for this deficit. In addition, some argue that the forces exerted during microsurgery are too low for humans to experience and therefore not appropriate to rely on. Despite data indicating that tactile feedback is non-essential, having such feature on surgical robots can provide benefits. Although soft tissue can show deformity during manipulation, this is not the case for rigid instruments used during the procedure. Several clinical studies noted that the lack of tactile feedback can result in bending needles, particularly when handling the needle using two robotic arms (19, 31, 43, 44). Furthermore, tactile feedback may become useful when implemented such that forces exerted are scaled on the surgeon's end. Artificially increased forces such that a surgeon can feel and judge these could potentially reduce any unnecessary trauma to delicate tissue. Nevertheless, whether the availability of tactile feedback can reduce the risk of soft-tissue damage needs to be thoroughly validated. Future studies may provide a better insight into tissue trauma between conventional manual microsurgery and robotic microsurgery with tactile feedback.

### 4.1.3. Cost

High costs of buying, using and maintaining surgical robotic systems have been a recurring theme throughout the literature. The cost of a single surgical robot can be in excess of $2 million (48), hence investing in surgical robots requires significant resources. Further direct and indirect costs arise that are essential to operate the system and provide a safe environment for robot-assisted surgery. Consumables required during a procedure can cost between $1,800 and $4,600 per instrument (49). Resources have to be allocated to provide training for operating theatre staff in order to familiarise them with surgical robots. Outside the operating room, further staffing is needed to reassure that these systems work reliably. Surgical robots are inherently complex systems that require specific expertise for repair and maintenance. Hence, hospitals that utilise surgical robots are required to negotiate service contracts with manufacturers that cost approximately an additional 10% of the system annually (49, 50). The spiralling costs associated with increased demands in staffing and consumables make the use of surgical robots less attractive.

Offering expensive treatment options can be favourable for hospitals if these are associated with improved outcome or increased income in long term. However, a little data exists that suggests that this is indeed the case for plastic reconstructive microsurgery. Right now, few arguments exist to justify investing significant resources into surgical robots. In addition, published data indicates that robotic-assisted microsurgery is associated with prolonged operating time compared to conventional microsurgery (9, 10, 15, 22, 34, 42). Subsequently, the number of patients that can be treated may decrease and waiting times suffer. Despite the claimed paradoxical cost reduction of surgical robots related to shorter hospitalisation and post-operative complications (15, 48), the overall benefits do not yet outweigh the capital required to justify its use in plastic and reconstructive microsurgery. Without an increased turnover of patients and improved cost-efficiency, very few plastic surgery departments will be willing to invest in robotic-assisted surgery at the moment.

### 4.1.4. Education

Surgical training often involves an apprenticeship model in which trainees initially observe a qualified professional and slowly gain skills through increasing their involvement during procedures. Surgical robots are often limited to a single surgeon controlling an entire system and therefore solely performs the whole procedure. As a result, there is little opportunity for assistants to get involved during robot-assisted operations. A lack of active involvement of surgeons may restrict their exposure to surgical robotics and limits opportunities to advance their skill set. There are two possible solutions to this dilemma, namely switch between surgeons during a procedure or make use of two or more full surgical robotic systems. While switching between different users is a relatively quick procedure, it is time consuming and delays may pose a threat to clinical outcomes during critical situations. Using multiple surgical robots may be a safer option during training young surgeons. This provides the lead surgeon with an assistant who can aid during the procedure, as well as allows trainees to gain skills necessary for robotic microsurgery. However, a single robotic system can cost in excess of $2 million, buying such system purely for training purposes is difficult to justify. Finally, it is important to appreciate that surgical robots should be considered as an additional tool, not as a replacement for conventional microsurgery. There are notable differences between the skills required for either form of microsurgery. Movements and handling of delicate tissue are significantly different, hence skills to successfully operate in such circumstances using a surgical robot are not directly transferable to conventional microsurgery. Future surgeons will need to be trained in both conventional and robotic-assisted microsurgery techniques to be capable of dealing with the wide variety of surgical problems that they will encounter throughout their career. Therefore, both robotic-assisted and conventional microsurgical experience should be incorporated into surgical training.

### 4.1.5. Surgical Workflow

Studies have suggested that in certain scenarios using surgical robots is less convenient compared to conventional manual microsurgery. Willems et al. showed that during microsurgery with sufficient access to the surgical field, conventional surgery requires less operating time compared to robotic-assisted microsurgery (45). Reviewing patients and planning procedures in advance to determine an optimal treatment plan is essential before any intervention. Nevertheless, a degree of uncertainty will always exists and predicting which operations offer good surgical access and which do not may be difficult. Consequently, there is a risk that surgeons may have to switch between robotic and conventional surgery during a procedure to achieve a desired result. Transitioning during a procedure is by all means possible, though it is a labourious and time-consuming process that depends on the familiarity of operating room staff with surgical robots. Any delays as a consequence of this process may lead to increased costs. Furthermore, any event that prolongs operating and anaesthetic time could increase the risk of complications. To optimise surgical workflow, surgical robots must account for uncertainty during microsurgery and need to be able to provide a smooth and quick transition between conventional and robotic microsurgery.

## 5. CONCLUSION

Criticising technology based on what it is not capable of doing and pointing out flaws may be easy. Yet, highlighting such deficiencies and reflecting on what aspects could be improved is an essential tool to advancing its practice. Numerous research has highlighted that surgical robots can offer substantial benefits when operating. Surgical robots allow surgeons to perform extremely fine manoeuvres within narrow spaces that are near impossible during conventional surgery. Despite numerous advances of surgical robotics and the associated improved clinical outcomes seen in several surgical specialties, the robotic systems that are currently available do not offer overall benefits over conventional reconstructive microsurgery. On one hand, current systems are not designed to capture the full scope of complex reconstructive surgical procedures. While at the same time, microsurgical procedures themselves are not designed to make use of the full potential of surgical robots. Instead of trying to adapt surgical robots to current practice, more success may be achieved by designing microsurgical procedures around surgical robots. Surgical robots offer theoretical benefits that could make complex microsurgery more convenient, yet there are significant barriers that have prevented integrating surgical robotics in common practice. To date, no systems exist that are specifically designed for plastic and reconstructive microsurgery. Without adequate microsurgical instrumentation and training, surgeons will be hesitant to adapt robotic systems in their operating theatre. Current microsurgical procedures are not designed to make use of the full potential of surgical robots. A lack of strong quantitive data can be considered as a limitation of this review, there is nevertheless strong evidence that, without the deficiencies mentioned being resolved, little change can be expected within the foreseeable future.

## AUTHOR CONTRIBUTIONS

YT: review design, data collection, data analysis and wrote the manuscript. PL: clinical advisor and data collection. JW: study supervision, review design and data interpretation. All authors reviewed and edited the manuscript.

## REFERENCES

1. Moorthy K, Munz Y, Dosis A, Hernandez J, Martin S, Bello F, et al. Dexterity enhancement with robotic surgery. *Surg Endosc* (2004) 18(5):790–5. doi: 10.1007/s00464-003-8922-2
2. Corcione F, Esposito C, Cuccurullo D, Settembre A, Miranda N, Amato F, et al. Advantages and limits of robot-assisted laparoscopic surgery: preliminary experience. *Surg Endosc* (2005) 19(1):117–9. doi: 10.1007/s00464-004-9004-9
3. Bell MC, Torgerson J, Seshadri-Kreaden U, Suttle AW, Hunt S. Comparison of outcomes and cost for endometrial cancer staging via traditional laparotomy, standard laparoscopy and robotic techniques. *Gynecol Oncol* (2008) 111(3):407–11. doi: 10.1016/j.ygyno.2008.08.022
4. Woo YJ, Nacke EA. Robotic minimally invasive mitral valve reconstruction yields less blood product transfusion and shorter length of stay. *Surgery* (2006) 140(2):263–7. doi: 10.1016/j.surg.2006.05.003
5. Shademan A, Decker RS, Opfermann JD, Leonard S, Krieger A, Kim PC. Supervised autonomous robotic soft tissue surgery. *Sci Transl Med* (2016) 8(337):ra64. doi: 10.1126/scitranslmed.aad9398
6. Lowrance WT, Eastham JA, Savage C, Maschino AC, Laudone VP, Dechet CB, et al. Contemporary open and robotic radical prostatectomy practice patterns among urologists in the United States. *J Urol* (2012) 187(6):2087–93. doi: 10.1016/j.juro.2012.01.061
7. Leow JJ, Chang SL, Meyer CP, Wang Y, Hanske J, Sammon JD, et al. Robot-assisted versus open radical prostatectomy: a contemporary analysis of an all-payer discharge database. *Eur Urol* (2016) 70(5):837–45. doi: 10.1016/j.eururo.2016.01.044
8. Bouquet de Joliniere J, Librino A, Dubuisson J-B, Khomsi F, Ben Ali N, Fadhlaoui A, et al. Robotic Surgery in Gynecology. *Front. Surg.* (2016) 3(2(). doi: 10.3389/fsurg.2016.00026
9. Li RA, Jensen J, Bowersox JC. Microvascular anastomoses performed in rats using a microsurgical telemanipulator. *Comput Aided Surg* (2000) 5(5):326–32. doi: 10.1002/1097-0150(2000)5:5<326::AID-IGS2>3.0.CO;2-0
10. Knight CG, Lorincz A, Cao A, Gidell K, Klein MD, Langenburg SE. Computer-assisted, robot-enhanced open microsurgery in an animal model. *J Laparoendosc Adv Surg Tech A* (2005) 15(2):182–5. doi: 10.1089/lap.2005.15.182
11. Katz RD, Rosson GD, Taylor JA, Singh NK. Robotics in microsurgery: use of a surgical robot to perform a free flap in a pig. *Microsurgery* (2005) 25(7):566–9. doi: 10.1002/micr.20160
12. Taleb C, Nectoux E, Liverneaux P. Limb replantation with two robots: a feasibility study in a pig model. *Microsurgery* (2009) 29(3):232–5. doi: 10.1002/micr.20602
13. Boyd B, Umansky J, Samson M, Boyd D, Stahl K. Robotic harvest of internal mammary vessels in breast reconstruction. *J Reconstr Microsurg* (2006) 22(4):261–6. doi: 10.1055/s-2006-939931
14. Bonawitz SC, Duvvuri U. Robot-assisted oropharyngeal reconstruction with free tissue transfer. *J Reconstr Microsurg* (2012) 28(7):485–90. doi: 10.1055/s-0032-1313758
15. Biron VL, O'Connell DA, Barber B, Clark JM, Andrews C, Jeffery CC, et al. Transoral robotic surgery with radial forearm free flap reconstruction: case control analysis. *J Otolaryngol Head Neck Surg* (2017) 46(1):20. doi: 10.1186/s40463-017-0196-0
16. Garcia JC, Lebailly F, Mantovani G, Mendonca LA, Garcia J, Liverneaux P. Telerobotic manipulation of the brachial plexus. *J Reconstr Microsurg* (2012) 28(7):491–4. doi: 10.1055/s-0032-1313761
17. Lequint T, Naito K, Chaigne D, Facca S, Liverneaux P. Mini-invasive robot-assisted surgery of the brachial plexus: a case of intraneural perineurioma. *J Reconstr Microsurg* (2012) 28(7):473–6. doi: 10.1055/s-0032-1313759
18. Garcia JC, Mantovani G, Gouzou S, Liveneaux P. Telerobotic anterior translocation of the ulnar nerve. *J Robot Surg* (2011) 5(2):153–6. doi: 10.1007/s11701-010-0226-7
19. Facca S, Liverneaux P. Robotic assisted microsurgery in hypothenar hammer syndrome: a case report. *Comput Aided Surg* (2010) 15(4-6):110–4. doi: 10.3109/10929088.2010.507942
20. Lai CS, Chen IC, Liu SA, Lu CT, Yen JH, Song DY. Robot-assisted free flap reconstruction of oropharyngeal cancer--a preliminary report. *Ann Plast Surg* (2015) 74 Suppl 2(2):S105–8. doi: 10.1097/SAP.0000000000000464
21. Miyamoto H, Leechavengvongs S, Atik T, Facca S, Liverneaux P. Nerve transfer to the deltoid muscle using the nerve to the long head of the triceps with the da Vinci robot: six cases. *J Reconstr Microsurg* (2014) 30(6):375–80. doi: 10.1055/s-0033-1361927
22. Nguyen D, Awad M, Farber S, Parikh R, Skolnick G, Woo A. Robotic-assisted cleft palate repair: a feasibility study. *Cleft Palate Craniofac J* (2016) 53(4):e119.
23. Selber JC. Transoral robotic reconstruction of oropharyngeal defects: a case series. *Plast Reconstr Surg* (2010) 126(6):1978–87. doi: 10.1097/PRS.0b013e3181f448e3
24. Tigan L, Miyamoto H, Hendriks S, Facca S, Liverneaux P. Interest of telemicrosurgery in peripheral nerve tumors: about a series of seven cases. *Chir Main* (2014) 33(1):13–16. doi: 10.1016/j.main.2013.10.177
25. Tsai YC, Liu SA, Lai CS, Chen YW, Lu CT, Yen JH, et al. Functional outcomes and complications of Robot-assisted free flap oropharyngeal reconstruction. *Ann Plast Surg* (2017) 78(3 Suppl 2):S82. doi: 10.1097/SAP.0000000000001010
26. Pedersen J, Song DH, Selber JC. Robotic, intraperitoneal harvest of the rectus abdominis muscle. *Plast Reconstr Surg* (2014) 134(5):1057–63. doi: 10.1097/PRS.0000000000000586
27. Jiang S, Ichihara S, Prunières G, Peterson B, Facca S, Xu WD, et al. Robot-assisted C7 nerve root transfer from the contralateral healthy side: a preliminary cadaver study. *Hand Surg Rehabil* (2016) 35(2):95–9. doi: 10.1016/j.hansur.2015.12.008
28. Maire N, Naito K, Lequint T, Facca S, Berner S, Liverneaux P. Robot-assisted free toe pulp transfer: feasibility study. *J Reconstr Microsurg* (2012) 28(7):481–4. doi: 10.1055/s-0032-1313760
29. Mantovani G, Liverneaux P, Garcia JC, Berner SH, Bednar MS, Mohr CJ. Endoscopic exploration and repair of brachial plexus with telerobotic manipulation: a cadaver trial. *J Neurosurg* (2011) 115(3):659–64. doi: 10.3171/2011.3.JNS10931
30. Porto de Melo PM, Garcia JC, Montero EF, Atik T, Robert EG, Facca S, et al. Feasibility of an endoscopic approach to the axillary nerve and the nerve to the long head of the triceps brachii with the help of the Da Vinci Robot. *Chir Main* (2013) 32(4):206–9. doi: 10.1016/j.main.2013.05.003
31. Robert E, Facca S, Atik T, Bodin F, Bruant-Rodier C, Liverneaux P. Vascular microanastomosis through an endoscopic approach: feasibility study on two cadaver forearms. *Chir Main* (2013) 32(3):136–40. doi: 10.1016/j.main.2013.01.002

32. Selber JC, Baumann DP, Holsinger CF. Robotic harvest of the latissimus dorsi muscle: laboratory and clinical experience. *J Reconstr Microsurg* (2012) 28(7):457–64. doi: 10.1055/s-0032-1315789
33. Patel NV, Pedersen JC. Robotic harvest of the rectus abdominis muscle: a preclinical investigation and case report. *J Reconstr Microsurg* (2012) 28(7):477–80. doi: 10.1055/s-0031-1287674
34. Karamanoukian RL, Bui T, Mcconnell MP, Evans GR, Karamanoukian HL. Transfer of training in robotic-assisted microvascular surgery. *Ann Plast Surg* (2006) 57(6):662–5. doi: 10.1097/01.sap.0000229245.36218.25
35. Karamanoukian RL, Finley DS, Evans GR, Karamanoukian HL. Feasibility of robotic-assisted microvascular anastomoses in plastic surgery. *J Reconstr Microsurg* (2006) 22(6):429–32. doi: 10.1055/s-2006-947697
36. Katz RD, Taylor JA, Rosson GD, Brown PR, Singh NK. Robotics in plastic and reconstructive surgery: use of a telemanipulator slave robot to perform microvascular anastomoses. *J Reconstr Microsurg* (2006) 22(1):53–8. doi: 10.1055/s-2006-931908
37. Latif MJ, Afthinos JN, Connery CP, Perin N, Bhora FY, Chwajol M, et al. Robotic intercostal nerve graft for reversal of thoracic sympathectomy: a large animal feasibility model. *Int J Med Robot* (2008) 4(3):258–62. doi: 10.1002/rcs.205
38. Le Roux PD, das H, Esquenazi S, Kelly PJ. Robot-assisted microsurgery: a feasibility study in the rat. *Neurosurgery* (2001) 48(3):584–9. doi: 10.1097/00006123-200103000-00026
39. Lee JY, Mattar T, Parisi TJ, Carlsen BT, Bishop AT, Shin AY. Learning curve of robotic-assisted microvascular anastomosis in the rat. *J Reconstr Microsurg* (2012) 28(7):451–6. doi: 10.1055/s-0031-1289166
40. Miyamoto H, Serradori T, Mikami Y, Selber J, Santelmo N, Facca S, et al. Robotic intercostal nerve harvest: a feasibility study in a pig model. *J Neurosurg* (2016) 124(1):264–8. doi: 10.3171/2015.1.JNS14603
41. Porto de Melo P, Miyamoto H, Serradori T, Ruggiero Mantovani G, Selber J, Facca S, et al. Robotic phrenic nerve harvest: a feasibility study in a pig model. *Chir Main* (2014) 33(5):356–60. doi: 10.1016/j.main.2014.07.006
42. Ramdhian RM, Bednar M, Mantovani GR, Facca SA, Liverneaux PA. Microsurgery and telemicrosurgery training: a comparative study. *J Reconstr Microsurg* (2011) 27(9):537–42. doi: 10.1055/s-0031-1285985
43. Taleb C, Nectoux E, Liverneaux PA. Telemicrosurgery: a feasibility study in a rat model. *Chir Main* (2008) 27(2-3):104–8. doi: 10.1016/j.main.2008.04.001
44. Nectoux E, Taleb C, Liverneaux P. Nerve repair in telemicrosurgery: an experimental study. *J Reconstr Microsurg* (2009) 25(4):261–5. doi: 10.1055/s-0028-1104562
45. Willems JI, Shin AM, Shin DM, Bishop AT, Shin AY. A comparison of robotically assisted microsurgery versus manual microsurgery in challenging situations. *Plast Reconstr Surg* (2016) 137(4):1317–24. doi: 10.1097/PRS.0000000000002030
46. Zhu J-H, Deng J, Liu X-J, Wang J, Guo Y-X, Guo C-B. Prospects of Robot-Assisted Mandibular Reconstruction with Fibula Flap: Comparison with a Computer-Assisted Navigation System and Freehand Technique. *J Reconstr Microsurg* (2016). doi: 10.1055/s-0036-1592141
47. Goldie SJ, Jackson MS, Soutar DS, Shaw-Dunn J. The functional intraoral Glasgow scale (FIGS) in retromolar trigone cancer patients. *J Plast Reconstr Aesthet Surg* (2006) 59(7):743–6. doi: 10.1016/j.bjps.2005.11.023
48. Barbash GI, Glied SA. New technology and health care costs--the case of robot-assisted surgery. *N Engl J Med* (2010) 363(8):701–4. doi: 10.1056/NEJMp1006602
49. Higgins RM, Frelich MJ, Bosler ME, Gould JC. Cost analysis of robotic versus laparoscopic general surgery procedures. *Surg Endosc* (2017) 31(1):185–92. doi: 10.1007/s00464-016-4954-2
50. Broome JT, Pomeroy S, Solorzano CC. Expense of robotic thyroidectomy: a cost analysis at a single institution. *Arch Surg* (2012) 147(12):1102–6. doi: 10.1001/archsurg.2012.1870

# 20

# Supermicrosurgery: History, Applications, Training and the Future

*Ido Badash [1], Daniel J. Gould [2] and Ketan M. Patel [2]**

*[1] Keck School of Medicine of USC, University of Southern California, Los Angeles, CA, United States, [2] Division of Plastic and Reconstructive Surgery, University of Southern California, Los Angeles, CA, United States*

Supermicrosurgery, a technique of dissection and anastomosis of small vessels ranging from 0.3 to 0.8 mm, has revolutionized the fields of lymphedema treatment and soft tissue reconstruction. The technique offers several distinct benefits to microsurgeons, including the ability to manipulate small vessels that were previously inaccessible, and to minimize donor-site morbidity by dissecting short pedicles in a suprafascial plane. Thus, supermicrosurgery has become increasingly popular in recent years, and its applications have greatly expanded since it was first introduced 20 years ago. While supermicrosurgery was originally developed for procedures involving salvage of the digit tip, the technique is now routinely used in a wide variety of microsurgical cases, including lymphovenous anastomoses, vascularized lymph node transfers and perforator-to-perforator anastomoses. With continued experimentation, standardization of supermicrosurgical training, and high quality studies focusing on the outcomes of these novel procedures, supermicrosurgery can become a routine and valuable component of every microsurgeon's practice.

**Keywords: supermicrosurgery, microsurgery, plastic surgery, free flap, perforator, soft tissue reconstruction, lymphedema, lymph node transfer**

***Edited by:***
*Jason K.F. Wong,*
*University of Manchester,*
*United Kingdom*

***Reviewed by:***
*Christopher G. Wallace,*
*Royal Devon and Exeter Hospital,*
*United Kingdom*
*Mark V. Schaverien,*
*University of Texas MD Anderson*
*Cancer Center, United States*

***Correspondence:***
*Ketan M. Patel*
*ketan.patel@med.usc.edu*

***Specialty section:***
*This article was submitted to*
*Visceral Surgery,*
*a section of the journal*
*Frontiers in Surgery*

## INTRODUCTION

Recent advances in technology and refinement of surgical techniques have ushered forth a new age in the field of reconstructive microsurgery. Microsurgical procedures have evolved from simple soft tissue reconstruction to more sophisticated applications of these techniques, including vascularized lymph node transfer (VLNT) and perforator-to-perforator anastomosis (1, 2). The outcomes and complication rates from microsurgery have improved over the past few decades, allowing today's microsurgeons to focus more on minimizing donor-site morbidity and maximizing the function and aesthetics of the reconstruction (3). Most importantly, today's reconstructive surgeons are able to execute procedures that were previously unachievable, such as anastomosis of vessels with a caliber less than a single millimeter. These advanced procedures have been grouped under the field of supermicrosurgery (4, 5).

Supermicrosurgery is defined as a technique of microneurovascular anastomosis for vessels and single nerve fascicles of 0.3 to 0.8 mm (4). The surgical technique utilizes highly delicate microsurgical instruments (30- to 80-micron needle micro-sutures) to accomplish small anastomoses (6). First introduced 20 years ago, the technique was pioneered by Koshima et al. in reconstructions involving vessel repair in the distal finger. Since then, the technique has been used in reconstructions that were previously limited by vessels of small caliber. For example, supermicrosurgery has allowed for the use of perforator-to-perforator freestyle flaps in diabetic foot wounds with compromised vasculature and lymphovenous anastomosis (LVA) for obstructive lymphedema (7, 8). Supermicrosurgical techniques have expanded the possibilities of what was previously achievable within the field of microsurgery.

This review summarizes the history of the development of supermicrosurgery, current applications of this technique, training methods and future directions for supermicrosurgery. We have searched the PubMed database for articles published in the English language. Keywords used included "supermicrosurgery," "perforator flaps," "perforator-to-perforator," "reconstructive microsurgery," "lymphedema," "microvascular anastomosis," and "microsurgery simulation." Original and review articles related to the applications of supermicrosurgery were reviewed. A total of 106 articles were reviewed and included, with levels of evidence ranging from I to V (**Table 1**) (9).

## HISTORY OF SUPERMICROSURGERY

The field of microsurgery dates back to the 1960s, when new surgical techniques and intraoperative magnification were introduced into vascular surgery through a series of landmark experimental procedures (10). The first microvascular surgery is reported to have occurred in 1960, when JH Jacobson and EL Suarez successfully joined two ends of a canine carotid artery together under a microscope (11). A number of pioneers around the world subsequently began developing the techniques and tools that would evolve into microvascular surgery. Eventually, this technology would be used to successfully to replant amputated digits and hands in patients for the first time (12). It was during this period that Harry J. Buncke performed his now famous experiments involving tissue transplantation in animal models, and developed many of the central principles of microsurgery that have led to his designation as the "founding father of microsurgery" (10).

Buncke and the other microsurgical pioneers of the 1960s, including John Cobbett, James Smith and Susumu Tamai, held the first ever panel on microsurgery at the Annual Meeting of the American Society of Plastic and Reconstructive Surgeons in New York City in 1967 (10). This meeting marked the first in-person exchange of microsurgical techniques, which included peripheral nerve repairs, digit transfers and tissue transplantation. Following the success of this meeting, the International Microsurgical Society was founded in 1970, and held the first international workshop for microvascular transplantation in the same year (10). Thus, over, the course of a decade, the field of microsurgery was born.

**TABLE 1** | Levels of Evidence for Therapeutic Studies.

| Level of Evidence | |
|---|---|
| I | Systematic review (with homogeneity) of randomized control trials (RCT); individual RCT (with narrow confidence intervals); all or none study. |
| II | Systematic review (with homogeneity) of cohort studies; individual cohort study (including low quality RCT, e.g. <80% follow-up); "outcomes" research; ecological study. |
| III | Systematic review (with homogeneity) of case-control studies; individual case-control study. |
| IV | Case series (and poor quality cohort and case-control study). |
| V | Expert opinion without explicit critical appraisal or based on physiology, bench research or "first principles". |

In 1987, a new era of microvascular reconstruction emerged when Taylor and Palmer provided a whole body perforator map that enabled surgeons to perform safe skin flaps using perforating vessels (13). Koshima et al. then published the first use of a perforator flap in 1989, the deep inferior epigastric skin flap, which heralded the development of a variety of different perforator flaps in the years after (14). The possibility of utilizing skin flaps based on "perforasomes" distributed throughout the body created a new paradigm in free flap reconstruction, allowing surgeons greater freedom when choosing which flaps to use (15).

Building on the concept of perforator flaps, Koshima reported the first use of flaps based on perforating vessels with a caliber less than 0.8 mm at the First International Course on Perforator Flap and Arterialized Skin Flaps in 1997. The possibility of utilizing such small vessels for anastomosis was significant, as this greatly expanded surgeon freedom in choosing free tissue flaps while also decreasing donor site morbidity through preservation of fascia, muscles, nerves and major vessels in the process of dissection. Koshima et al. called this technique "supramicrosurgery" for the first time in their description of the paraumbilical perforator flap in 1998 (16). In 2007, Koshima referred to the technique as "supermicrosurgery" at the first international meeting on microsurgical innovative technology, and published a definition of the procedure in 2010 (5). A consensus was reached on the name of "supermicrosurgery" at the First European Conference on Supermicrosurgery held in Barcelona in March 2010 (4). The technique was quickly adopted by surgeons around the world, and several studies began reporting successful use of perforator flaps and other microvascular procedures utilizing vessels of small caliber (<0.8 mm) (17–21). The use of supermicrosurgery thus developed as the next step in the evolution of microvascular reconstruction.

Over the next decade, supermicrosurgical techniques became increasingly incorporated into the surgical toolkit of microsurgeons. Supermicrosurgery has revolutionized the management of lymphedema, and the technique has also helped salvage fingertip replantations and free flap reconstructions (22–24). Furthermore, the advent of supermicrosurgery and subsequent flap customization with freestyle flaps has allowed reconstruction to not only address soft-tissue coverage, but also functional recovery, chronic infected wound control, and cosmetic improvement (19). The utility of supermicrosurgery allows for another level of operating freedom from which to craft reconstructions. The following sections outline some of the current applications and controversies in its use.

## CURRENT APPLICATIONS

### Lymphedema Treatment

Supermicrosurgery has revolutionized the field of lymphedema, a chronic condition of the lymphatic system resulting in the collection of protein-rich fluid in the interstitial space that significantly impairs patient quality of life (25–30). Until recently, lymphedema was predominantly managed with nonsurgical physiotherapy involving

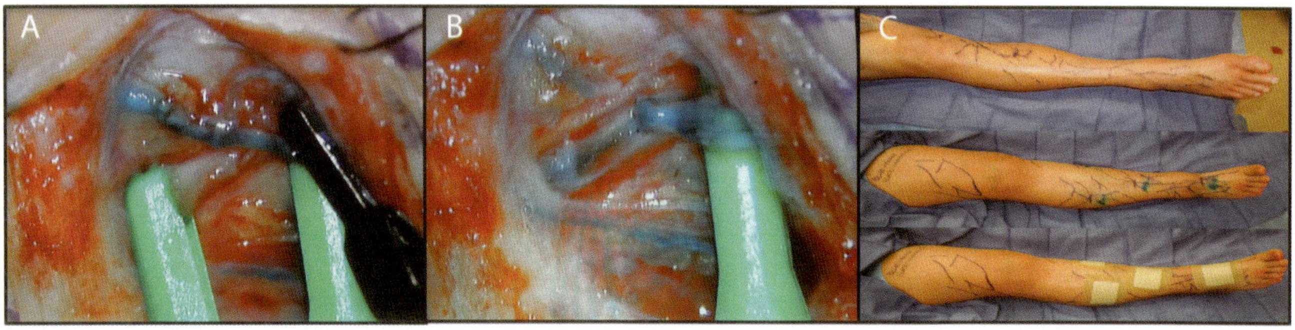


**FIGURE 1** | Lymphovenous anastomosis by end-to-side technique. The lymphatic vessel and vein are shown clamped **(A)**. After anastomosis, the outflow vein and lymphatic vessel are unclamped to demonstrate flow **(B)**. Many lymphovenous anastomoses are performed on each limb in sequence in order to improve lymphatic outflow **(C)**.

compression wrapping, manual drainage and exercise, although liposuction and debulking surgery have also been used with varying degrees of success (29). The advent of supermicrosurgery introduced the procedures of LVA and supermicrosurgical VLNT, which are becoming increasingly utilized treatment options for this condition (1, 8, 31).

LVA involves the creation of a microsurgical connection between subcutaneous lymphatic vessels and venules in order to bypass lymphatic drainage in the distal extremity. The anastomosis may be performed through either an end-to-end, end-to-side, or side-to-end technique (32) (**Figure 1**). Lymphatic vessels in the distal extremity are used since distal lymphatics are less affected by lymphedema and are thus more readily available for bypass. Additionally, subcutaneous lymphatics and venules are the preferred vessels for LVA, as venous pressure is lower in subcutaneous venules and results in less venous backflow (3). Successful LVA requires supermicrosurgical techniques, as lymphatic vessels have a small vessel caliber often measuring less than 0.5 mm. Thus, while LVA was originally reported in the 1960s, it has only been performed consistently and successfully since the advent of supermicrosurgery (25).

Koshima et al. first reported their experience performing LVA using supermicrosurgery in 1996 (33). Since then, the technique has been utilized for lymphedema treatment in various institutions worldwide and has gained significant traction as a major option for surgical management of lymphedema (34). Recent innovations in imaging techniques have allowed surgeons to better evaluate lymphatic vessel patency and function, permitting more reliable planning and improved long-term patency of the anastomosis (25). For example, a study by Campisi et al. investigating 1,800 patients with peripheral lymphedema treated with LVA found subjective improvement in 87% of patients and objective volume changes in 83%. Importantly, of the patients followed up in their study, 85% were able to discontinue the use of conservative measures, with an average follow-up time of 10 years and a 69% average reduction in excess volume (35). Other studies have similarly reported positive quantitative and qualitative improvements in lymphedema following LVA (31, 32, 36–39). The introduction of additional techniques and refinement of the procedure will likely continue to improve outcomes in the future (39).

Nonetheless, the use of LVA for lymphedema treatment remains controversial. Although some study results have been encouraging, other studies have reported less favorable outcomes, including a lack of volume reduction or benefits over nonoperative management (40). LVA is a challenging technique that requires a high level of technical skill to perform, the benefits are not always visible, and an objective method for the evaluation of results is still lacking (34). These drawbacks, combined with the small number of high quality studies and lack of clinical algorithms for lymphedema treatment, have led to skepticism regarding the efficacy and role of the LVA technique. For now, it is thought that the best indication for LVA is early stage lymphedema resistant to nonoperative treatment (25, 41).

Beyond LVA, VLNT has also been successfully performed for the treatment of lymphedema. In VLNT, a free tissue flap containing vascularized lymph nodes is transferred from one of various donor sites around the body to either a soft tissue defect or a non-anatomic area on the edematous limb in order to reconstitute lymphatic flow (1, 40, 42). Commonly used donor sites and associated lymph nodes include the supraclavicular (**Figure 2**), groin (**Figure 3**), submental, axillary, and thoracic flaps (42). The use of supermicrosurgery allows for the transfer of lymphoadipose flaps with small perforating vessels less than 0.8 mm in caliber, as well as manipulation of venules and lymphatic vessels within or near the implanted tissue (4, 43). Supermicrosurgery has been increasingly used for VLNT, as the technique permits the use of thinner flaps to reduce donor-site morbidity and may improve lymphatic drainage (44).

Two theories currently exist for how VLNT treats lymphedema. One theory is that lymphangiogenesis occurs via growth factors produced by the transplanted lymph nodes, and that newly sprouted lymphatic vessels are able to reconstitute lymphatic pathways (1, 45). Another theory posits that the transferred vascularized lymph node acts a lymphatic pump: the combination of pulsations at the arterial anastomosis acting as a pump and the suction effect of the flap's venous output create a driving force for lymphatic drainage through the transplanted lymph node (1, 44, 46). The lack of current histological, imaging or physiologic proof of these mechanisms in action prevents definitive validation of either

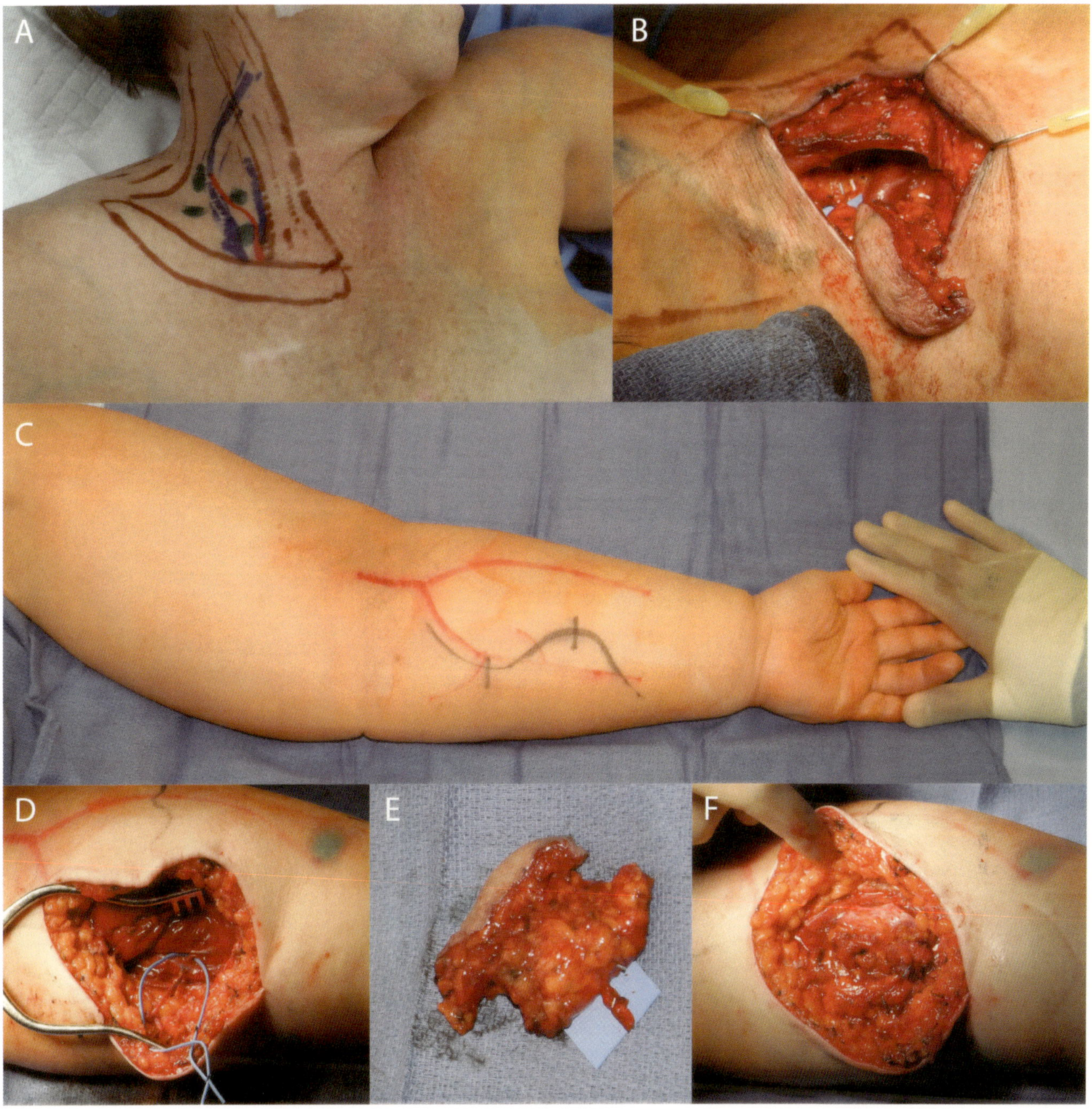


**FIGURE 2 |** Supraclavicular flap. Skin markings for the supraclavicular donor site of the vascularized lymph node transfer to the upper extremity **(A)**. Nodes were confirmed with lymphoscintigraphy and ICG. **(B)** shows the flap in place after harvest. **(C)** shows the recipient edematous upper extremity. **(D)** shows the dissected recipient artery and vein. **(E)** shows the dissected flap, and **(F)** shows the flap after inset and de-epithelialization.

theory. However, Chong et al. have recently developed a method for visualizing lymphatic vessel contractility in mice through the use of infra-red imaging, which may be used to uncover the underlying mechanism behind VLNT in the future (47).

Many studies have validated the use of simple microsurgical VLNT for the treatment of lymphedema, with some showing superior outcomes over LVA (1, 48–51). Despite its efficacy, VLNT does not always result in optimal lymphatic outflow and also constitutes free flap surgery, which can involve significant donor-site morbidity. However, advancement and refinement in technique aim to reduce these drawbacks. Visconti et al. have described the successful use of a new cervical lymph node-adipo-cutaenous flap in rats using supermicrosurgical perforator-to-perforator anastomosis, and Yamamoto et al. have recently reported the use of VLNT using both perforator-to-perforator anastomosis and efferent lymphaticolymphatic anastomosis between donor and

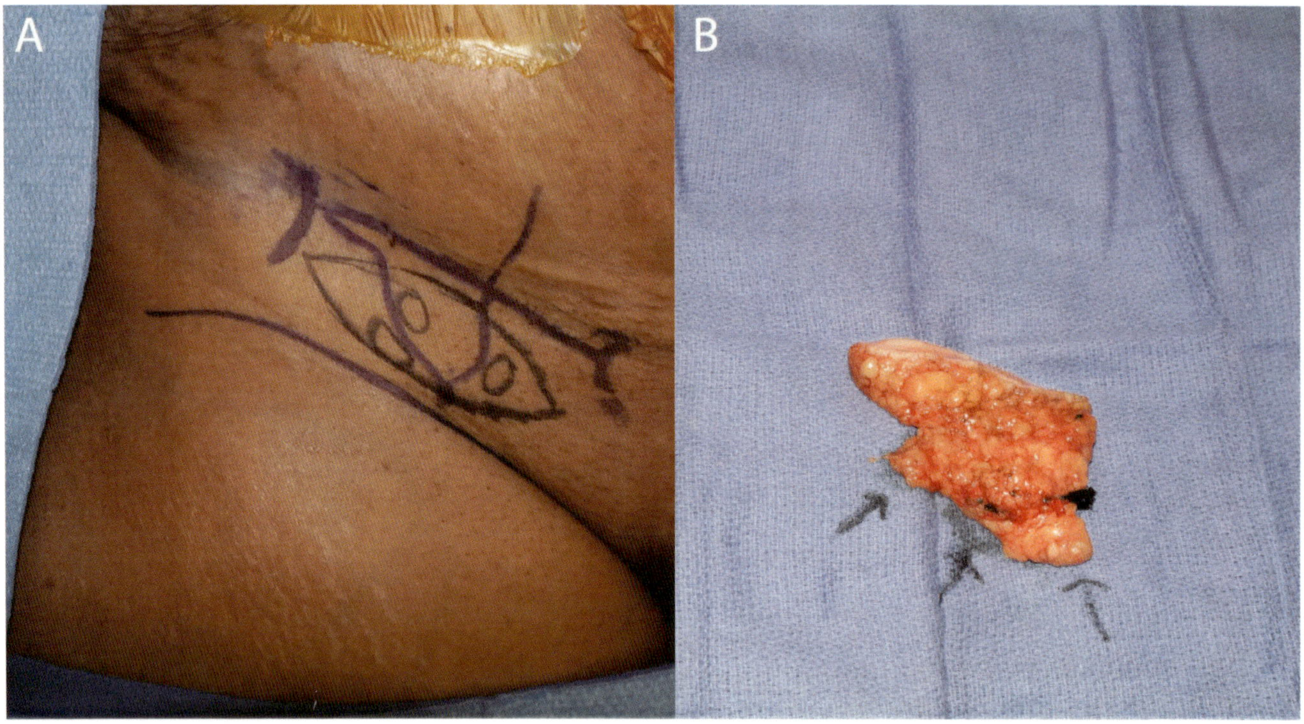


**FIGURE 3 |** Skin markings for the groin-based lymphatic flap with nodes identified by lymphoscintigraphy and ICG **(A)**. The dissected flap is shown with arrows indicating lymph nodes **(B)**.

recipient lymphatic vessels (52, 53). Moreover, some surgeons combine LVA with VLNT, anastomosing efferent lymphatic vessels to outflow veins within or near the flap in order to improve lymphatic drainage of the implanted tissue (52). Continued experimentation with techniques to improve lymphatic drainage and additional research on optimal donor and recipient sites will likely improve patient outcomes in the future and support more routine use of this procedure for the treatment of lymphedema.

## Soft Tissue Reconstruction

Although functional and aesthetic outcomes have improved with the use of perforator flaps for microsurgical free tissue reconstruction, the procedure still risks compromising the major vessels, involves long operating times, and can cause significant donor-site morbidity and scarring (54–56). The supermicrosurgical technique of raising a true perforator flap and performing perforator-to-perforator anastomosis at the recipient site can help solve many of these issues. As a result, supermicrosurgery has been increasingly used in lower extremity, craniofacial, hand, and breast reconstruction (17, 19, 57, 58).

The main advantage of supermicrosurgical reconstruction is that it allows for the use of *true* perforators for anastomosis, defined by Wei et al. as cutaneous vessels that pierce the deep fascia on their course to ultimately reach the skin (59). The utilization of a supermicrosurgical approach creates a very thin flap by dissecting only the most superficial perforators; **Figure 4** demonstrates the use of a thin Superficial Circumflex Iliac Perforator (SCIP) flap to reconstruct a small defect over the Achilles tendon. These thin true perforator flaps reduce donor-site morbidity, as cutting in a suprafascial plane helps preserve muscle, fascia, cutaneous nerves and major vessels (60). Additionally, since the pedicles for these true perforator flaps are shorter, dissection is less time-consuming and time spent in the operating room is reduced (4). Finally, the elucidation of the perforasome theory, mapping of perforators throughout the body, and the utilization of preoperative imaging for locating perforators have provided surgeons with much greater flexibility in regards to choosing a specific donor site that best suits the reconstruction (54). Several kinds of perforator flaps harvested for supermicrosurgical anastomosis have been described, including the thoracodorsal, lateral thoracic, superficial circumflex iliac, paraumbilical, anterolateral thigh and gluteal artery perforator flaps (60).

The use of a perforator as a recipient vessel also offers several advantages. First, the large number of perforators available within even small regions of the body allows for an increase in selection of choices for a recipient vessel (15). This is particularly useful when the larger vessels are present within the zone of injury, or when thorough dissection would be required to expose a deep vessel, thus increasing the risk of recipient-site morbidity. Perforator-to-perforator anastomosis is also useful for patients with significant atherosclerosis or other conditions resulting in fewer major vessels supplying the leg. For example, supermicrosurgery has been increasingly utilized in diabetic foot reconstruction by using the collateral vessels in the zone of ischemia as recipient vessels (7, 61). In this case, recipient perforators may be used to perform free flap

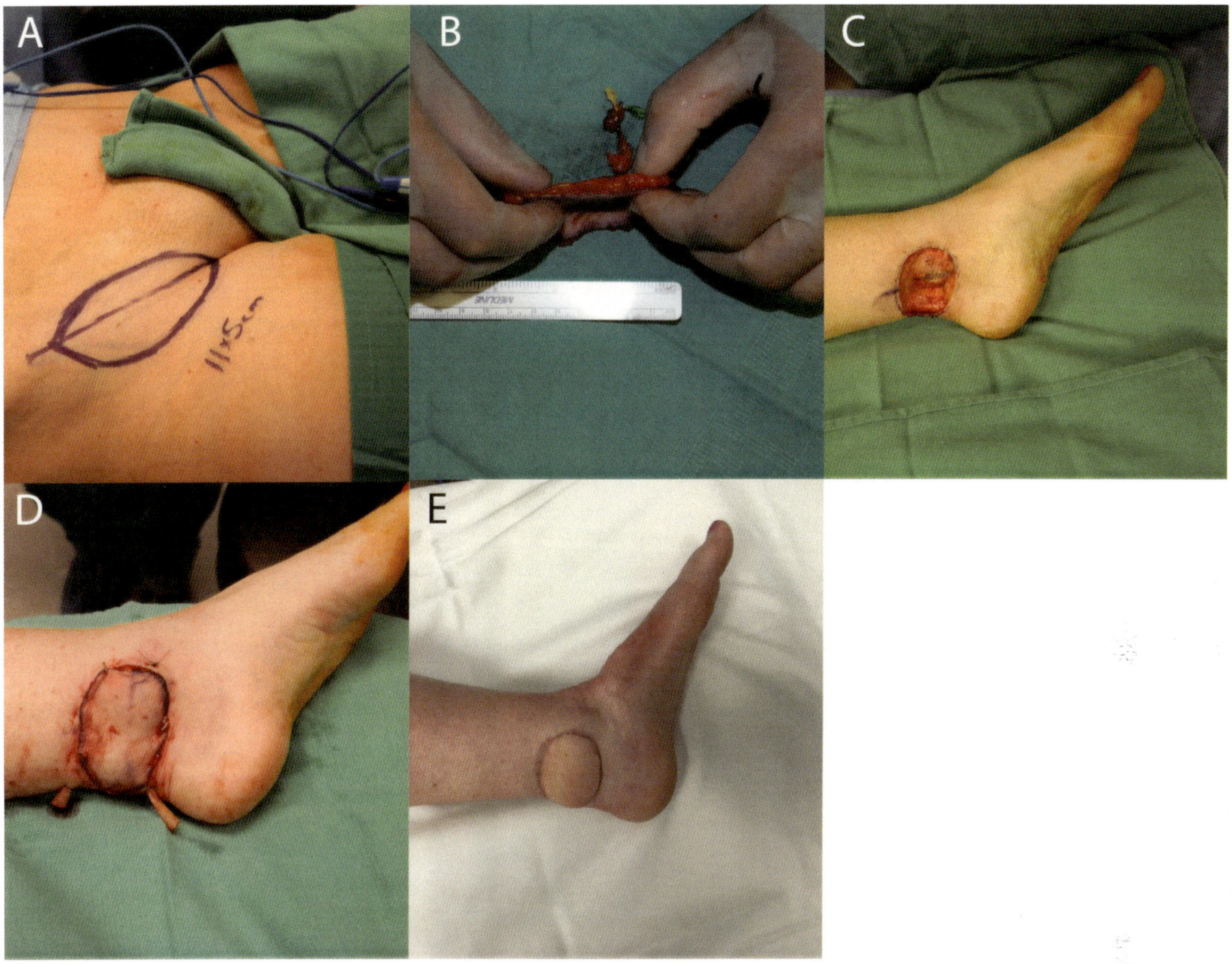


**FIGURE 4 | (A)** shows markings for the SCIP flap, and **(B)** shows the thin dissected flap. **(C)** demonstrates the recipient wound bed, and **(D)** demonstrates the recipient site with the flap in place. **(E)** shows the same foot 3 months postoperatively.

coverage without compromising distal flow (**Figure 5**). Finally, perforator-to-perforator anastomosis also has implications for flap salvage, providing additional options for bypassing areas of congestion or thrombosis (23, 62, 63).

Despite the benefits offered by supermicrosurgical soft tissue reconstruction, the technique has its limitations. First, there is a presumed increased probability of developing thrombosis of the small perforator vessels, which predisposes to flap necrosis (64). Additionally, many institutions are not equipped with the technology required to perform supermicrosurgery, including powerful microscopes capable of 50x magnification, fine surgical instruments, and imaging technologies necessary for perforator mapping, including multidetector-row computer tomography, magnetic resonance imaging, and near-infrared fluorescence imaging with indocyanine green (65–67). Finally, the technique takes significant time to master due to the short length of the flap pedicle and the difficulty in preforming anastomosis of small vessels.

## Hand Surgery

One area that has received substantial attention in supermicrosurgical research is hand surgery. Supermicrosurgery is ideal for reconstructions of the hand, as the delicate anatomic structure of fingertips necessitates the use of very fine surgical instruments and sutures. Furthermore, for safe reconstruction of the distal digits, supermicrosurgical skills are required, as the vessel calibers in this location are typically smaller than 0.5 mm (68). Supermicrosurgery has been successfully used for fingertip replantation, toe-tip transfers, free nail flaps and free perforator flaps (24, 68–70).

With the advent of supermicrosurgery, fingertip replantation is now used in digital amputations in order to permit the restoration of function, length and aesthetics while avoiding painful stump neuromas (71). Positive outcomes for fingertip replantation have been validated in the literature; for example, a study by Hattori et al. found that patients with successful replantation had a greater range of motion, less pain, better disabilities of the arm, shoulder and hand (DASH) score, and were more satisfied compared to the patients

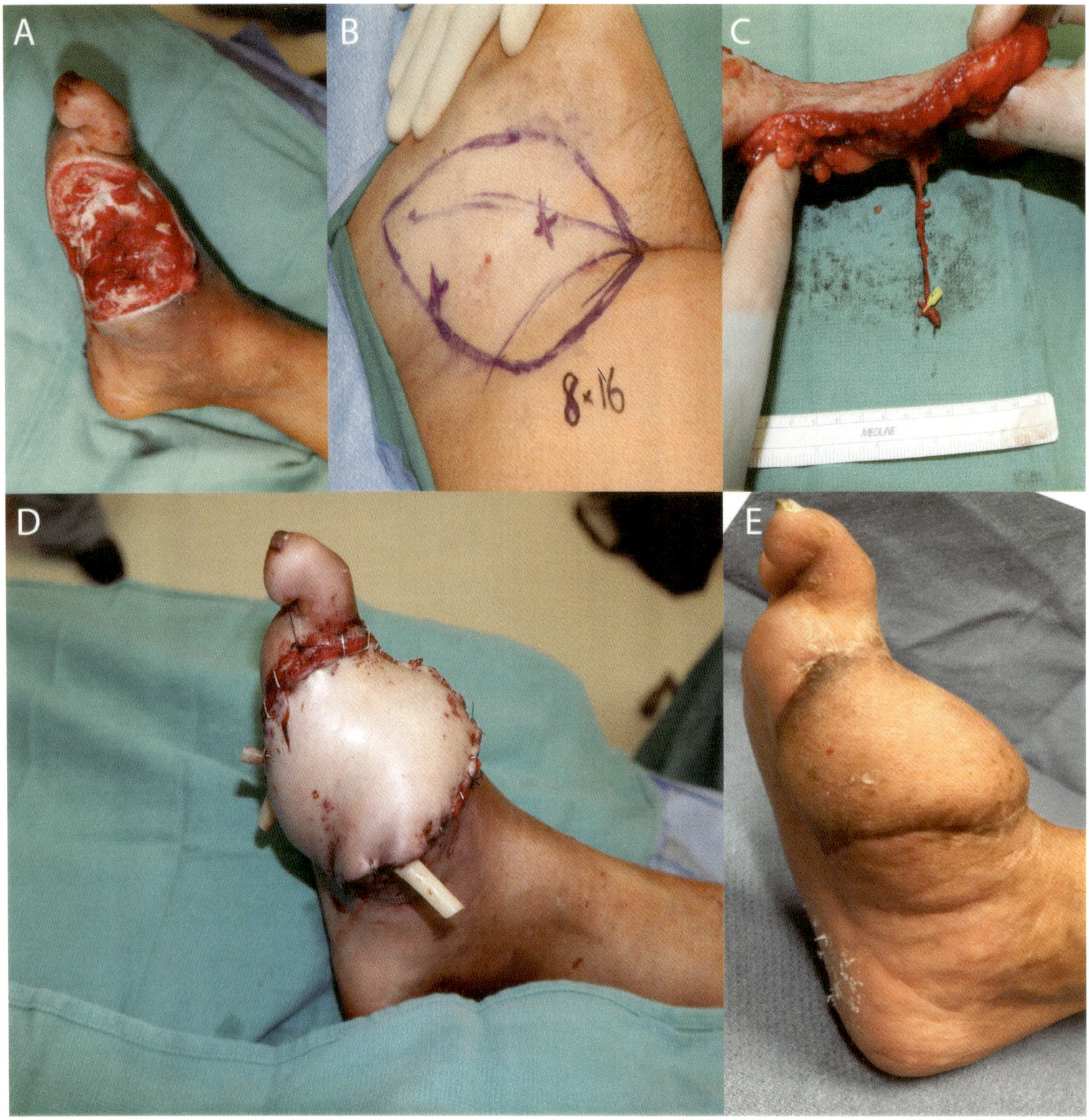


**FIGURE 5 |** Salvage of a diabetic wound. The patient presented with an infected great toe amputation, and underwent 3 staged debridements with osteotomy. **(A)** shows the defect before soft tissue reconstruction, **(B)** demonstrates the markings for SCIP flap, **(C)** shows the dissected flap and vessels, and **(D)** shows the flap after inset. **(E)** demonstrates the flap 6 months postoperatively.

undergoing amputation and revision (72). Still, many hand surgeons perceive that these technically challenging, lengthy procedures provide little functional improvement over revision amputations, and the success rate of replantations may decrease in crush injuries in which the amputated fingertips are severely damaged (68).

Fingertip reconstruction with free tissue flaps, including various perforator, nail and toe flaps has also been made possible through the use of supermicrosurgery (69, 73, 74). These procedures are usually reserved for situations where the distal fingertip is not available or too severely injured to be used for replantation. The development and refinement of new flaps, such as the dorsoradial perforator (DRAP), superficial palmar branch of the radial artery (SUPBRA), and medialis pedis free flaps, have allowed for a single stage fingertip reconstruction under regional anesthesia with minimal donor site scarring. These perforator flaps are innervated and can restore some sensory function, as well as preserving aesthetic outcomes including skin texture and color (69, 75, 76). As supermicrosurgery becomes increasingly incorporated into the field of hand surgery, the introduction of additional flaps and improvement of current techniques may allow for flap reconstruction to completely restore digital function in cases where replantation is not possible.

## Other Applications

A major benefit of supermicrosurgery is the ability to manipulate structures on a much finer scale, allowing for precise and organic reconstructions of very delicate body parts. For example, successful replantation of partially amputated nasal segments have been performed with high rates of success (77, 78). Additionally, reconstruction of the upper eyelid has been performed using an ear helix flap through supermicrosurgical techniques, and successful tongue reconstruction has also been previously reported using supermicrosurgery (18, 79). Finally, urethral reconstructions may be performed with supermicrosurgery, using either appendix transfers or more traditional free flaps (80, 81). These procedures highlight the importance of supermicrosurgical procedures in further expanding the reaches of microvascular surgery, allowing for virtually every part of the body to be successfully reconstructed.

Microvascular aesthetic surgery has also been enriched with the advent of supermicrosurgical techniques. In particular, perforator adiposal free flaps have been well-described for the use of facial and breast augmentation, with aesthetic outcomes reportedly greater than free fat injection and the conventional dermal fat flap (5). The use of flaps for aesthetic procedures also affords the surgeon significant flexibility in the procedure; for example, the paraumbilical perforator adiposal flap for breast reconstruction can be easily defatted if the bulky fat needs to be reduced, a variety of perforating vessels may be used for this technique, and many flaps can be raised and tailored to the specific needs of patients depending on the shape and size of the defect (82). According to Koshima et al., utilizing supermicrosurgery to raise a paraumbilical perforator flap for facial and breast augmentation is particularly useful in young women who may become pregnant in the future, due to minimal donor-site morbidity of the abdomen, and for children who have the potential for further skeletal growth (82).

Supermicrosurgery has also contributed to innovations in microneural repair. In 2010, Koshima et al. introduced a new method for peripheral nerve repair utilizing supermicrosurgical techniques, which he called the fascicular turnover flap. The procedure first involves the separation and coaptation of a single nerve fascicle from either the proximal or distal end of a nerve gap. The nerve fascicle is then turned over the nerve gap and positioned against the contralateral nerve end, and the fascicular flap and contralateral nerve trunk are sutured. For larger nerve gaps, bilateral turnover fascicular flaps from both the proximal and distal nerve trunks can be sutured along the middle portion of the nerve gap (83). It is believed that axonal flow is eventually reconstituted via axonal sprouting (83, 84). Although no controls were used in their experiments, Koshima et al. reported excellent sensory recovery for the fascicular turnover flap in digital nerve repair, as well as a quicker operating time and less invasive procedure compared with the vascularized nerve graft method (4, 5, 83, 85).

# TRAINING IN SUPERMICROSURGERY

Although most plastic surgery residency programs teach microsurgical techniques, supermicrosurgery requires a higher skill level for eye–microscope–hand coordination, more dexterous handling of tissues, and more refined motor skills than microsurgery (86). These technical skills need to be trained and extensively practiced in order to be appropriately utilized in the operating room.

Surgical simulation training aids in the development of critical psychomotor, technical and judgment skills through repetition, and by providing the opportunity to learn from one's errors without causing major harm (87). As supermicrosurgery is a new technique practiced by a minority of surgeons, there is an increased need for surgical simulators and training models to facilitate rapid acquisition of skills. Currently, several simulators exist for training supermicrosurgical techniques, including synthetic and biologic nonliving simulators, as well as live animal models (64).

Synthetic models are recommended for acquiring fundamental supermicrosurgical skills, such as learning microscopic adjustments and the handling of surgical tools. The most basic models include practice cards containing affixed silicon tubes measuring less than 0.8 mm in diameter which may be used for practicing anastomosis of supermicrosurgery-caliber vessels (88). These practice cards are attached to the stage of a microscope, and can be manipulated with the microsurgical instruments that are used clinically. More high-fidelity biologic cadaveric models, such as the chicken thigh model introduced by Chen et al., can be used for advanced skill acquisition once basic skills have been achieved and the trainee is comfortable using the microscope and associated instruments (86). In the chicken thigh model, branches of the ischiatic artery and vein have diameters ranging between 0.3–0.5 mm, allowing for practice on biologic submillimeter vessels. A major benefit of nonliving biologic models is that the trainee can receive tactile feedback that is nearly identical to procedures performed in human patients. These models are cost-effective and do not require pre- or postoperative care (86).

Once supermicrosurgical skills have been sufficiently developed using nonliving models, the trainee can progress to practicing on live animal models. Several living rat models featuring an assortment of submillimeter vessels are available for the practice of supermicrosurgical techniques (89–92). Different models allow for the practice of a large variety of techniques, ranging from simple perforator-to-perforator anastomoses to complete flap transfers. Once the surgeon is proficient at performing these skills on live animal models, he or she may be ready to utilize these techniques in the care of patients.

## ROBOTIC-ASSISTED SURGERY AS AN ENABLING TECHNOLOGY

One of the greatest challenges with supermicrosurgery is the high level of dexterity and surgical control required for successful anastomosis. Robotic-assisted surgery (RAS), defined as surgery that is performed by a human surgeon through the use of a robotic instrument, may facilitate use of this technique. Although RAS is already used to perform very delicate surgeries requiring manipulation of small structures, there is currently only 1 study in the literature describing a successful supermicrosurgical procedure performed with the Da Vinci surgical system (93).

RAS offers several unique benefits that may assist surgeons with performing the technique and enhance supermicrosurgical procedures. First, the Da Vinci allows highly precise control of instruments that may be continuously adjusted throughout the procedure, which increases the exactness of the operator's movements. Additionally, the Da Vinci surgical system allows the surgeon to work on anatomic areas that may be difficult to access in conventional surgery; this may offer the surgeon greater ergonomic comfort during surgery and allows for additional operating angles. Finally, RAS allows for complete repression of ordinary hand tremors, further increasing the precision of surgical movements (93). Therefore, RAS enables accessibility to the utilization of supermicrosurgery.

However, use of RAS requires increased operating time, is expensive, and the repertoire of movements and actions performed through RAS are more limited than those that can be performed by human hands. Therefore, the use of RAS by experienced surgeons will likely be reserved for procedures that require extremely delicate supermicrosurgical skills beyond those needed for more routine procedures, and for performing remote-controlled surgeries from distant sites (93). Nonetheless, RAS represents an exciting new frontier for supermicrosurgery and may be the key to manipulating even smaller anatomic structures in the future.

## FUTURE DIRECTIONS

### Organ Transplantation

Studies are underway investigating limb transplantation, uterine transplantation, and eye transplantation in animal models using supermicrosurgical techniques (92, 94, 95). Kisu et al. have recently reported the use of supermicrosurgery in a successful uterine transplantation in cynomolgus monkeys through anastomosis of the internal iliac artery and superficial uterine vein with their corresponding recipient vessels (94). The success of this procedure highlights the importance of supermicrosurgery for transplantation of organs with small feeding vessels that were previously not amenable to microsurgery. A similar principle was illustrated in the limb transplantation procedures performed in a rat animal model by Sucher et al. (92). It is perceivable that bioengineered body parts could also rely heavily on supermicrosurgical techniques in the future.

### Customized Reconstruction

An exciting consequence of the increased use of supermicrosurgery in soft tissue reconstruction will be the possibility of raising customized flaps tailored to fit individual reconstructive needs. Since supermicrosugery allows surgeons to use thin flaps from all over the body with minimal donor-site morbidity, it is becoming increasingly possible to design flaps based on the specific color, size, three-dimensional shape, blood supply and innervation patterns desired. Therefore, further refinement of supermicrosurgical procedures and experimentation with new flap types may allow surgeons to perform highly customized reconstructions that improve both aesthetic and functional outcomes in patients with complex reconstructive needs (4).

The concept of "like-with-like" reconstruction has already begun to gain traction with the advent of perforator flaps, but supermicrosurgery opens the doors for truly individualized free-style perforator flaps based on needs of the reconstruction. There are a few studies in the literature describing experimentation with customized perforator flaps designed to exactly reconstruct soft tissue defects (96, 97). For example, Jin et al. have recently reported their experience using supermicrosurgery to perform like-with-like buccal reconstruction with the SCIP flap; the authors report designing flaps with surface areas and volumes tailored to fulfill both the cosmetic and functional requirements of the recipient oral defect. Using this procedure, the authors described excellent aesthetic and functional outcomes in the buccal region, successful like-with-like reconstruction, and minimal donor-site scarring (96).

Stacked perforator free flaps represent another opportunity for supermicrosurgery to solve complex reconstructive problems. "Stacking" of flaps involves the transfer of tissue from multiple donor sites into a single recipient site, a technique which has previously been described for breast reconstruction in patients that require additional volume to achieve an optimum result. Stacked deep inferior epigastric perforator (DIEP) flaps, profunda artery perforator flaps, superficial inferior epigastric artery (SIEA) flaps, and several other combinations have been used for this purpose (98, 99). Although these procedures have generally produced successful reconstructive results, they still involve significant recipient and donor-site morbidity, especially if bilateral donor sites are used. Supermicrosurgery may enhance the utility of stacked flaps by allowing more freedom in choosing donor and recipient vessels for anastomosis; for example, one can envision using small intercostal or internal mammary perforators as recipient vessels for stacked perforator flap inset using perforator-to-perforator anastomosis, or using the feeding perforating vessel of the primary free flap as the recipient vessel for a second flap through intra-flap anastomosis (99–102). These techniques may reduce donor and recipient site morbidity by eliminating the need for large vessel dissection.

Supermicrosurgery may also be applied to the concept of chimeric flaps, which consist of separate flaps of various different tissue types that are connected to one another through a single vascular pedicle. They can be further broken down into those chimeric flaps which are connected by their intrinsic vasculature and prefabricated flaps which are connected through microanastomosis. By allowing for the transfer of different tissue types and the independent inset of each component, chimeric flaps create a large degree of spatial freedom in order to restore volume and contour of complex 3-dimensional defects (103). Supermicrosurgery allows for the dissection and use of unique intrinsic chimeric flaps relying on small feeding vessels that are not amenable to traditional microsurgery in order to reconstruct complex defects; for example, Yamamoto et al. have previously described the use of a quadruple-component intrinsic chimeric SCIP flap that included portions of the Sartorius muscle, deep fascia, inguinal lymph node and skin/fat for a complex ankle reconstruction (104). Fernandez Garrido et al. similarly described the use of a chimeric SCIP flap with a piece of external oblique muscle fascia tailored to reconstruct a dorsal foot defect (105). With further refinement of technique, supermicrosurgery may allow for the prefabrication of highly customized, multi-component chimeric flaps using tissues from all over the body, without the limitation of feeding vessel size, that can be precisely tailored to a patient's reconstructive needs.

### Extreme Salvage

An important application of supermicrosurgery has been the ability to salvage extremities in the setting of significant systemic or local disease. With the use of supermicrosurgical techniques, extreme limb salvage can be performed in the setting of conditions that have previously limited simple microsurgical free tissue transfer, including renal failure, post-transplant patients on immunosuppressant medications, severe diabetic microvascular disease, advanced peripheral vascular disease with severe ischemia, and a history of amputation. In these cases, wound healing is impaired, circulation is poor and major vessels are often calcified, making microsurgery extremely difficult (61, 106). Through supermicrosurgery, small collateral vessels that have formed in the setting of chronic ischemia, or small perforators left over after major lower extremity trauma, can be used as recipient vessels for free tissue anastomosis without compromising distal flow (19, 61). Thus, even extremely sick patients with poor vascular flow from the major vessels due to injury or advanced ischemia can be given the opportunity for reconstruction as long as they have a small artery with an adequate pulse. For example, Suh et al. showed that patients with ischemic diabetic foot ulcers and significant comorbidities, including renal failure, immunosuppression, and previous amputation, can nonetheless undergo lower extremity reconstruction using small recipient end arteries or perforators in a different angiosome territory, with a reported overall limb salvage rate of 90.5% (7). Supermicrosurgery presents the best option for patients with severe injuries and multiple comorbidities to avoid extremity amputation.

## CONCLUSIONS

Supermicrosurgery has greatly expanded the scope of procedures that can be performed under a microscope. Since the anastomosis of small vessels is a central component of many surgeries, supermicrosurgery has had an immense impact on a wide variety of different procedures, from lymphedema management to soft tissue reconstruction, digit replantation and aesthetic surgery. Importantly, supermicrosurgery is a brand new field, and a consensus was only met on its name in 2010 (4). Therefore, it is certain that the field will continue to see additional innovations, refinements and adoption in the coming years. The goal is that with further innovations and refinement of technique, the supermicrosurgical armamentarium will expand, operating times will shorten, the learning curve will decrease and patient outcomes will improve.

There is now a need for outcome-based research investigating functional outcomes and patient satisfaction following supermicrosurgery. Using the results of such studies, it will be possible to formally adopt supermicrosurgery in clinical decision-making algorithms when facing challenging cases in reconstruction. The development of additional simulation models and training programs dedicated to supermicrosurgery will be necessary to increase widespread adoption of these techniques.

## AUTHOR CONTRIBUTIONS

IB, DG, and KP all contributed to the concept, literature review, generation of figures, manuscript drafting and editing of this review. All authors verified the contents of the final manuscript and maintain that the information contained therein is accurate and true.

## REFERENCES

1. Raju A, Chang DW. Vascularized lymph node transfer for treatment of lymphedema: a comprehensive literature review. *Ann Surg* (2015) 261(5):1013–23. doi: 10.1097/SLA.0000000000000763
2. Tashiro K, Harima M, Yamamoto T, Narushima M, Koshima I. Locating recipient perforators for perforator-to-perforator anastomosis using color doppler ultrasonography. *J Plast Reconstr Aesthet Surg* (2014) 67(12):1680–3. doi: 10.1016/j.bjps.2014.08.047
3. Park JE, Chang DW. Advances and innovations in microsurgery. *Plast Reconstr Surg* (2016) 138(5):915e–24. doi: 10.1097/PRS.0000000000002715
4. Masia J, Olivares L, Koshima I, Teo TC, Suominen S, van Landuyt K, et al. Barcelona consensus on supermicrosurgery. *J Reconstr Microsurg* (2014) 30(1):53 8. doi: 10.1055/s-0033-1354742
5. Koshima I, Yamamoto T, Narushima M, Mihara M, Iida T. Perforator flaps and supermicrosurgery. *Clin Plast Surg* (2010) 37(4):683–9. doi: 10.1016/j.cps.2010.06.009
6. Yamamoto T, Yamamoto N, Ishiura R. Thirty-micron needle for precise supermicrosurgery. *Microsurgery* (2017) 37(6):735–6. doi: 10.1002/micr.30165
7. Suh HS, Oh TS, Lee HS, Lee SH, Cho YP, Park JR, et al. A new approach for reconstruction of diabetic foot wounds using the angiosome and supermicrosurgery concept. *Plast Reconstr Surg* (2016) 138(4):702e–9. doi: 10.1097/PRS.0000000000002401

8. Mihara M, Hara H, Tange S, Zhou HP, Kawahara M, Shimizu Y, et al. Multisite lymphaticovenular bypass using supermicrosurgery technique for lymphedema management in lower lymphedema cases. *Plast Reconstr Surg* (2016) 138(1):262–72. doi: 10.1097/PRS.0000000000002254
9. Burns PB, Rohrich RJ, Chung KC. The levels of evidence and their role in evidence-based medicine. *Plast Reconstr Surg* (2011) 128(1):305–10. doi: 10.1097/PRS.0b013e318219c171
10. Tamai S. History of microsurgery. *Plast Reconstr Surg* (2009) 124(6 Suppl):e282–94. doi: 10.1097/PRS.0b013e3181bf825e
11. Jacobson JH, Suarez EL. Microsurgery in anastomosis of small vessels. *Surg Forum* (1960) 11:243–5.
12. Malt RA, Mckhann C. Replantation of severed arms. *JAMA* (1964) 189:716–22. doi: 10.1001/jama.1964.03070100010002
13. Taylor GI, Palmer JH. The vascular territories (angiosomes) of the body: experimental study and clinical applications. *Br J Plast Surg* (1987) 40(2):113–41. doi: 10.1016/0007-1226(87)90185-8
14. Koshima I, Soeda S. Inferior epigastric artery skin flaps without rectus abdominis muscle. *Br J Plast Surg* (1989) 42(6):645–8. doi: 10.1016/0007-1226(89)90075-1
15. Saint-Cyr M, Wong C, Schaverien M, Mojallal A, Rohrich RJ. The perforasome theory: vascular anatomy and clinical implications. *Plast Reconstr Surg* (2009) 124(5):1529–44. doi: 10.1097/PRS.0b013e3181b98a6c
16. Koshima I, Inagawa K, Urushibara K, Moriguchi T. Paraumbilical perforator flap without deep inferior epigastric vessels. *Plast Reconstr Surg* (1998) 102(4):1052–7. doi: 10.1097/00006534-199809020-00020
17. Kompatscher P, Manestar M, Schuster A, Lang A, Beer GM. The thoracoacromial vessels as recipient vessels in microsurgery and supermicrosurgery: an anatomical and sonographic study. *Plast Reconstr Surg* (2005) 115(1):77–83.
18. Kim JS, Choi TH, Kim NG, Lee KS, Han KH, Son DG, et al. The replantation of an amputated tongue by supermicrosurgery. *J Plast Reconstr Aesthet Surg* (2007) 60(10):1152–5. doi: 10.1016/j.bjps.2007.01.009
19. Hong JP. The use of supermicrosurgery in lower extremity reconstruction: the next step in evolution. *Plast Reconstr Surg* (2009) 123(1):230–5. doi: 10.1097/PRS.0b013e3181904dc4
20. Koshima I, Nanba Y, Tsutsui T, Takahashi Y. Medial plantar perforator flaps with supermicrosurgery. *Clin Plast Surg* (2003) 30(3):447–55. doi: 10.1016/S0094-1298(03)00044-0
21. Koshima I, Nanba Y, Tsutsui T, Takahashi Y, Itoh S, Fujitsu M. Minimal invasive lymphaticovenular anastomosis under local anesthesia for leg lymphedema: is it effective for stage III and IV? *Ann Plast Surg* (2004) 53(3):261–6.
22. Felmerer G, Sattler T, Lohrmann C, Tobbia D. Treatment of various secondary lymphedemas by microsurgical lymph vessel transplantation. *Microsurgery* (2012) 32(3):171–7. doi: 10.1002/micr.20968
23. Hong JP, Koshima I. Using perforators as recipient vessels (supermicrosurgery) for free flap reconstruction of the knee region. *Ann Plast Surg* (2010) 64(3):291–3. doi: 10.1097/SAP.0b013e3181ac4263
24. Kim JS, Yang JW, Lee DC, Ki SH, Roh SY. Challenges in fingertip replantation. *Semin Plast Surg* (2013) 27(4):165–73. doi: 10.1055/s-0033-1360583
25. Patel KM, Manrique O, Sosin M, Hashmi MA, Poysophon P, Henderson R. Lymphatic mapping and lymphedema surgery in the breast cancer patient. *Gland Surg* (2015) 4(3):244–56. doi: 10.3978/j.issn.2227-684X.2015.03.02
26. Symvoulakis EK, Anyfantakis DI, Lionis C. Primary lower limb lymphedema: a focus on its functional, social and emotional impact. *Int J Med Sci* (2010) 7(6):353–7. doi: 10.7150/ijms.7.353
27. Johansson K, Holmström H, Nilsson I, Ingvar C, Albertsson M, Ekdahl C. Breast cancer patients' experiences of lymphoedema. *Scand J Caring Sci* (2003) 17(1):35–42. doi: 10.1046/j.1471-6712.2003.00119.x
28. Passik SD, Mcdonald MV. Psychosocial aspects of upper extremity lymphedema in women treated for breast carcinoma. *Cancer* (1998) 83(12 Suppl American):2817–20. doi: 10.1002/(SICI)1097-0142(19981215)83:12B+<2817::AID-CNCR32>3.0.CO;2-2
29. Ahmed RL, Prizment A, Lazovich D, Schmitz KH, Folsom AR. Lymphedema and quality of life in breast cancer survivors: the Iowa women's health study. *J Clin Oncol* (2008) 26(35):5689–96. doi: 10.1200/JCO.2008.16.4731
30. Taghian NR, Miller CL, Jammallo LS, O'Toole J, Skolny MN. Lymphedema following breast cancer treatment and impact on quality of life: a review. *Crit Rev Oncol Hematol* (2014) 92(3):227–34. doi: 10.1016/j.critrevonc.2014.06.004
31. Demirtas Y, Ozturk N, Yapici O, Topalan M. Comparison of primary and secondary lower-extremity lymphedema treated with supermicrosurgical lymphaticovenous anastomosis and lymphaticovenous implantation. *J Reconstr Microsurg* (2010) 26(2):137–43. doi: 10.1055/s-0029-1243299
32. Yamamoto T, Yoshimatsu H, Yamamoto N, Narushima M, Iida T, Koshima I. Side-to-end Lymphaticovenular anastomosis through temporary lymphatic expansion. *PLoS ONE* (2013) 8(3):e59523. doi: 10.1371/journal.pone.0059523
33. Koshima I, Inagawa K, Urushibara K, Moriguchi T. Supermicrosurgical lymphaticovenular anastomosis for the treatment of lymphedema in the upper extremities. *J Reconstr Microsurg* (2000) 16(6):437–42. doi: 10.1055/s-2006-947150
34. Auba C, Marre D, Rodríguez-Losada G, Hontanilla B. Lymphaticovenular anastomoses for lymphedema treatment: 18 months postoperative outcomes. *Microsurgery* (2012) 32(4):261–8. doi: 10.1002/micr.20980
35. Campisi C, Bellini C, Campisi C, Accogli S, Bonioli E, Boccardo F. Microsurgery for lymphedema: clinical research and long-term results. *Microsurgery* (2010) 30(4):256–60. doi: 10.1002/micr.20737
36. Chang DW. Lymphaticovenular bypass for lymphedema management in breast cancer patients: a prospective study. *Plast Reconstr Surg* (2010) 126(3):752–8. doi: 10.1097/PRS.0b013e3181e5f6a9
37. Campisi C, Davini D, Bellini C, Taddei G, Villa G, Fulcheri E, et al. Lymphatic microsurgery for the treatment of lymphedema. *Microsurgery* (2006) 26(1):65–9. doi: 10.1002/micr.20214
38. Chang DW, Suami H, Skoracki R. A prospective analysis of 100 consecutive lymphovenous bypass cases for treatment of extremity lymphedema. *Plast Reconstr Surg* (2013) 132(5):1305–14. doi: 10.1097/PRS.0b013e3182a4d626
39. Matsutani H, Hayashi A, Yamamoto T. All-star lymphatic supermicrosurgery: multiple lymph flow diversion using end-to-end, end-to-side, side-to-end, and side-to-side lymphaticovenular anastomoses in a surgical field. *Journal of Plastic, Reconstructive & Aesthetic Surgery* (2015) 68(5):e107–108. doi: 10.1016/j.bjps.2015.02.022
40. Silva AK, Chang DW. Vascularized lymph node transfer and lymphovenous bypass: novel treatment strategies for symptomatic lymphedema. *J Surg Oncol* (2016) 113(8):932–9. doi: 10.1002/jso.24171
41. Damstra RJ, Voesten HG, van Schelven WD, van der Lei B, Anastomosis Lvenous. Lymphatic venous anastomosis (LVA) for treatment of secondary arm lymphedema. A prospective study of 11 LVA procedures in 10 patients with breast cancer related lymphedema and a critical review of the literature. *Breast Cancer Res Treat* (2009) 113(2):199–206. doi: 10.1007/s10549-008-9932-5
42. Scaglioni MF, Arvanitakis M, Chen YC, Giovanoli P, Chia-Shen Yang J, Chang EI. Comprehensive review of vascularized lymph node transfers for lymphedema: outcomes and complications. *Microsurgery* (2018) 38(2):222-229–. doi: 10.1002/micr.30079
43. Becker C, Assouad J, Riquet M, Hidden G. Postmastectomy Lymphedema. *Ann Surg* (2006) 243(3):313–5. doi: 10.1097/01.sla.0000201258.10304.16
44. Lin CH, Ali R, Chen SC, Wallace C, Chang YC, Chen HC, et al. Vascularized groin lymph node transfer using the wrist as a recipient site for management of postmastectomy upper extremity lymphedema. *Plast Reconstr Surg* (2009) 123(4):1265–75. doi: 10.1097/PRS.0b013e31819e6529
45. Becker C, Vasile JV, Levine JL, Batista BN, Studinger RM, Chen CM, et al. Microlymphatic surgery for the treatment of iatrogenic lymphedema. *Clin Plast Surg* (2012) 39(4):385–98. doi: 10.1016/j.cps.2012.08.002
46. Cheng MH, Huang JJ, Huang JJ, Nguyen DH, Saint-Cyr M, Zenn MR, et al. A novel approach to the treatment of lower extremity lymphedema by transferring a vascularized submental lymph node flap to the ankle. *Gynecol Oncol* (2012) 126(1):93–8. doi: 10.1016/j.ygyno.2012.04.017
47. Chong C, Scholkmann F, Bachmann SB, Luciani P, Leroux JC, Detmar M, et al. In vivo visualization and quantification of collecting lymphatic vessel contractility using near-infrared imaging. *Sci Rep* (2016) 6(6):srep22930. doi: 10.1038/srep22930
48. Tobbia D, Semple J, Baker A, Dumont D, Johnston M. Experimental assessment of autologous lymph node transplantation as treatment of postsurgical lymphedema. *Plast Reconstr Surg* (2009) 124(3):777–86. doi: 10.1097/PRS.0b013e3181b03787
49. Batista BN, Germain M, Faria JC, Becker C. Lymph node flap transfer for patients with secondary lower limb lymphedema. *Microsurgery* (2017) 37(1):29–33. doi: 10.1002/micr.22404
50. Akita S, Mitsukawa N, Kuriyama M, Kubota Y, Hasegawa M, Tokumoto H, et al. Comparison of vascularized supraclavicular lymph node

transfer and lymphaticovenular anastomosis for advanced stage lower extremity lymphedema. *Ann Plast Surg* (2015) 74(5):1–9. doi: 10.1097/SAP.0000000000000513
51. Granzow JW, Soderberg JM, Kaji AH, Dauphine C. An effective system of surgical treatment of lymphedema. *Ann Surg Oncol* (2014) 21(4):1189–94. doi: 10.1245/s10434-014-3515-y
52. Yamamoto T, Yoshimatsu H, Yamamoto N. Complete lymph flow reconstruction: a free vascularized lymph node true perforator flap transfer with efferent lymphaticolymphatic anastomosis. *J Plast Reconstr Aesthet Surg* (2016) 69(9):1227–33. doi: 10.1016/j.bjps.2016.06.028
53. Visconti G, Brunelli C, Mulè A, Franceschini G, Chen HC, Masetti R, et al. Septum-based cervical lymph-node free flap in rat: a new model. *J Surg Res* (2016) 201(1):1–12. doi: 10.1016/j.jss.2015.09.027
54. Engel H, Gazyakan E, Cheng MH, Piel D, Germann G, Giessler G. Customized reconstruction with the free anterolateral thigh perforator flap. *Microsurgery* (2008) 28(7):489–94. doi: 10.1002/micr.20538
55. di Candia M, Lie K, Kumiponjera D, Simcock J, Cormack GC, Malata CM. Versatility of the anterolateral thigh free flap: the four seasons flap. *Eplasty* (2012) 12:e21.
56. Weckx A, Loomans N, Lenssen O. Perforator free flaps in head and neck reconstruction: a single-center low-volume experience. *Oral Surg Oral Med Oral Pathol Oral Radiol* (2017) 123(4):429–35. doi: 10.1016/j.oooo.2016.11.010
57. Choi DH, Goh T, Cho JY, Hong JP. Thin superficial circumflex iliac artery perforator flap and supermicrosurgery technique for face reconstruction. *J Craniofac Surg* (2014) 25(6):1–3. doi: 10.1097/SCS.0000000000001093
58. Yoon CS, Noh HJ, Malzone G, Suh HS, Choi DH, Hong JP. Posterior interosseous artery perforator-free flap: treating intermediate-size hand and foot defects. *J Plast Reconstr Aesthet Surg* (2014) 67(6):808–14. doi: 10.1016/j.bjps.2014.03.007
59. Wei FC, Jain V, Suominen S, Chen HC. Confusion among perforator flaps: what is a true perforator flap? *Plast Reconstr Surg* (2001) 107(3):874–6. doi: 10.1097/00006534-200103000-00037
60. Ozkan O, Koshima I, Gonda K. A supermicrosurgical flap model in the rat: a free true abdominal perforator flap with a short pedicle. *Plast Reconstr Surg* (2006) 117(2):479–85. doi: 10.1097/01.prs.0000197215.94170.b8
61. Suh HS, Oh TS, Hong JP. Innovations in diabetic foot reconstruction using supermicrosurgery. *Diabetes Metab Res Rev* (2016) 32(Suppl 1):275–80. doi: 10.1002/dmrr.2755
62. Hwang KT, Kim WH, Kim JT, Kim YH. Perforator flap salvage using supermicrosurgical division and diversion of the pedicle. *J Plast Reconstr Aesthet Surg* (2013) 66(4):585–7. doi: 10.1016/j.bjps.2012.09.021
63. Defazio MV, Abbate OA, Lakhiani C, Song DH. Pedicle-to-perforator bypass using supermicrosurgical technique for deep inferior epigastric artery perforator flap salvage. *Plast Reconstr Surg Glob Open* (2017) 5(10):e1542. doi: 10.1097/GOX.0000000000001542
64. Bas CE, Cwykiel J, Siemionow M. A new supermicrosurgery training model of saphenous artery and great saphenous vein anastomosis for development of advanced microsurgical skills. *J Reconstr Microsurg* (2017) 33(6):426–34. doi: 10.1055/s-0037-1599101
65. Lee BT, Matsui A, Hutteman M, Lin SJ, Winer JH, Laurence RG, et al. Intraoperative near-infrared fluorescence imaging in perforator flap reconstruction: current research and early clinical experience. *J Reconstr Microsurg* (2010) 26(1):059–65. doi: 10.1055/s-0029-1244805
66. Masia J, Navarro C, Clavero JA, Alomar X. Noncontrast magnetic resonance imaging for preoperative perforator mapping. *Clin Plast Surg* (2011) 38(2):253–61. doi: 10.1016/j.cps.2011.03.004
67. Wei FC, Al Deek NF, Lin Tay SK. Principles and Techniques of Microvascular Surgery. In: Neligan PC, Gurtner GC, editors. *Plastic Surgery*. . 4th ed. Canada: Elsevier Health Sciences (2018). p. Vol. 1: Principles. 444–72.
68. Yoshimatsu H, Yamamoto T, Iwamoto T, Hayashi A, Narushima M, Iida T, et al. The role of non-enhanced angiography in toe tip transfer with small diameter pedicle. *Microsurgery* (2015) 35(5):364–9. doi: 10.1002/micr.22353
69. Song D, Pafitanis G, Yang P, Narushima M, Li Z, Liu L, et al. Innervated dorsoradial perforator free flap: a reliable supermicrosurgery fingertip reconstruction technique. *J Plast Reconstr Aesthet Surg* (2017) 70(8):1001–8. doi: 10.1016/j.bjps.2017.05.038
70. Fujitsu M. Pulp flap replantation of the amputated fingertip. *Plast Reconstr Surg* (2011) 127(3):77e–8. doi: 10.1097/PRS.0b013e3182063451
71. Dagum AB. Fingertip Amputations: Supermicrosurgery and Replantation. In: Rozmaryn LM, editor. *Fingertip Injuries: Diagnosis, Management and Reconstruction*. New York, NY: Springer International Publishing (2015). p. p. 83–95.
72. Hattori Y, Doi K, Ikeda K, Estrella EP. A retrospective study of functional outcomes after successful replantation versus amputation closure for single fingertip amputations. *J Hand Surg Am* (2006) 31(5):811–8. doi: 10.1016/j.jhsa.2006.02.020
73. Regmi S, Gu JX, Zhang NC, Liu HJ. A systematic review of outcomes and complications of primary fingertip reconstruction using reverse-flow homodigital Island flaps. *Aesthetic Plast Surg* (2016) 40(2):277–83. doi: 10.1007/s00266-016-0624-y
74. Song D, Deng X, Chen Y, Xie S, Zhou X. Thinned chimeric radial collateral artery perforator flap in complex distal thumb reconstruction. *Arch Orthop Trauma Surg* (2015) 135(11):1623–31. doi: 10.1007/s00402-015-2324-5
75. Rodriguez-Vegas M. Medialis pedis flap in the reconstruction of palmar skin defects of the digits: clarifying the anatomy of the medial plantar artery. *Ann Plast Surg* (2014) 72(5):542–52. doi: 10.1097/SAP.0b013e318268a901
76. Iwuagwu FC, Orkar SK, Siddiqui A. Reconstruction of volar skin and soft tissue defects of the digits including the pulp: experience with the free SUPBRA flap. *J Plast Reconstr Aesthet Surg* (2015) 68(1):26–34. doi: 10.1016/j.bjps.2014.08.064
77. Kim S, Jeong H, Choi TH, Kim JS. Successful re-plantation of an amputated nasal segment by supermicrosurgery: a case report and review of the literature. *J Plast Reconstr Aesthet Surg* (2010) 63(4):e380–83. doi: 10.1016/j.bjps.2009.10.012
78. Stupka I, Dvorak Z, Vesely J, Novak P, Perrotta RE, Lombardo GA. Reconstruction of a nose bitten and eaten by a dog: a ten-year follow-up of a bitten-off nose replantation performed on an eleven-year-old boy. *Ann Plast Surg* (2015) 75(6):585–7. doi: 10.1097/SAP.0000000000000643
79. Koshima I, Urushibara K, Okuyama H, Moriguchi T. Ear helix flap for reconstruction of total loss of the upper eyelid. *Br J Plast Surg* (1999) 52(4):314–6. doi: 10.1054/bjps.1998.3055
80. Bayramiçli M, Akdeniz ZD. Urethra reconstruction with lateral pectoral flap in female-to-male transsexual patients. *J Plast Reconstr Aesthet Surg* (2016) 69(11):1558–60. doi: 10.1016/j.bjps.2016.05.030
81. Koshima I, Inagawa K, Okuyama N, Moriguchi T. Free vascularized appendix transfer for reconstruction of penile urethras with severe fibrosis. *Plast Reconstr Surg* (1999) 103(3):964–9. doi: 10.1097/00006534-199903000-00030
82. Koshima I, Inagawa K, Yamamoto M, Moriguchi T. New microsurgical breast reconstruction using free paraumbilical perforator adiposal flaps. *Plast Reconstr Surg* (2000) 106(1):61–5. doi: 10.1097/00006534-200007000-00011
83. Koshima I, Narushima M, Mihara M, Uchida G, Nakagawa M. Fascicular turnover flap for nerve gaps. *J Plast Reconstr Aesthet Surg* (2010) 63(6):1008–14. doi: 10.1016/j.bjps.2009.02.083
84. Geuna S, Papalia I, Ronchi G, D'Alcontres FS, Natsis K, Papadopulos NA, et al. The reasons for end-to-side coaptation: how does lateral axon sprouting work? *Neural Regen Res* (2017) 12(4):529–33. doi: 10.4103/1673-5374.205081
85. Ito T, Nakagawa R, Ishiura R, Yamamoto T, Narushima M. Nerve reconstruction after sural nerve biopsy with supermicrosurgical fascicular turnover flap. *J Plast Reconstr Aesthet Surg* (2016) 69(1):146. doi: 10.1016/j.bjps.2015.08.005
86. Chen WF, Eid A, Yamamoto T, Keith J, Nimmons GL, Lawrence WT. A novel supermicrosurgery training model: the chicken thigh. *J Plast Reconstr Aesthet Surg* (2014) 67(7):973–8. doi: 10.1016/j.bjps.2014.03.024
87. Gallagher AG, Ritter EM, Champion H, Higgins G, Fried MP, Moses G, et al. Virtual reality simulation for the operating room. *Ann Surg* (2005) 241(2):364–72. doi: 10.1097/01.sla.0000151982.85062.80
88. Matsumura N, Horie Y, Shibata T, Kubo M, Hayashi N, Endo S. Basic training model for supermicrosurgery: a novel practice card model. *J Reconstr Microsurg* (2011) 27(6):377–82. doi: 10.1055/s-0031-1281518
89. Liu HL. Microvascular anastomosis of submillimeter vessels-a training model in rats. *J Hand Microsurg* (2013) 5(1):14–17. doi: 10.1007/s12593-013-0089-z
90. Yamashita S, Sugiyama N, Hasegawa K, Namba Y, Kimata Y. A novel model for supermicrosurgery training: the superficial inferior epigastric artery flap in rats. *J Reconstr Microsurg* (2008) 24(8):537–43. doi: 10.1055/s-0028-1088226

91. Sakrak T, Köse AA, Karabağli Y, Koçman AE, Ozbayoğlu AC, Cetịn C. Rat tail revascularization model for advanced microsurgery training and research. *J Reconstr Microsurg* (2011) 27(7):391–6. doi: 10.1055/s-0031-1281519
92. Sucher R, Lin CH, Zanoun R, Atsina KK, Weinstock M, Pulikkotil B, et al. Mouse hind limb transplantation: a new composite tissue allotransplantation model using nonsuture supermicrosurgery. *Transplantation* (2010) 90(12):1374–80. doi: 10.1097/TP.0b013e3181ff4fc3
93. Maire N, Naito K, Lequint T, Facca S, Berner S, Liverneaux P. Robot-assisted free toe pulp transfer: feasibility study. *J Reconstr Microsurg* (2012) 28(7):481–4. doi: 10.1055/s-0032-1313760
94. Kisu I, Mihara M, Banno K, Hara H, Yamamoto T, Araki J, et al. A new surgical technique of uterine auto-transplantation in cynomolgus monkey: preliminary report about two cases. *Arch Gynecol Obstet* (2012) 285(1):129–37. doi: 10.1007/s00404-011-1901-2
95. So KF, Kf S. The optic nerve transplantation and whole eyeball transplantation in the zebrafish. *Invest Ophthalmol Vis Sci* (2016) 57(4):2139. doi: 10.1167/iovs.16-19107
96. Jin S, He Y, Tian Z, Feng S, Zhang Y. Superficial circumflex iliac artery perforator flap aided by color Doppler sonography mapping for like-with-like buccal reconstruction. *Oral Surg Oral Med Oral Pathol Oral Radiol* (2015) 119(2):170–6. doi: 10.1016/j.oooo.2014.10.024
97. Ono S, Sebastin SJ, Ohi H, Chung KC. Microsurgical flaps in repair and reconstruction of the hand. *Hand Clin* (2017) 33(3):425–41. doi: 10.1016/j.hcl.2017.04.001
98. Angrigiani C, Rancati A, Artero G, Khouri RK, Walocko FM. Stacked thoracodorsal artery perforator flaps for unilateral breast reconstruction. *Plast Reconstr Surg* (2016) 138(6):969e–72. doi: 10.1097/PRS.0000000000002740
99. Stalder MW, Lam J, Allen RJ, Sadeghi A. Using the retrograde internal mammary system for stacked perforator flap breast reconstruction: 71 breast reconstructions in 53 consecutive patients. *Plast Reconstr Surg* (2016) 137(2):265e. doi: 10.1097/01.prs.0000475743.08559.b6
100. Rosson GD, Holton LH, Silverman RP, Singh NK, Nahabedian MY. Internal mammary perforators: a cadaver study. *J Reconstr Microsurg* (2005) 21(4):239–42. doi: 10.1055/s-2005-871750
101. Patel NG, Rozen WM, Chow WT, Chowdhry M, Fitzgerald O'Connor E, Sharma H, et al. Stacked and bipedicled abdominal free flaps for breast reconstruction: considerations for shaping. *Gland Surg* (2016) 5(2):115–21. doi: 10.3978/j.issn.2227-684X.2016.02.03
102. Dellacroce FJ, Sullivan SK, Trahan C. Stacked deep inferior epigastric perforator flap breast reconstruction: a review of 110 flaps in 55 cases over 3 years. *Plast Reconstr Surg* (2011) 127(3):1093–9. doi: 10.1097/PRS.0b013e318205f223
103. Hallock GG. The chimera flap: a quarter century odyssey. *Ann Plast Surg* (2017) 78(2):223–9. doi: 10.1097/SAP.0000000000000884
104. Yamamoto T, Saito T, Ishiura R, Iida T. Quadruple-component superficial circumflex iliac artery perforator (SCIP) flap: A chimeric SCIP flap for complex ankle reconstruction of an exposed artificial joint after total ankle arthroplasty. *J Plast Reconstr Aesthet Surg* (2016) 69(9):1260–5. doi: 10.1016/j.bjps.2016.06.010
105. Fernandez Garrido M, Qiu SS, Vega Garcia C, Pons Playa G, Masiá Ayala J. Chimeric Superficial Circumflex Iliac Perforator Flap Including External Oblique Fascia: A Refinement of Conventional Harvesting. *Plast Reconstr Surg Glob Open* (2016) 4(6):e766. doi: 10.1097/GOX.0000000000000757
106. Fitzgerald O'Connor EJ, Vesely M, Holt PJ, Jones KG, Thompson MM, Hinchliffe RJ. A systematic review of free tissue transfer in the management of non-traumatic lower extremity wounds in patients with diabetes. *Eur J Vasc Endovasc Surg* (2011) 41(3):391–9. doi: 10.1016/j.ejvs.2010.11.013

21

# Current Strategies and Future Directions to Optimize ACL Reconstruction in Adolescent Patients

*Dustin Jon Richter*[1], *Roger Lyon*[1,2], *Scott Van Valin*[1,2] *and Xue-Cheng Liu*[1,2]*

*[1] Department of Orthopaedic Surgery, Medical College of Wisconsin, Milwaukee, WI, United States,* *[2] Department of Orthopaedic Surgery, Children's Hospital of Wisconsin, Milwaukee, WI, United States*

The incidence of anterior cruciate ligament (ACL) injuries in the pediatric population has risen in recent years. These injuries have historically presented a management dilemma in skeletally immature patients with open physes and significant growth remaining at time of injury. While those nearing skeletal maturity may be treated with traditional, transphyseal adult techniques, these same procedures risk iatrogenic damage to the growth plates and resultant growth disturbances in younger patients with open physes. Moreover, conservative management is non-optimal as significant instabilities of the knee remain. Despite the development of physeal-sparing reconstructive techniques for younger patients, there remains debate over which procedure may be most suitable on a patient to patient basis. Meanwhile, the drivers behind clinical and functional outcomes following ACL reconstruction remain poorly understood. Therefore, current strategies are not yet capable of optimizing surgical ACL reconstruction on an individualized basis with absolute confidence. Instead, aims to improve surgical treatment of ACL tears in skeletally immature patients will rely on additional approaches in the near future. Namely, finite element models have emerged as a tool to model complex knee joint biomechanics. The inclusion of several individualized variables such as bone age, three dimensional geometries around the knee joint, tunnel positioning, and graft tension collectively present a possible means of better understanding and even predicting how to enhance surgical decision-making. Such a tool would serve surgeons in optimizing ACL reconstruction in the skeletally immature individuals, in order to improve clinical outcomes as well as reduce the rate of post-operative complications.

**Keywords: anterior cruciate ligament, injury, reconstruction, adolescents, modeling**

***Edited by:***
*Klane K. White, University of Washington, United States*

***Reviewed by:***
*Dominick Tuason, Pediatric Orthopaedic Associates of New Jersey, United States*
*Thorsten Rudroff, Colorado State University, United States*
*James Wylie, University of Utah, United States*

***Correspondence:**
*Xue-Cheng Liu*
*xliu@chw.org*

***Specialty section:***
*This article was submitted to Pediatric Orthopedics, a section of the journal Frontiers in Surgery*

## INTRODUCTION

Historically, anterior cruciate ligament (ACL) injuries were thought to be rare in the pediatric population. Instead, tibial eminence avulsion fractures were thought to be more common, as a result of the characteristically non-ossified bone found in adolescents (1). Recent studies however, indicate the incidence of ACL tears in the pediatric population has increased over the last 20 years, with the highest

**List of abbreviations:** ACL, anterior cruciate ligament; AM, Anteromedial; PL, Posterolateral.

incidence occurring during high school years (2). Increased rates of ACL injuries are linked to both improved diagnostic techniques, as well as increased awareness within the medical community (3).

In the past, skeletally immature patients with ACL tears faced a management dilemma (4). In particular, the physes of the knee are of greatest anatomic concern due to the theoretical risk of physeal damage and growth disturbance. The distal femoral and proximal tibial physes contribute to 37 and 25% of overall limb length, respectively (5). As a result, pubertal status is of the utmost concern when evaluating surgical candidates' risk of physeal disruption. In particular, sex differences between the age of typical skeletal maturity must be considered. In general, it is well-recognized females reach complete puberty including growth spurt and closure of the physes before their male counterparts. Skeletal maturity is reached at approximately age 14 years in girls, and age 16 in boys. Importantly, however, the amount of growth around the knee that remains after 12–13 years in girls and 14 years in boys is negligible (6). Therefore, until these ages are reached, surgeons must be aware of the growing physes when considering conservative versus operative management, and ultimately which ACL reconstruction strategy to utilize. Meanwhile, it must be kept in mind that each individual does not adhere to these guidelines, which means each case must be carefully analyzed in the setting of the particular patient and their growth status.

As previously mentioned, operative management restores stability of the knee but risks iatrogenic damage to the physis, which may ultimately lead to leg-length discrepancies and angular deformities of the lower extremity (7). Conversely, conservative management consisting of activity modification, rehabilitation exercises, and bracing avoids disruption of the physis, but has been associated with residual instability of the knee (8). These prolonged instabilities have been shown to lead to further complications and injuries, primarily meniscal tears and chondral degeneration (4). Therefore, the current consensus treatment for ACL tears in pediatric patients involves early surgical intervention restoring stability of the knee, which has now been associated with superior outcomes in comparison to conservative management (9).

However, ideal surgical techniques remain controversial due to insufficient data correlating these various techniques to clinical outcomes while taking into account the timing of surgery and rehabilitation regimes (8). The two primary surgical procedures in contention include transphyseal and physeal-sparing techniques. Anatomic, transphyseal reconstruction involves drilling tunnels though both the tibial and femoral physes, and is generally regarded with caution due to the risk of physeal disruption and growth disturbance. Physeal-sparing techniques, however, avoid drilling directly through the physis with modified all-epiphseal tunnels.

The tunnels used in transphyseal reconstructions account for little of the total cross sectional area of the physis. In addition, it has not been proven equivocally that drilling through the physis results in detectable valgus/varus deformities or growth disruption (2). Additionally, the question of which surgical procedure is optimal for each patient is complicated by variables such as the amount of remaining growth at time of surgery, and individual variations in geometry of the knee. Given advancements in finite element modeling capable of simulating biomechanical behavior of the knee joint (10), more sophisticated methods to optimize ACL reconstructions in skeletally immature patients on an individualized basis certainly seems an attainable goal in the relatively near future.

## Summary of Current Surgical Procedures

A summary of the following current surgical procedures is provided in **Table 1**. Previous studies have shown the ACL is composed of two main bundles consisting of the anteromedial (AM) and posterolateral (PL) constituents (15, 16). It has been determined the AM bundle assumes most of the strain in higher flexion angles, while the PL bundle takes up more strain in lower flexion angles (17). Together, the two bundles comprise the ACL, which prevents anterior tibial translation in addition to rotational stresses. Single bundle transtibial ACL reconstructions are often considered a traditional technique for restoring stability lost due to ACL rupture. While biomechanical studies have shown this technique can restore anterior-posterior stability, rotational kinematics are often not completely restored (18). Double bundle transtibial ACL reconstructions have been utilized to better restore stability and more normal knee kinematics (19). While this initially appears far more advantageous than the single bundle reconstructions, double bundle techniques are more technical procedures requiring longer operative times and more substantial bone loss. Overall, while some studies find double bundle reconstructions to provide better results, many other studies have failed to find significant differences in clinical outcomes (20). More recently, independent tunnel drilling for the femoral tunnel has been developed and accepted as a technique to more accurately replicate the anatomic femoral origin of the ACL (21).

As previously described, physeal-sparing techniques avoid disruption of the physes to decrease risk of growth abnormalities. In turn, this decreases the risk of leg length discrepancies and angular deformities. These procedures, however, are not without their disadvantages. Lawrence et al. describes an all-epiphyseal technique with a lateral femoral and oblique tibial tunnel, creating an acute angle the graft must traverse. Ultimately, this may lead to wear and unnecessary stress on the graft, increasing risk of re-rupture (12). To avoid this problem, an extraphyseal technique described by Janarv et al. places the graft in an "over-the-top" femoral position (13). While this technique avoids the graft being subjected to an acute angle, it is inherently non-anatomic and may not fully restore normal knee kinematics and stability.

Finally, partial physeal-sparing techniques (14) have been developed with the hopes of maintaining aspects of an anatomical reconstruction while minimizing risk of growth disturbance. In these procedures, a transphyseal tibial tunnel is drilled, but the femoral tunnel remains all-epiphyseal. As the femoral physis accounts for a larger proportion of limb growth, the avoidance of disrupting this physis is thought to minimize significant growth disturbances.

An additional procedure, which has just recently been developed, includes a hybrid physeal-sparing technique for ACL reconstruction. This technique provides an anatomic reconstruction that minimizes the risk of physeal damage but is also reproducible and less technical than the aforementioned physeal-sparing techniques. Willson et al. posits this technique provides high success rates with low morbidity in adolescents nearing skeletal maturity (22).

**TABLE 1** | Summary of Surgical Procedures.

| Surgical Procedure | Description | Advantages | Disadvantages |
|---|---|---|---|
| Anatomic Transtibial Single Bundle Reconstruction (11) | A femoral and tibial tunnel are drilled across the femoral and tibial physes, respectively, with a single-bundle graft which mostly reproduces the anteromedial (AM) bundle of the ACL. | Simple reconstruction which several studies have shown restore nearly normal knee kinematics. | Growth disturbances and angular deformities. Post-surgical stability and rotational laxity have been shown to be inferior to double bundle reconstructions. |
| Anatomic Transtibial Double Bundle Reconstruction (11) | Reconstructs AM and posterolateral (PL) bundles of anatomic ACL tendon separately. | The bundles are tensioned separately, resulting in even more natural tension patterns and restoring both anterior-posterior and rotational laxity. | Growth disturbances and angular deformities. Possible changes in knee joint kinematics may contribute to development of osteoarthritis (OA). Rupture of contralateral intact knee. |
| All epiphyseal technique of Lawrence et al. (12) | A lateral epiphyseal femoral tunnel and oblique epiphyseal tibial tunnel are drilled, avoiding the physes. The graft is secured in the tunnels via bioabsorbable screws. | Avoids disruption of open physes, decreasing chance of growth disturbances, leg length discrepancies and angular deformities. | The acute angle created by the tunnels may increase strain on the graft and increase risk of re-rupture. Growth disturbance by unidentified mechanism. |
| All epiphyseal technique of Janarv et al. (13) | A tibial epiphyseal tunnel is drilled, and the graft is placed posteriorly and over the femoral condyle in an "over-top" position on the femur and secured to the femoral metaphysis. | Avoids disruption of open physes, decreasing chance of growth disturbances, leg length discrepancies and angular deformities. | This non-anatomic reconstruction may not restore natural knee kinematics as well as anatomic reconstructions. Growth disturbance by unidentified mechanism. |
| Partial Physeal-Sparing Technique (14) | A transphyseal tibial tunnel disrupts the tibial physis, but the graft is fixed to the metaphysis of the lateral femur sparing the femoral physis. | Reduced risk of growth disruption, as femoral physis accounts for larger proportion of growth of lower limb. | Growth disturbance by disruption of tibial physis or unidentified mechanism. |

In sum, the variety of surgical procedures each provide a set of advantages and disadvantages which must be considered in pediatric patients with ACL ruptures. When choosing which procedure is optimal for a particular patient, factors including skeletal age and 3D geometry of the knee both affect surgical outcome. In regard to skeletal age, a current consensus has been well-described in the literature (23). In pre-pubescent patients with open physes and a great deal of anticipated growth remaining, physeal-sparing techniques are considered the most appropriate approach. To contrast, in adolescents with closed or closing physes, adult transphyseal techniques are regarded most highly due to the relatively low risk of iatrogenic damage and growth disturbances. However, many patients fall somewhere in the middle of this spectrum, and uncertainties often arise in skeletally-immature patients.

## Summary of Current Post Surgical Complications

As depicted in **Table 2**, a wide range of complications arises from both traditional transphyseal and physeal-sparing reconstructions. The main concern when performing ACL reconstructions has historically been disruption of the physes, leading to growth arrest. Ultimately, this disruption of growth leads to either leg length discrepancies or angular deformities of the leg (7). More

**TABLE 2** | Summary of Post-Surgical Complications.

| Author/s | Surgical Procedure | Number of Subjects | Mean Age (Years) | Mean Follow-Up (Months) | Complications | Current Solution |
|---|---|---|---|---|---|---|
| Kumar et al. (24) | Transphyseal reconstruction | 32 | 11.3 | 72.3 | 1 re-rupture | Repair rupture with additional ACL reconstruction |
| | | | | | 1 valgus deformity | Surgical intervention to absolve angular deformity |
| Kocher et al. (25) | Transphyseal reconstruction | 59 | 14.7 | 43 | 2 re-ruptures | Repair rupture with additional ACL reconstruction |
| Edwards and Grana (26) | Transphyseal reconstruction | 20 | 13.7 | 34 | 2 re-ruptures<br>1 persistent laxity | Repair rupture or lax graft with additional ACL reconstruction |
| Chotel et al. (27) | Physeal-Sparing | 2 | 8.5 | 24 | 2 limb overgrowths | Percutaneous epiphysiodesis |
| Shifflet et al. (28) | Physeal-Sparing | 4 | 12.1 | 54 | 4 cases of growth arrest | Surgical intervention to correct limb length discrepancy |
| Kocher et al. (29) | Physeal-Sparing | 44 | 10.3 | 44 | 2 re-ruptures | Repair rupture with additional ACL reconstruction |
| | | | | | 4 repeat meniscal tears | Meniscal repair |

recently, studies have suggested limb overgrowth leading to growth discrepancies may be underreported, and also pose a major clinical problem following ACL reconstruction in adolescents (30). Additional complications include re-rupture of the ACL graft, or even contralateral ACL tear. In fact, recent evidence suggests contralateral ACL tear may be more common than ACL graft rupture in patients following ACL reconstruction (31).

In response to these complications, further surgical intervention or other procedures such as percutaneous epiphysiodesis are often required. Additional procedures not only result in additional financial burden for patients and their families, but also require additional recovery time and further delay until return to normal activities. Moreover, few if any prevention or predictive measures are currently in place to minimize the risk of these adverse outcomes. In addition, patients experience a wide range of functional outcomes affecting their daily lives and ability to reengage in sports or similar activities. These outcomes are assessed via common knee scores such as the International Knee Documentation (IKDC) subjective evaluation and Lysholm knee scores (32). Ideally, surgeons would strive for preventative strategies to minimize the risk of post-operative complications and to maximize clinical knee scores representing functional outcomes. However, the many mechanisms contributing to complications have either not been elucidated or are not clearly understood.

For example, in a systematic review by Collins et al., (33) physeal-sparing techniques counter-intuitively accounted for 25% of angular deformities and 47% of limb length discrepancy cases. This is unexpected, as it has long been thought sparing the physis decreases the risk of growth abnormalities. Furthermore, Collins et al. discovered limb overgrowth accounted for 62% of cases involving limb length discrepancy. Historically, growth arrest due to disruption of the physis has been the main concern after ACL reconstruction. Therefore, it suggests growth abnormalities are most likely under reported in the current literature, in addition to a gross lack of understanding underlying the precise causes and mechanisms leading to growth abnormalities following ACL reconstruction.

Meanwhile, it has been shown the 3D geometry of the distal femoral condyles has significant effects on knee joint kinematics (34). Therefore, it is likely individual differences in condylar shape and contour affect post-operative outcomes, in addition to the aforementioned skeletal age. As will next be discussed, current surgical procedures fail to address individual differences in condylar geometry during the procedure. Ultimately, this may lead to differences in tunnel orientations, angles, and positions between patients, which further contribute to post-operative complications and outcomes.

## CURRENT STANDARD OF CARE DOES NOT ADDRESS INDIVIDUAL 3D GEOMETRY OF THE KNEE

Pena et al. have previously shown the angle of the femoral tunnel primarily affects tension of the graft, while the tibial tunnel significantly affects laxity and meniscal stresses (35). For example, tibial drill-guide angles between 55 and 65 degrees have been proposed as optimal angles for proper stress redistribution (36). Moreover, the graft tension is vitally important as enough tension is required to maintain stability, while a mechanism has been proposed where too much tension leads to physeal compression and ultimately damage (33). Furthermore, changes in tunnel positioning may take place in skeletally immature patients as growth around the knee potentially impacts reconstruction, which likely has direct impacts on *in vivo* graft tension as well. Of significance, a previous study has utilized multidector-row CT to demonstrate bone tunnel changes over time. Specifically, changes in angular geometry and actual movement of the articular outlets of tibial and femoral tunnels were measured at 1 year postoperatively compared to 3 weeks following the procedure (37). Therefore, it can be assumed tunnel position, angles, and draft tension cumulatively affect knee kinematics and functional outcomes.

Currently, a standard 7-mm-offset femoral tunnel guide is used to set the femoral guide pin in most conventional transphyseal ACL reconstructions. However, several studies such as Chung et al. (38) have suggested using a 10-mm-offset tunnel guide better enables the placement of a more anatomically positioned femoral tunnel which leads to greater stability, fewer complications, and better overall functional outcomes. This suggests very small differences in the positioning or placement of the guide pin have the potential to have tangible effects on clinical outcomes following ACL reconstructions. Meanwhile, it remains to be investigated how variation in individual distal femoral condyle 3D geometry and contour may affect positioning of the tunnel guide and guide pin. Based on Chung et al. suggesting even slight variation in the offset guide has important effects on tunnel positioning mimicking anatomical ACL placement, it is logical that small variations in distal femoral condyle geometry may affect tunnel angle and positioning as well. Although this remains to be investigated throughout the literature, anatomical variation in 3D geometry at the distal condyle likely effects tunnel placement, and in turn, has implications for vitally important clinical outcomes.

### Current Standard of Care Does Not Address Biomechanics of ACL Grafts

As previously illustrated, graft tension has important consequences on stability, functional outcomes, and complications such as graft rupture. However, the ideal graft tension which is determined during reconstruction remains a topic of contention within the surgical community. Most surgeons apply a "sufficient magnitude" of tension between 40 to 90 n to the graft at full extension (39). Kondo et al. illustrated how different tensioning strategies influenced functional outcomes such as knee flexion at 2 years of follow-up (40). Therefore, the great deal of variation in current graft tensioning protocols lends itself as a possible candidate to explain poorly understood differences in clinical outcomes. Additional factors compound the complexity of graft tension. For example, different graft types including patellar ligaments and hamstring tendons have been shown to exhibit different biomechanical properties such as strength and elasticity in long term follow-up studies (41).

Due to the ability of graft tension to affect functional outcomes, the need to better understand the many variables affecting tension after ACL reconstruction becomes imperative. Due to the fact that femoral condylar contour affects knee kinematics, it is plausible to conceive the 3D geometry has effects on long term graft tension. If these effects could be predicted through a computational model, graft tensioning protocols could be optimized to set initial graft tension more precisely to reduce post-surgical complications. Importantly, recent studies have validated the finite element modeling of such phenomena. Specifically, Pena et al. have demonstrated the plausibility of such modeling by using finite element analysis to study the effect of graft stiffness and graft tensioning on ACL reconstruction (42).

### Finite Element Models Capable of Simulating Biomechanical Behavior of Knee Joint

For decades, the biomechanics of the knee joint have been simulated by numerical means. Nonetheless, the intricate ability of the knee joint to provide both stability under high loads and simultaneous mobility continues to provide a challenging task to accurately model. Recently, modern non-linear, finite element models based on MRI have been shown to represent the knee with a "high degree of anatomical realism" (10). These models have since been developed to predict progressive aspects such degenerative pathology or surgical reconstruction. Most importantly, several studies have proven the ability of finite element analysis to model surgical repair and replacement strategies in relation to the knee (43–45). A review by Galbusera et al. highlights the progression and current utility of these models (10). Thus the simulation of the knee following surgical reconstruction is now achievable through the widespread validation of non-linear finite element packages and modern software with powerful capabilities to simulate the complex biomechanics of knee ligaments.

As previously illustrated, several factors pose the potential to be incorporated into finite element models to aid in the optimization of ACL reconstruction. For example, tunnel placement is of the foremost importance, but if and how it is affected by individual three-dimensional geometry of the knee would be a powerful modeling capability. Furthermore, skeletally immature patients pose the problem of growth around the knee taking place following reconstruction, which may resultantly alter tunnel positioning. Therefore, if bone age was to be incorporated into finite element models, the possibility of predicting tunnel position shifts could perhaps be anticipated to allow for optimal final tunnel location upon completion of growth around the knee. Finally, the many variables associated with graft tension such as tunnel angles, length, graft type, and tension set during the procedure, all have the potential to serve as valuable variables to better predict functional and clinical outcomes.

## CLINICAL SIGNIFICANCE

The clinical significance of a predictive computational model capable of optimizing surgical outcomes are robust and far-reaching. Such an algorithm would not only allow surgeons to plan individualized procedures with unprecedented insight and ability, but would significantly increase functional outcomes while minimizing the risk of complications. With a greater understanding and ability to predict the effects of individual 3D geometry of the knee joint on tunnel positioning and graft tension, surgical techniques could be adjusted for individuals using pre-operative MRI data. Such a powerful tool may additionally be able to shorten surgical times based on pre-operative planning, reduce recovery time, and shorten rehabilitation regimens as patients experienced optimized reconstructions allowing for fast and complication-free recoveries.

The usefulness and validity of 3D-imaging of the knee was first established years ago by utilizing CT evaluation of tunnel placement (46). More recently, several studies have begun to highlight the utility of finite element modeling. For example, finite element analysis has been utilized to investigate the effects of tunnel orientation and stress distribution in ACL grafts (47), as well as to investigate the optimization of graft placement in ACL reconstruction (48). These studies provide early evidence of finite-element analysis aiding in the optimization of ACL reconstruction. The main limitation to these models is obviously the potential cost, which would potentially pose a barrier to widespread use on an individualized basis. Nonetheless, the development of select, cornerstone models in well-designed studies may be enough to glean useful information that can be applied to individual cases.

## CONCLUSIONS

Within the pediatric population, ACL injuries are becoming increasingly common. Current consensus suggests early reconstruction restores joint stability and is associated with superior long-term outcomes in comparison to solely conservative management. While physeal-sparing techniques have been developed for younger patients with significant growth remaining, these procedures have not eliminated the risks of post-operative complications and still pose distinct disadvantages. Therefore, in an effort to optimize ACL reconstruction in skeletally immature patients, the development and incorporation of finite element models poses a possible future direction. These models may potentially guide surgeons in choosing surgical techniques by including several individualized variables to allow optimal tunnel positioning, graft tension, and resulting biomechanics of the knee. Through these methods, the goal to continually strive to improve outcomes and reduce complications may be achieved.

## AUTHOR CONTRIBUTION

All authors have met the criteria for authorship. They have made substantial contribution, have read and approved of the final submitted work, as well as agree to be accountable for all aspects of the work ensuring questions related to accuracy or integrity are appropriately investigated and resolved.

## REFERENCES


1. Kocher MS, Garg S, Micheli LJ, Beck NA, Lawrence JTR, Nordin JD. Physeal sparing reconstruction of the anterior cruciate ligament in skeletally immature prepubescent children and adolescents. *J Bone Joint Surg Am* (2005) 87(11):2371–9. doi: 10.2106/JBJS.D.02802
2. Beck NA, Lawrence JTR, Nordin JD, Defor TA, Tompkins M. ACL tears in school-aged children and Adolescents over 20 years. *Pediatrics* (2017) 139(3):e20161877. doi: 10.1542/peds.2016-1877
3. Adirim TA, Cheng TL. Overview of injuries in the young athlete. *Sports Med* (2003) 33(1):75–81. doi: 10.2165/00007256-200333010-00006
4. Mohtadi N, Grant J. Managing anterior cruciate ligament deficiency in the skeletally immature individual: a systematic review of the literature. *Clin J Sport Med* (2006) 16(6):457–64. doi: 10.1097/01.jsm.0000248844.39498.1f
5. Fabricant PD, Kocher MS. Anterior cruciate ligament injuries in children and adolescents. *Orthop Clin North Am* (2016) 47(4):777–88. doi: 10.1016/j.ocl.2016.05.004
6. Kelly PM, Diméglio A. Lower-limb growth: how predictable are predictions? *J Child Orthop* (2008) 2(6):407–15. doi: 10.1007/s11832-008-0119-8
7. Kaeding CC, Flanigan D, Donaldson C. Surgical techniques and outcomes after anterior cruciate ligament reconstruction in preadolescent patients. *Arthroscopy* (2010) 26(11):1530–8. doi: 10.1016/j.arthro.2010.04.065
8. Al-Hadithy N, Dodds AL, Akhtar KS, Gupte CM. Current concepts of the management of anterior cruciate ligament injuries in children. *Bone Joint J* (2013) 95-B(11):1562–9. doi: 10.1302/0301-620X.95B11.31778
9. Davis DL, Chen L, Ehinger M. A study of epiphyses in the young prepubescent knee using magnetic resonance imaging: evaluation of parameters for anterior cruciate ligament reconstruction. *Orthop J Sports Med* (2014) 2(4):2325967114530090. doi: 10.1177/2325967114530090
10. Galbusera F, Freutel M, Dürselen L, D'Aiuto M, Croce D, Villa T, et al. Material models and properties in the finite element analysis of knee ligaments: a literature review. *Front Bioeng Biotechnol* (2014) 2:54. doi: 10.3389/fbioe.2014.00054
11. van Eck CF, Lesniak BP, Schreiber VM, Fu FH. Anatomic single- and double-bundle anterior cruciate ligament reconstruction flowchart. *Arthroscopy* (2010) 26(2):258–68. doi: 10.1016/j.arthro.2009.07.027
12. Lawrence JT, Bowers AL, Belding J, Cody SR, Ganley TJ. All-epiphyseal anterior cruciate ligament reconstruction in skeletally immature patients. *Clin Orthop Relat Res* (2010) 468(7):1971–7. doi: 10.1007/s11999-010-1255-2
13. Janarv PM, Nyström A, Werner S, Hirsch G. Anterior cruciate ligament injuries in skeletally immature patients. *J Pediatr Orthop* (1996) 16(5):673–7.
14. Lipscomb AB, Anderson AF. Tears of the anterior cruciate ligament in adolescents. *J Bone Joint Surg Am* (1986) 68(1):19–28. doi: 10.2106/00004623-198668010-00004
15. Girgis FG, Marshall JL, Monajem A. The cruciate ligaments of the knee joint. Anatomical, functional and experimental analysis. *Clin Orthop Relat Res* (1975) 106(106):216–31.
16. Yasuda K, van Eck CF, Hoshino Y, Fu FH, Tashman S. Anatomic single- and double-bundle anterior cruciate ligament reconstruction, part 1: Basic science. *Am J Sports Med* (2011) 39(8):1789–800. doi: 10.1177/0363546511402659
17. Sakane M, Fox RJ, Woo SL, Livesay GA, Li G, Fu FH. In situ forces in the anterior cruciate ligament and its bundles in response to anterior tibial loads. *J Orthop Res* (1997) 15(2):285–93. doi: 10.1002/jor.1100150219
18. Fu FH, Jordan SS. The lateral intercondylar ridge--a key to anatomic anterior cruciate ligament reconstruction. *J Bone Joint Surg Am* (2007) 89(10):2103–4. doi: 10.2106/JBJS.G.00851
19. Abebe ES, Moorman CT, Dziedzic TS, Spritzer CE, Cothran RL, Taylor DC, et al. Femoral tunnel placement during anterior cruciate ligament reconstruction: an in vivo imaging analysis comparing transtibial and 2-incision tibial tunnel-independent techniques. *Am J Sports Med* (2009) 37(10):1904–11. doi: 10.1177/0363546509340768
20. Xu M, Gao S, Zeng C, Han R, Sun J, Li H, et al. Outcomes of anterior cruciate ligament reconstruction using single-bundle versus double-bundle technique: meta-analysis of 19 randomized controlled trials. *Arthroscopy* (2013) 29(2):357–65. doi: 10.1016/j.arthro.2012.08.024
21. Giron F, Cuomo P, Edwards A, Bull AM, Amis AA, Aglietti P. Double-bundle "anatomic" anterior cruciate ligament reconstruction: a cadaveric study of tunnel positioning with a transtibial technique. *Arthroscopy* (2007) 23(1):7–13. doi: 10.1016/j.arthro.2006.08.008
22. Willson RG, Kostyun RO, Milewski MD, Nissen CW. Anterior cruciate ligament reconstruction in skeletally immature patients: early results using a hybrid physeal-sparing technique. *Orthop J Sports Med* (2018) 6(2):2325967118755330):2325967118755533. doi: 10.1177/2325967118755330
23. Lang PJ, Sugimoto D, Micheli LJ. Prevention, treatment, and rehabilitation of anterior cruciate ligament injuries in children. *Open Access J Sports Med* (2017) 8:133–41. doi: 10.2147/OAJSM.S133940
24. Kumar S, Ahearne D, Hunt DM. Transphyseal anterior cruciate ligament reconstruction in the skeletally immature: follow-up to a minimum of sixteen years of age. *J Bone Joint Surg Am* (2013) 95(1):e1. doi: 10.2106/JBJS.K.01707
25. Kocher MS, Smith JT, Zoric BJ, Lee B, Micheli LJ. Transphyseal anterior cruciate ligament reconstruction in skeletally immature pubescent adolescents. *J Bone Joint Surg Am* (2007) 89(12):2632–9. doi: 10.2106/JBJS.F.01560
26. Edwards PH, Grana WA. Anterior cruciate ligament reconstruction in the immature athlete: long-term results of intra-articular reconstruction. *Am J Knee Surg* (2001) 14(4):232–7.
27. Chotel F, Henry J, Seil R, Chouteau J, Moyen B, Bérard J. Growth disturbances without growth arrest after ACL reconstruction in children. *Knee Surg Sports Traumatol Arthrosc* (2010) 18(11):1496–500. doi: 10.1007/s00167-010-1069-5
28. Shifflett GD, Green DW, Widmann RF, Marx RG. Growth Arrest Following ACL Reconstruction With Hamstring Autograft in Skeletally Immature Patients: A Review of 4 Cases. *J Pediatr Orthop* (2016) 36(4):355–61. doi: 10.1097/BPO.0000000000000466
29. Kocher MS, Garg S, Micheli LJ. Physeal sparing reconstruction of the anterior cruciate ligament in skeletally immature prepubescent children and adolescents. Surgical technique. *J Bone Joint Surg Am* (2006) 88(Suppl 1 Pt 2):283–93. doi: 10.2106/00004623-200609001-00012
30. Koch PP, Fucentese SF, Blatter SC. Complications after epiphyseal reconstruction of the anterior cruciate ligament in prepubescent children. *Knee Surg Sports Traumatol Arthrosc* (2016) 24(9):2736–40. doi: 10.1007/s00167-014-3396-4
31. Magnussen RA, Meschbach NT, Kaeding CC, Wright RW, Spindler KP. ACL Graft and Contralateral ACL Tear Risk within Ten Years Following Reconstruction: A Systematic Review. *JBJS Rev* (2015) 3(1):1. doi: 10.2106/JBJS.RVW.N.00052
32. Collins NJ, Misra D, Felson DT, Crossley KM, Roos EM. Measures of knee function: International Knee Documentation Committee (IKDC) Subjective Knee Evaluation Form, Knee Injury and Osteoarthritis Outcome Score (KOOS), Knee Injury and Osteoarthritis Outcome Score Physical Function Short Form (KOOS-PS), Knee Outcome Survey Activities of Daily Living Scale (KOS-ADL), Lysholm Knee Scoring Scale, Oxford Knee Score (OKS), Western Ontario and McMaster Universities Osteoarthritis Index (WOMAC), Activity Rating Scale (ARS), and Tegner Activity Score (TAS). *Arthritis Care Res (Hoboken).* (2011) 63(Suppl 11):S208–28. doi: 10.1002/acr.20632
33. Collins MJ, Arns TA, Leroux T, Black A, Mascarenhas R, Bach BR, et al. Growth Abnormalities Following Anterior Cruciate Ligament Reconstruction in the Skeletally Immature Patient: A Systematic Review. *Arthroscopy* (2016) 32(8):1714–23. doi: 10.1016/j.arthro.2016.02.025
34. Siebold R, Axe J, Irrgang JJ, Li K, Li K, Tashman S, , et al. A computerized analysis of femoral condyle radii in ACL intact and contralateral ACL reconstructed knees using 3D CT. *Knee Surg Sports Traumatol Arthrosc* (2010) 18(1):26–31. doi: 10.1007/s00167-009-0969-8
35. Peña E, Calvo B, Martinez MA, Palanca D, Doblaré M. Influence of the tunnel angle in ACL reconstructions on the biomechanics of the knee joint. *Clin Biomech* (2006) 21(5):508–16. doi: 10.1016/j.clinbiomech.2005.12.013
36. Yao J, Wen CY, Zhang M, Cheung JT, Yan C, Chiu KY, et al. Effect of tibial drill-guide angle on the mechanical environment at bone tunnel aperture after anatomic single-bundle anterior cruciate ligament reconstruction. *Int Orthop* (2014) 38(5):973–81. doi: 10.1007/s00264-014-2290-5
37. Araki D, Kuroda R, Matsumoto T, Nagamune K, Matsushita T, Hoshino Y, et al. Three-dimensional analysis of bone tunnel changes after anatomic double-bundle anterior cruciate ligament reconstruction using multidetector-row computed tomography. *Am J Sports Med* (2014) 42(9):2234–41. doi: 10.1177/0363546514540274
38. Chung JY, Ha CW, Lee DH, Park YG, Park YB, Awe SI. Anatomic placement of the femoral tunnel by a modified transtibial technique using a large-offset

femoral tunnel guide: A cadaveric study. *Knee* (2016) 23(4):659–65. doi: 10.1016/j.knee.2015.10.001

39. Cunningham R, West JR, Greis PE, Burks RT. A survey of the tension applied to a doubled hamstring tendon graft for reconstruction of the anterior cruciate ligament. *Arthroscopy* (2002) 18(9):983–8. doi: 10.1053/jars.2002.36102
40. Kondo E, Yasuda K, Kitamura N, Onodera J, Yokota M, Yagi T, et al. Effects of initial graft tension on clinical outcome after anatomic double-bundle anterior cruciate ligament reconstruction: comparison of two graft tension protocols. *BMC Musculoskelet Disord* (2016) 17:65. doi: 10.1186/s12891-016-0909-y
41. Biuk E, Zelic Z, Rapan S, Curic G, Biuk D, Radic R. Analysis of biomechanical properties of patellar ligament graft and quadruple hamstring tendon graft. *Injury* (2015) 46(Suppl 6):S14–17. doi.
42. Pena E, Martinez MA, Calvo B, Palanca D, Doblare M. A finite element simulation of the effect of graft stiffness and graft tensioning in ACL reconstruction. *Clin Biomech* (2005) 20(6):636–44.
43. Yoon KH, Kim YH, Ha JH, Kim K, Park WM. Biomechanical evaluation of double bundle augmentation of posterior cruciate ligament using finite element analysis. *Clin. Biomech.* (2010) 25:1042–6.
44. Fitzpatrick CK, Komistek RD, Rullkoetter PJ. Developing simulations to reproduce in vivo fluoroscopy kinematics in total knee replacement patients. *J Biomech* (2014) 47(10):2398–405. doi: 10.1016/j.jbiomech.2014.04.024
45. Innocenti B, Bilgen ÖF, Labey L, van Lenthe GH, Sloten JV, Catani F. Load sharing and ligament strains in balanced, overstuffed and understuffed UKA. A validated finite element analysis. *J Arthroplasty* (2014) 29(7):1491–8. doi: 10.1016/j.arth.2014.01.020
46. Forsythe B, Kopf S, Wong AK, et al. The location of femoral and tibial tunnels in anatomic double-bundle anterior cruciate ligament reconstruction analyzed by three-dimensional computed tomography models. *J Bone Joint Surg Am* (2010) 92(6):1418–26.
47. van der Bracht H, Tampere T, Beekman P, et al. Peak stresses shift from femoral tunnel aperture to tibial tunnel aperture in lateral tibial tunnel ACL reconstructions: a 3D graft-bending angle measurement and finite-element analysis. *Knee Surg Sports Traumatol Arthrosc* (2018) 26(2):508–17.
48. Westermann RW, Wolf BR, Elkins J. Optimizing graft placement in anterior cruciate ligament reconstruction: A finite element analysis. *J Knee Surg* (2017) 30(2):97–106.

# Arthroscopic Viewing Position Affects Anterior Cruciate Ligament Reconstruction Femoral Tunnel Length Measurements

*Sheeba M. Joseph [1], Michael R. Karns [1,2], Derrick M. Knapik [1,2]* and James E. Voos [1,2]*

[1] Department of Orthopaedic Surgery, University Hospitals Cleveland Medical Center, Cleveland, OH, United States, [2] Sports Medicine Institute, University Hospitals Cleveland Medical Center, Cleveland, OH, United States

**Purpose:** To purpose of this study was to compare arthroscopic anterior cruciate ligament (ACL) reconstruction femoral tunnel length measurements from the anterolateral portal between the standard notch view using a 30° arthroscope versus a "top-down" view utilizing a 70° arthroscope to visual the far side of the femoral tunnel aperture.

**Methods:** Arthroscopic femoral tunnel length measurements using calibrated reamers from the standard notch versus the "top-down" view were obtained and reviewed in 54 skeletally mature patients undergoing ACL reconstruction with no prior bony knee surgery. Patient age, height, weight, sex, and surgery laterality were also recorded. Measurements of femoral tunnel length were repeated using both views for inter-observer and intra-observer correlation.

**Results:** Inter-observer and intra-observer intra-class correlation coefficients for the standard notch view and "top-down" views were excellent, with higher reliability values appreciated using the "top down" view. Mean overall femoral tunnel length measurements obtained using the standard notch view were significantly longer than measurements from the "top-down" view ($p < 0.001$).

**Conclusions:** The standard notch view provides significantly longer femoral tunnel length measurements in comparison to the "top-down" view.

**Edited by:**
*Vassilios S. Nikolaou, University General Hospital Attikon, Greece*

**Reviewed by:**
*Michael-Alexander Malachias, National and Kapodistrian University of Athens, Greece*
*Leonidas Roumeliotis, National and Kapodistrian University of Athens, Greece*

***Correspondence:**
*Derrick M. Knapik*
*derrick.knapik@gmail.com*

**Specialty section:**
*This article was submitted to Orthopedic Surgery, a section of the journal Frontiers in Surgery*

**Keywords: ACL reconstruction, arthroscopy, femoral tunnel length, seventy-degree arthroscopy, graft-tunnel mismatch**

## INTRODUCTION

As of 2015, over 200,000 anterior cruciate ligament (ACL) reconstructions are performed each year in the United States.(1–3) To improve patient outcomes and return to play rates, advances in surgical techniques have sought to achieve more anatomic reconstructions.(4) As such, multiple techniques have been developed to enhance the surgeon's ability to create the femoral tunnel at the anatomic origin of the ACL including drilling from an accessory medial portal with the knee in a hyper-flexed (~120°) position.(5, 6) However, drilling the femoral tunnel at such a low, posterior position in the hyper-flexed knee using rigid reamers increases the risks for short tunnels, posterior cortical blowout, and common peroneal nerve injury if the guide pins exits inferior to the biceps femoris.(7–10) Several commercially available flexible reamer systems have been developed permitting drilling of an anatomically placed femoral tunnel closer to 90° of knee flexion, resulting in longer tunnel lengths and safer distances from the common peroneal nerve.(11, 12)

Achieving anatomic femoral tunnel placement and subsequent graft insertion demands adequate visualization of the intercondylar notch wall of the lateral femoral condyle. Osaki et al examined the femoral tunnel aperture within the intercondylar notch and demonstrated a discrepancies of up to 5 mm using an outside-in drilling technique and 4.2 mm with a trans-portal drilling technique between tunnel lengths measured at the center versus the shortest aspects of the femoral tunnel aperture.(13) The authors attributed their findings to the obliquity of the femoral tunnel relative to the lateral femoral intercondylar notch wall. Accordingly, the anatomy and inevitable oblique orientation for femoral tunnel drilling may result in overestimation of tunnel length if the near side (i.e., distal aspect) of the aperture is referenced versus referencing the far side (i.e., proximal aspect) of the aperture. Such tunnel length inaccuracy may lead to a proud plug with use of a bone-tendon-bone graft or an insufficient graft within the tunnel using soft-tissue only grafts.(14)

Visualizing the entire femoral ACL footprint can be challenging from a standard anterolateral-viewing portal using a 30° arthroscope. Several authors have described improved visualization of the femoral ACL footprint using a 70° arthroscope from the lateral portal.(14, 15) Moreover, use of the 70° arthroscope using the standard anterolateral viewing portal enables the surgeons to achieve a "top-down" view of the femoral reamer when using the trans-portal technique for drilling the femoral tunnel, serving as the senior author's preferred technique during ACL reconstruction. Unlike the standard notch view obtained with a 30° arthroscope from the anterolateral portal, this "top-down" view permits visualization of the far side (i.e., proximal aspect) of the ACL femoral tunnel aperture. The purpose of the study is to compare femoral tunnel length measurements using the "top-down" view with a 70° arthroscope to reference the far side of the femoral tunnel aperture versus measurements from the standard notch view using a 30° arthroscope to reference the near side. The authors hypothesized that femoral tunnel length measurements obtained from the "top-down" view would be more accurate than measurements obtained using the standard notch view.

## METHODS

The study protocol was pre-approved by the author's Institutional Review Board. Arthroscopic images of skeletally mature patients with closed physes undergoing primary ACL reconstruction by a single fellowship-trained Orthopaedic sports surgeon between July 1, 2014 and December 31, 2016 were retrospectively reviewed for study inclusion. As such, no formal patient consent was required. Skeletally immature patients and those with prior bony knee surgery were excluded. Demographic data including patient age, sex, height, weight and laterality of surgery were recorded.

### Surgical Technique

A standard 30° arthroscope was used for the diagnostic arthroscopy and to address any chondral or meniscal pathology. It is the senior author's preference to use a 70° arthroscope for the ACL reconstruction portion of the operation to view the intercondylar notch and ACL footprint, perform tunnel drilling, and visualize graft insertion. At the time of femoral tunnel drilling using a flexible reamer (Clancy Flexible Reamer, Smith and Nephew, Memphis, TN) the 70° arthroscope is placed in the standard anterolateral portal looking laterally at the reamer. The surgeon stopped the reamer and obtained the first of two images of the reamer within the tunnel. Despite using a 70° arthroscope, the image obtained is identical to that obtained with a 30° arthroscope given then positioning of the light cord/camera lens. (**Figure 1A,B**) Care was taken to ensure a hash mark number label was clearly visible on the reamer in the image as reference for measurements of tunnel depth. The second image was obtained by rotating the camera 90° to achieve the "top-down" view, which orients the visual field looking down on the reamer to visualize the far side (i.e., back-side) of the reamer and femoral tunnel aperture. (**Figure 1C,D**) Care was again taken to ensure inclusion of a hash mark number label on the reamer for reference of tunnel depth.

### Measurements and Calculations

The flexible reamer's links between each 5 mm labeled hash mark were measured using a digital caliper with accuracy to 0.01 mm (Mitutoyo, Mitutoyo Corp., Model Japan). A single metal link was measured to be 1.01 mm long. (**Figure 2A**) The length of a single link and the two adjacent gaps on either side was measured as 1.89 mm long. (**Figure 2B**) These two measurements were rounded to the nearest 0.1 mm. Thus, the length of the space between two links was determined by subtracting the length of a single link (1.0 mm) and then dividing the remaining length by two, given the presence of two inter-link gaps. [i.e., (1.9–1.0 mm)/2 = 0.45 mm]. (**Figure 2C**) Thus, the femoral tunnel length could be accurately calculated from arthroscopic images by referencing the visualized hash mark number label and subtracting the link lengths (1.0 mm) and the inter-link gap lengths (0.45 mm) until the point at which the reamer intersected with the femoral tunnel wall aperture. The femoral tunnel length measurements were determined from the surgical arthroscopic images using the standard notch view and the "top-down" view for each patient.

### Statistical Analysis

An a priori power analysis was conduced to determine the minimum number of patients necessary to detect a significant difference in femoral tunnel length measurements between views. Using an initial set of 20 measurements ($n$ = 10 patients), SD was assumed to be 0.63 mm. With an alpha-level of 0.05 and power set to 95%, the minimum number of patients needed to detect a 0.5 mm difference was calculated to be 54 patients.(16)

All data were analyzed for normality using the Shapiro-Wilk test. An intraclass correlation coefficient (ICC) for femoral tunnel length measurements was calculated by the senior author at two separate time points (minimum: 2 weeks apart) in all patients ($n$ = 54 patients; $n$ = 108 images) while an interclass class correlation coefficient was calculated in 26 patients ($n$ = 52 images) between two authors. Following established recommendations,

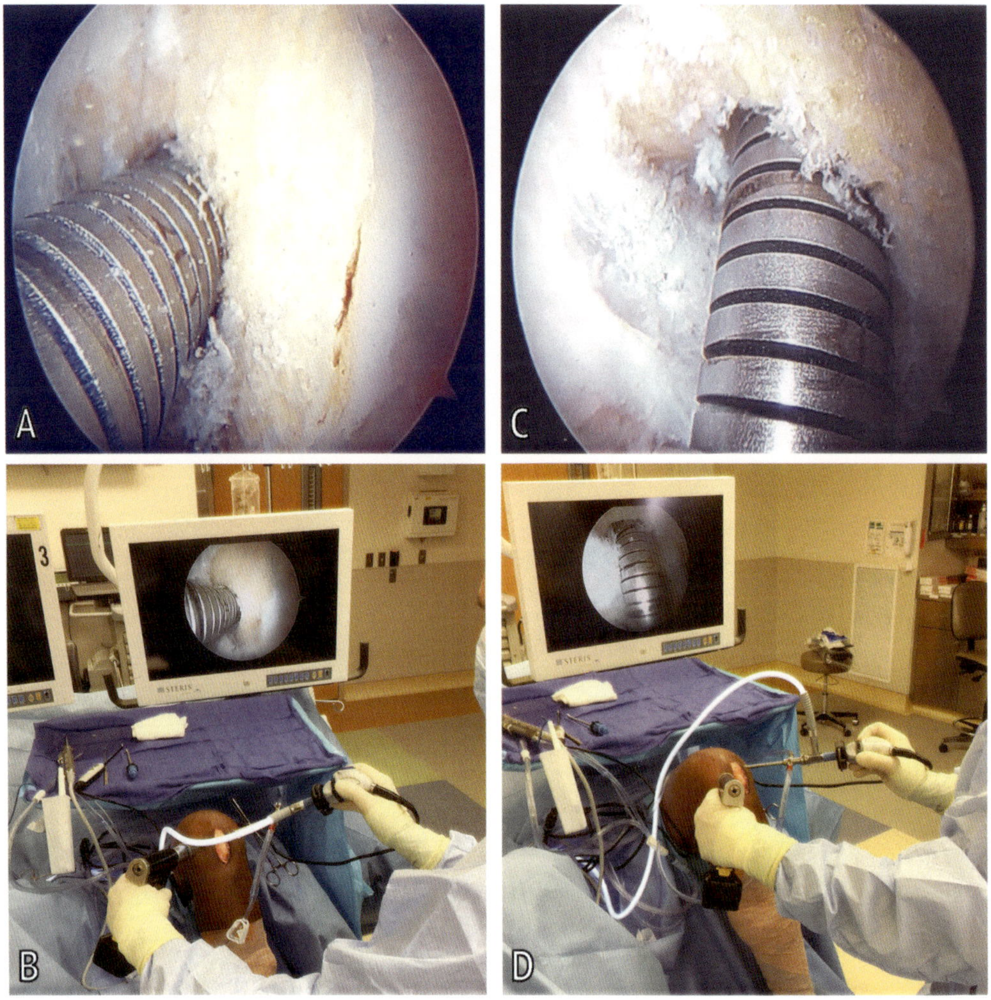


**FIGURE 1** | Arthroscopic images of a left knee during femoral tunnel reaming to obtain femoral tunnel reamer measurements. **(A)** Standard notch view **(B)** Surgeon hand and camera position for obtaining standard notch view **(C)** Top-down view **(D)** Surgeon hand and camera position for obtaining top-down view.

an ICC of <0.4 was determined to be poor, 0.4–0.75 to be fair to good, and >0.75 to be excellent.(17, 18) Paired samples *t*-test was used to test the null hypothesis that no significant difference would be present between measurements obtained via the standard notch view versus measurements obtained via the "top-down" view. An independent sample *t*-test was used to compare dichotomous variables (patient sex, laterality of surgery) in paired measurements obtained from the two views. Pearson's correlations were used to compare age, height, and weight to the difference in paired measurements obtained from the two views. A *p*-value of <0.05 was used to determine statistical significance. All statistical analysis was performed using SPSS (Version 23, IBM, Armonk, New York) software.

## RESULTS

A total of 60 patients underwent ACL reconstruction during the study period with imaging and documentation of both standard-notch and "top-down" views for femoral tunnel length measurement. Six patients were excluded due to bony debris obscuring the reamer's hash mark number labels, preventing accurate tunnel length measurement in at least one of the views. Mean age of the 54 patients included for final analysis was 26 ± 9.8 years (range, 15 to 51 years) with a mean height and weight of 69 ± 4.4 inches (range, 58–77 inches) and 84.0 ± 18.7 kilograms (range, 54.0–136 kilograms), respectively. The study group included 19 females and 35 males. Twenty-seven patients underwent surgery to the left knee while 27 had surgery on the right knee.

Measurements of both the standard notch view and "top down" view produced excellent intra-observer (0.0877, 0.932; respectively) and inter-observer (0.916, 0.960; respectively) values. Femoral tunnel length measurements obtained via the standard notch view were significantly longer than those obtained via the "top-down" view ($p < 0.001$; mean 2.24 ± 0.868 mm longer) (**Figures 3 and 4**). Univariate analysis showed that the difference in femoral tunnel length measurements obtained via the standard notch-view versus the top-down view did not

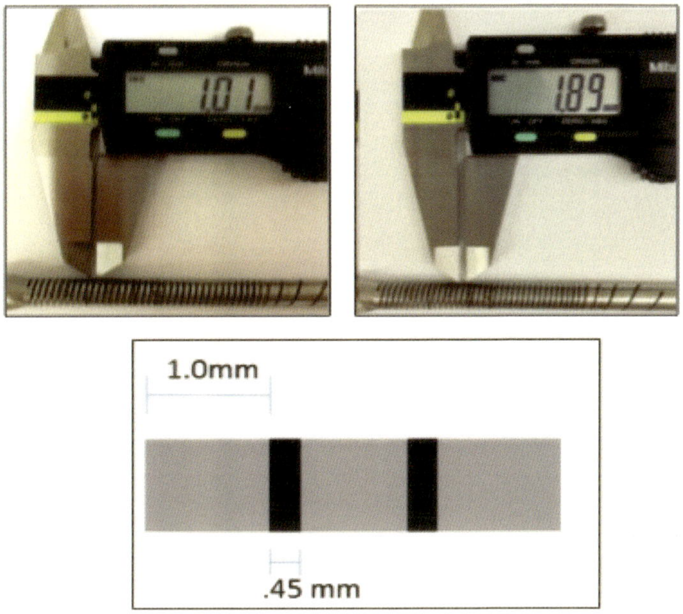


**FIGURE 2** | Digital caliper measurement of flexible reamer links and gaps for femoral tunnel length measurements.

vary significantly with age (r = 0.12, $p$ = 0.40), height (r = 0.013, $p$ = 0.92), or weight (r = 0.042, $p$ = 0.76). There was no significant difference in mean femoral tunnel length measurements between females (mean, 2.27 ± 0.666 mm) and males (mean, 2.22 ± 0.974 mm) ($p$ = 0.852). Furthermore, no significant difference in femoral tunnel length measurements was appreciated based on surgical laterality (mean, 2.08 ± 0.776 mm for left versus 2.40 ± 0.94457 mm for right; $p$ = 0.179).

## DISCUSSION

The purpose of this investigation was to better understand different in femoral tunnel length measurements during ACL reconstruction comparing the standard notch view using a 30° arthroscope versus the "top down" view with a 70° arthroscope. The authors found that in 54 subjects undergoing ACL reconstruction, measurements of femoral tunnel length via the standard notch view were significantly longer than those obtained using a "top down" view. Patient sex, age, height, weight and surgical laterality had no significant impact on mean femoral tunnel length measurements. Data from this investigation adds to the growing body of research regarding femoral tunnel aperture morphology and its clinical implications during ACL reconstruction.(13, 19, 20)

Multiple studies have implicated non-anatomic femoral tunnel placement as the reason for ACL reconstruction failure and instability post-operatively (21–23) as current efforts towards achieving optimal stability and outcomes have focused on anatomic ACL reconstruction techniques.(4, 24) Obtaining anatomic femoral tunnel placement and subsequent tunnel length measurement relies on adequate visualization of the native ACL footprint. Numerous techniques have been proposed for gaining better visualization of the lateral femoral condylar wall within the notch, including a modified mid-patellar portal (25) and a central accessory medial portal.(26) By using a 70° arthroscope through the standard anterolateral portal, the "top-down" view described in this study provides the surgeon with an unobstructed view of the far side of the femoral tunnel aperture without the need for extra portals. By providing a perpendicular

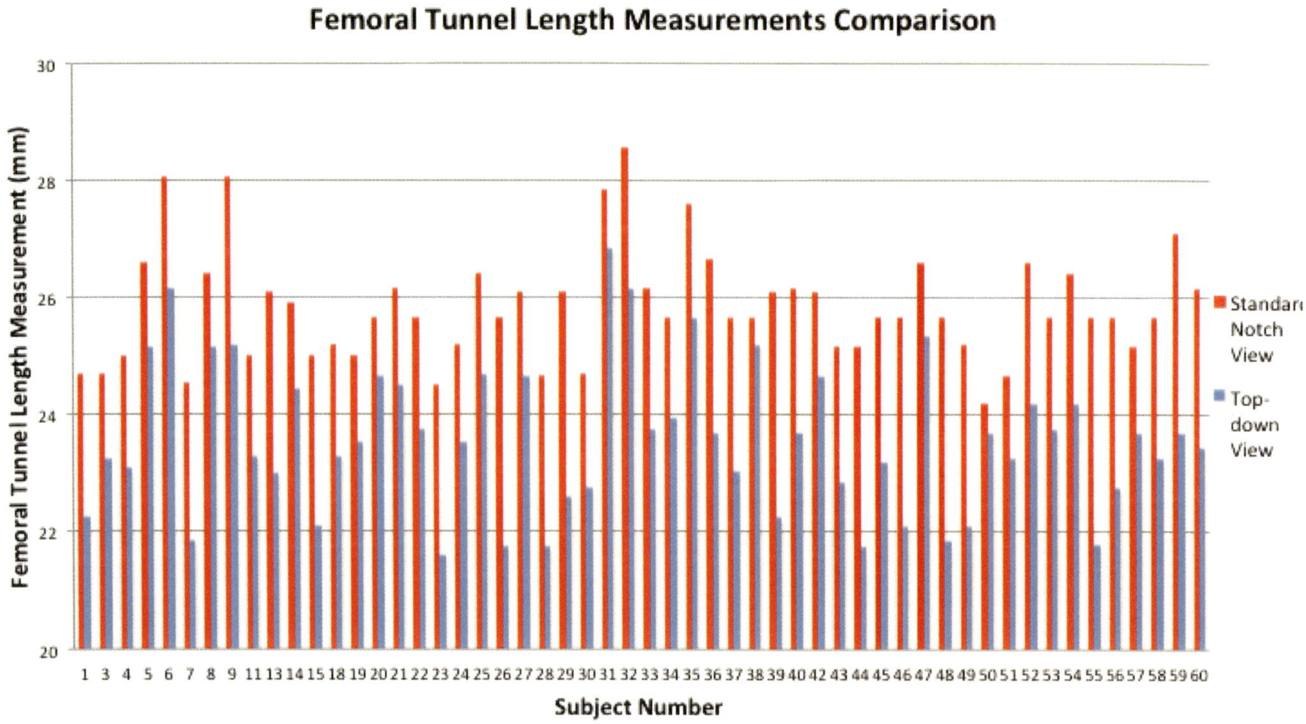


**FIGURE 3 |** Comparison of femoral tunnel length measurements obtained by the standard notch view and the top-down view.

view of the reamer at the femoral tunnel aperture, the authors found excellent intra- and inter-observer reliability values, indicative of the high reproducibility of measurements using the "top down" view. In their investigation utilizing a 3-dimensional knee model, Hoshino et al. further demonstrated the ability to reduce distortion and consequent inaccurate measurement readings using the 70° arthroscope when compared views obtained using 0° and 30° arthroscopes.(27)

Compared to the standard notch view, the "top down" view avoids over-estimation of femoral tunnel length measurements. This effectively mitigates potential complications associated with graft-tunnel length mismatch, which has been shown to be crucial in order to ensure optimal outcomes following ACL reconstruction.(28, 29) When using a bone-patellar tendon-bone graft or osseous grafts such as an Achilles or quadriceps tendon, over-estimation of the femoral tunnel length may lead to a proud bone plug within the notch and/or inadequate bone-plug interface at the tibial tunnel, compromising the integrity of interference screw fixation (30), leading to intra-operative or postoperative complications.(31) Arguably, a buffer distance may be built into graft length and tunnel drilling calculations. However, having a femoral bone plug that ends flush with the femoral tunnel aperture within the notch avoids potential complications associated with a recessed femoral bone plug such as the "windshield wiper effect," thought to result in tunnel widening and graft abrasion.(32, 33)

Moreover, for a soft-tissue graft, overestimation of femoral tunnel length can lead to placement of an inadequate amount of the graft within the femoral tunnel.(34) Lee et al. demonstrated that such grafts incompletely fill femoral tunnel apertures and tend to rest off-center within the tunnel.(35) Accordingly, a discordant measurement of osseous tunnel length versus graft length may be amplified with the graft's final eccentric resting position. Previous investigations have examined the temporal changes in the cross-sectional area of the femoral tunnel aperture, enlarging with time (36) with slower remodeling of the bone-tendon interface at the intra-articular aperture.(37) The consequences of these natural history changes in ACL

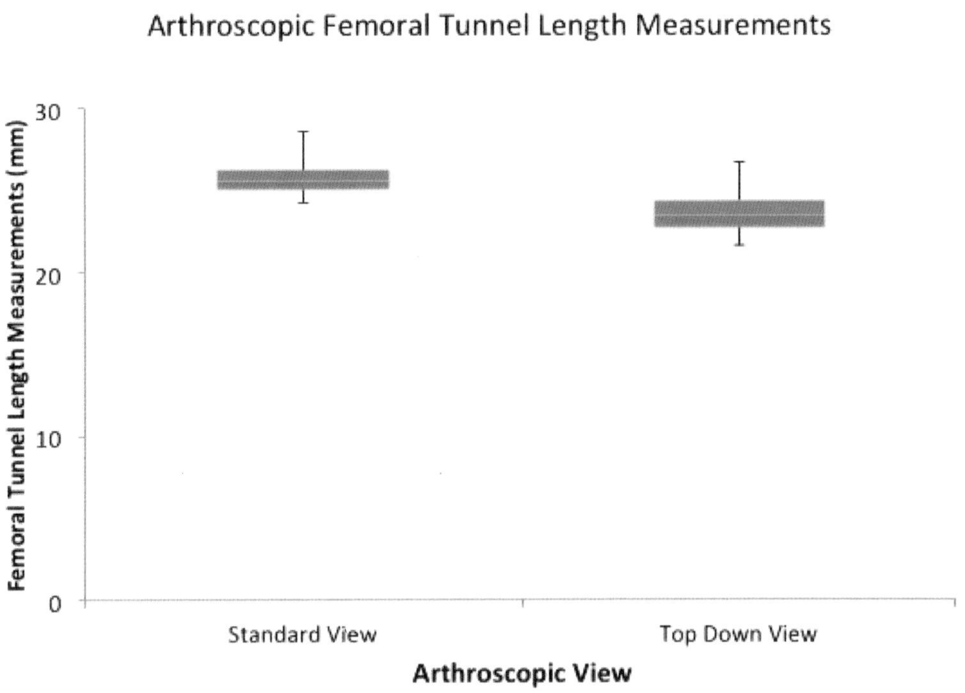


**FIGURE 4** | Box plots of femoral tunnel length measurements in millimeters by arthroscopic technique. Upper and lower hinges represent 25 and 75% quartiles; middle represent median or 50% quartile.

reconstruction grafts are magnified with increased motion at the tunnel aperture, resulting in lower rates of healing at sites of motion.(38)

This study was not without limitations. A single surgeon obtained all arthroscopic photographs used to measure femoral tunnel length during surgery. While use of the 70° arthroscope is the senior author's preference, inviting the potential for observer bias, the excellent inter-observer reliability values obtained demonstrate the validity of the methods utilized and results obtained. However, additional studies utilizing multiple different surgeons is warranted to further validate the conclusions and surgical technique of the "top down" view. Second, if suspensory fixation techniques with an adjustable loop fixation function are utilized, then concerns about graft-tunnel mismatch become less pertinent since the loop portion of the graft-button construct is adjustable following passage of the graft.(20) Lastly, post-operative functional outcome scores and complications rates were not analyzed, as such despite the reported significant difference in femoral tunnel length overestimation using the standard notch view, the clinical relevance of this finding cannot be extrapolated and is beyond the scope of this investigation.

## CONCLUSIONS

The "top-down" view using a 70° arthroscope provides a viable alternative to the standard notch view with a 30° arthroscope for visualizing the anatomic ACL footprint. The "top down" view helps avoid tunnel length overestimation by referencing the backside of the reamer for tunnel length measurements, especially in cases where lateral femoral intercondylar notch wall obliquity is high or the tunnel drilling obliquity is high. By providing a more accurate assessment of femoral tunnel length, the surgeon can plan appropriately for final tunnel length preparation and graft length preparation, facilitating more advantageous ACL reconstruction by avoiding complications associated with graft-tunnel length mismatch. Future long-term prospective studies examining functional outcomes and complication rates following ACL reconstruction utilizing the "top-down" view with a 70° arthroscope versus the standard notch view with a 30° arthroscope are necessary to better understand the clinical impact of technique on outcomes following reconstruction.

## AUTHOR CONTRIBUTIONS

SMJ: project conception and design, measurements, data analysis, manuscript preparation. MRK: project conception and design, measurements, data analysis. DMK: data analysis and manuscript preparation. JEV: project conception and design, obtained surgical images, manuscript preparation.

## REFERENCES

1. Buller LT, Best MJ, Baraga MG, Kaplan LD. Trends in anterior cruciate ligament reconstruction in the United States. *Orthop J Sports Med* (2015) 3(1):2325967114563664):. doi: 10.1177/2325967114563664
2. Evans CL, Miller MD, Diduch DR. Revision anterior cruciate ligament surgery: one-stage versus two-stage technique. *Insall & Scott: Surgery of the Knee*. Vol. 1. 6th ed. Elsevier (2018). p. 685–701.
3. Mall NA, Chalmers PN, Moric M, Tanaka MJ, Cole BJ, Bach BR, et al. Incidence and trends of anterior cruciate ligament reconstruction in the United States. *Am J Sports Med* (2014) 42(10):2363–70. doi: 10.1177/0363546514542796
4. Dhawan A, Gallo RA, Lynch SA. Anatomic tunnel placement in anterior cruciate ligament reconstruction. *J Am Acad Orthop Surg* (2016) 24(7):443–54. doi: 10.5435/JAAOS-D-14-00465
5. Harner CD, Honkamp NJ, Ranawat AS. Anteromedial portal technique for creating the anterior cruciate ligament femoral tunnel. *Arthroscopy* (2008) 24(1):113–5. doi: 10.1016/j.arthro.2007.07.019
6. Tompkins M, Milewski MD, Brockmeier SF, Gaskin CM, Hart JM, Miller MD. Anatomic femoral tunnel drilling in anterior cruciate ligament reconstruction: use of an accessory medial portal versus traditional transtibial drilling. *Am J Sports Med* (2012) 40(6):1313–21. doi: 10.1177/0363546512443047
7. Bedi A, Raphael B, Maderazo A, Pavlov H, Williams RJ. Transtibial versus anteromedial portal drilling for anterior cruciate ligament reconstruction: a cadaveric study of femoral tunnel length and obliquity. *Arthroscopy* (2010) 26(3):342–50. doi: 10.1016/j.arthro.2009.12.006
8. Lee DH, Kim HJ, Ahn HS, Bin SI. Comparison of femoral tunnel length and obliquity between transtibial, anteromedial portal, and outside-in surgical techniques in single-bundle anterior cruciate ligament reconstruction: a meta-analysis. *Arthroscopy* (2016) 32(1):142–50. doi: 10.1016/j.arthro.2015.07.026
9. Lubowitz JH. Anteromedial portal technique for the anterior cruciate ligament femoral socket: pitfalls and solutions. *Arthroscopy* (2009) 25(1):95–101. doi: 10.1016/j.arthro.2008.10.012
10. Lubowitz JH, Konicek J. Anterior cruciate ligament femoral tunnel length: cadaveric analysis comparing anteromedial portal versus outside-in technique. *Arthroscopy* (2010) 26(10):1357–62. doi: 10.1016/j.arthro.2010.02.014
11. Fitzgerald J, Saluan P, Richter DL, Huff N, Schenck RC. Anterior cruciate ligament reconstruction using a flexible reamer system: technique and pitfalls. *Orthop J Sports Med* (2015) 3(7):2325967115592875. doi: 10.1177/2325967115592875
12. Silver AG, Kaar SG, Grisell MK, Reagan JM, Farrow LD. Comparison between rigid and flexible systems for drilling the femoral tunnel through an anteromedial portal in anterior cruciate ligament reconstruction. *Arthroscopy* (2010) 26(6):790–5. doi: 10.1016/j.arthro.2009.10.012
13. Osaki K, Okazaki K, Matsubara H, Kuwashima U, Murakami K, Iwamoto Y. Asymmetry in femoral tunnel socket length during anterior cruciate ligament reconstruction with transportal, outside-in, and modified transtibial techniques. *Arthroscopy* (2015) 31(12):2365–70. doi: 10.1016/j.arthro.2015.06.026
14. Bucher TA, Naim S, Mandalia V. The use of the 70° arthroscope for anatomic femoral and tibial tunnel placement and tunnel viewing in anterior cruciate ligament reconstruction. *Arthrosc Tech* (2014) 3(1):e79–81. doi: 10.1016/j.eats.2013.08.001
15. Bedi A, Dines J, Dines DM, Kelly BT, O'Brien SJ, Altchek DW, et al. Use of the 70° arthroscope for improved visualization with common arthroscopic procedures. *Arthroscopy* (2010) 26(12):1684–96. doi: 10.1016/j.arthro.2010.04.070
16. Faul F, Erdfelder E, Lang AG, Buchner A. G*Power 3: a flexible statistical power analysis program for the social, behavioral, and biomedical sciences. *Behav Res Methods* (2007) 39(2):175–91. doi: 10.3758/BF03193146
17. Fleiss J. *The design and analysis of clinical experiments*. New York: Wiley (1986).
18. Shrout PE, Fleiss JL. Intraclass correlations: uses in assessing rater reliability. *Psychol Bull* (1979) 86(2):420–8. doi: 10.1037/0033-2909.86.2.420
19. Hensler D, Working ZM, Illingworth KD, Thorhauer ED, Tashman S, Fu FH. Medial portal drilling: effects on the femoral tunnel aperture morphology during anterior cruciate ligament reconstruction. *J Bone Joint Surg Am* (2011) 93(22):2063–71. doi: 10.2106/JBJS.J.01705
20. Okazaki K, Osaki K, Nishikawa K, Matsubara H, Tashiro Y, Iwamoto Y. Overestimation of femoral tunnel length during anterior cruciate ligament reconstruction using the retrograde outside-in drilling technique. *Arch Orthop Trauma Surg* (2016) 136(8):1159–63. doi: 10.1007/s00402-016-2492-y
21. Wright RW, Huston LJ, Spindler KP, Dunn WR, Haas AK, Allen CR, et al. Descriptive epidemiology of the Multicenter ACL Revision Study (MARS) cohort. *Am J Sports Med* (2010) 38(10):1979–86. doi: 10.1177/0363546510378645
22. Morgan JA, Dahm D, Levy B,Stuart MJ MARS Study Group. Femoral tunnel malposition in ACL revision reconstruction. *J Knee Surg* (2012) 25(5):361–8. doi: 10.1055/s-0031-1299662
23. Samitier G, Marcano AI, Alentorn-Geli E, Cugat R, Farmer KW, Moser MW. Failure of anterior cruciate ligament reconstruction. *Arch Bone Jt Surg* (2015) 3(4):220–40.
24. Pinczewski LA, Salmon LJ, Jackson WF, von Bormann RB, Haslam PG, Tashiro S. Radiological landmarks for placement of the tunnels in single-bundle reconstruction of the anterior cruciate ligament. *J Bone Joint Surg Br* (2008) 90(2):172–9. doi: 10.1302/0301-620X.90B2.20104
25. Calvisi V, Lupparelli S, Giuliani P. A view from above: a modified Patel's medial midpatellar portal for anterior cruciate ligament arthroscopic surgery. *Arthroscopy* (2007) 23(3):324.e1–5. doi: 10.1016/j.arthro.2006.07.040
26. Cohen SB, Fu FH. Three-portal technique for anterior cruciate ligament reconstruction: use of a central medial portal. *Arthroscopy* (2007) 23(3):325.e1–5. doi: 10.1016/j.arthro.2006.07.030
27. Hoshino Y, Rothrauff BB, Hensler D, Fu FH, Musahl V. Arthroscopic image distortion-part II: the effect of lens angle and portal location in a 3D knee model. *Knee Surg Sports Traumatol Arthrosc* (2016) 24(6):2072–8. doi: 10.1007/s00167-014-3268-y
28. Grawe B, Smerina A, Allen A. Avoiding graft-tunnel length mismatch in anterior cruciate ligament reconstruction: the single-bone plug technique. *Arthrosc Tech* (2014) 3(3):e417–20. doi: 10.1016/j.eats.2014.04.003

29. Kopf S, Forsythe B, Wong AK, Tashman S, Anderst W, Irrgang JJ, et al. Nonanatomic tunnel position in traditional transtibial single-bundle anterior cruciate ligament reconstruction evaluated by three-dimensional computed tomography. *J Bone Joint Surg Am* (2010) 92(6):1427–31. doi: 10.2106/JBJS.I.00655
30. Brown JA, Brophy RH, Franco J, Marquand A, Solomon TC, Watanabe D, et al. Avoiding allograft length mismatch during anterior cruciate ligament reconstruction: patient height as an indicator of appropriate graft length. *Am J Sports Med* (2007) 35(6):986–9. doi: 10.1177/0363546506298584
31. Yanke A, Ellman MB, Sherman SL, Bach BR. Graft-tunnel mismatch in bone-tendon-bone ACL reconstruction: preventation and treatment. *Tech Orthop* (2012) 27(2):153–7.
32. Gill TJ, Steadman JR. Anterior cruciate ligament reconstruction the two-incision technique. *Orthop Clin North Am* (2002) 33(4):727–35.
33. Yanke A, Ellman MB, Sherman SL, Bach BRJ. Graft-tunnel mismatch in bone-tendon-bone ACL reconstruction: techniques in orthopaedics. *Tech Orthop* (2012) 27(2):153–7.
34. Zantop T, Ferretti M, Bell KM, Brucker PU, Gilbertson L, Fu FH. Effect of tunnel-graft length on the biomechanics of anterior cruciate ligament-reconstructed knees: intra-articular study in a goat model. *Am J Sports Med* (2008) 36(11):2158–66. doi: 10.1177/0363546508320572
35. Lee BH, Bansal S, Park SH, Wang JH. Eccentric graft positioning within the femoral tunnel aperture in anatomic double-bundle anterior cruciate ligament reconstruction using the transportal and outside-in techniques. *Am J Sports Med* (2015) 43(5):1180–8. doi: 10.1177/0363546514568278
36. Tachibana Y, Mae T, Shino K, Kanamoto T, Sugamoto K, Yoshikawa H, et al. Morphological changes in femoral tunnels after anatomic anterior cruciate ligament reconstruction. *Knee Surg Sports Traumatol Arthrosc* (2015) 23(12):3591–600. doi: 10.1007/s00167-014-3252-6
37. Bedi A, Kawamura S, Ying L, Rodeo SA. Differences in tendon graft healing between the intra-articular and extra-articular ends of a bone tunnel. *Hss J* (2009) 5(1):51–7. doi: 10.1007/s11420-008-9096-1
38. Rodeo SA, Kawamura S, Kim HJ, Dynybil C, Ying L. Tendon healing in a bone tunnel differs at the tunnel entrance versus the tunnel exit: an effect of graft-tunnel motion? *Am J Sports Med* (2006) 34(11):1790–800. doi: 10.1177/0363546506290059

# Permissions

All chapters in this book were first published in FIS, by Frontiers; hereby published with permission under the Creative Commons Attribution License or equivalent. Every chapter published in this book has been scrutinized by our experts. Their significance has been extensively debated. The topics covered herein carry significant findings which will fuel the growth of the discipline. They may even be implemented as practical applications or may be referred to as a beginning point for another development.

The contributors of this book come from diverse backgrounds, making this book a truly international effort. This book will bring forth new frontiers with its revolutionizing research information and detailed analysis of the nascent developments around the world.

We would like to thank all the contributing authors for lending their expertise to make the book truly unique. They have played a crucial role in the development of this book. Without their invaluable contributions this book wouldn't have been possible. They have made vital efforts to compile up to date information on the varied aspects of this subject to make this book a valuable addition to the collection of many professionals and students.

This book was conceptualized with the vision of imparting up-to-date information and advanced data in this field. To ensure the same, a matchless editorial board was set up. Every individual on the board went through rigorous rounds of assessment to prove their worth. After which they invested a large part of their time researching and compiling the most relevant data for our readers.

The editorial board has been involved in producing this book since its inception. They have spent rigorous hours researching and exploring the diverse topics which have resulted in the successful publishing of this book. They have passed on their knowledge of decades through this book. To expedite this challenging task, the publisher supported the team at every step. A small team of assistant editors was also appointed to further simplify the editing procedure and attain best results for the readers.

Apart from the editorial board, the designing team has also invested a significant amount of their time in understanding the subject and creating the most relevant covers. They scrutinized every image to scout for the most suitable representation of the subject and create an appropriate cover for the book.

The publishing team has been an ardent support to the editorial, designing and production team. Their endless efforts to recruit the best for this project, has resulted in the accomplishment of this book. They are a veteran in the field of academics and their pool of knowledge is as vast as their experience in printing. Their expertise and guidance has proved useful at every step. Their uncompromising quality standards have made this book an exceptional effort. Their encouragement from time to time has been an inspiration for everyone.

The publisher and the editorial board hope that this book will prove to be a valuable piece of knowledge for researchers, students, practitioners and scholars across the globe.

# List of Contributors

**Robert T. Spychal**
3D PRINT Laboratory, Department of Surgery, Peninsula Health, Frankston, VIC, Australia

**Michael P. Chae, Warren M. Rozen and David J. Hunter-Smith**
3D PRINT Laboratory, Department of Surgery, Peninsula Health, Frankston, VIC, Australia
Monash University Plastic and Reconstructive Surgery Group (Peninsula Clinical School), Peninsula Health, Frankston, VIC, Australia

**Michael W. Findlay**
3D PRINT Laboratory, Department of Surgery, Peninsula Health, Frankston, VIC, Australia
Department of Surgery, Stanford University, Stanford, CA, USA

**Paul G. McMenamin**
Department of Anatomy and Developmental Biology, Centre for Human Anatomy Education, School of Biomedical Sciences, Faculty of Medicine, Nursing and Health Sciences, Monash University, Clayton, VIC, Australia

**René Gueguen**
Faculty of Medicine and UFR STAPS, University of Lorraine, EA 3450, Development, Adaptation and Handicap, Villers-lès-Nancy, France

**Laetitia Peultier-Celli and Philippe Perrin**
Faculty of Medicine and UFR STAPS, University of Lorraine, EA 3450, Development, Adaptation and Handicap, Villers-lès-Nancy, France
Laboratory for the Analysis of Posture, Equilibrium and Motor Function (LAPEM), University Hospital of Nancy, Vandoeuvre-lès-Nancy, France

**Jean Paysant**
Faculty of Medicine and UFR STAPS, University of Lorraine, EA 3450, Development, Adaptation and Handicap, Villers-lès-Nancy, France
Regional Institute of Physical Medicine and Rehabilitation, Nancy Cedex, France

**Didier Mainard**
Department of Orthopedics and Trauma Surgery, University Hospital of Nancy, Nancy, France

**Frank Wein and Nicolas Paris**
Department of Orthopedics Surgery, Médipôle Gentilly-Saint Jacques, Maxéville, France

**Patrick Boisseau and Alexandre Ferry**
Institut de Formation en Masso-Kinésithérapie, Nancy, France

**Isabelle Chary-Valckenaere**
Department of Rheumatology, University Hospital of Nancy, Vandoeuvre-lès-Nancy, France
IMoPA, UMR 7365 CNRS, Vandoeuvre-lès-Nancy, France

**Daniel Schmauss and Hans-Günther Machens**
Department of Plastic Surgery and Hand Surgery, Klinikum rechts der Isar, Technische Universität München, Munich Germany

**Yves Harder**
Department of Plastic Surgery and Hand Surgery, Klinikum rechts der Isar, Technische Universität München, Munich Germany
Department of Plastic, Reconstructive and Aesthetic Surgery, Ospedale Regionale di Lugano, Ente Ospedaliero Cantonale, Lugano, Switzerland

**Andrej Ring, Pascal Kirchhoff, Ole Goertz, Bjorn Behr, Adrien Daigeler, Marcus Lehnhardt and Kamran Harati**
Department for Plastic and Hand Surgery, Burn Center/Sarcoma Reference Center, Ruhr-University Bochum, Bochum, Germany

**Marco Romeo**
Department of Plastic and Reconstructive Surgery, Hospital de Guadalajara, Guadalajara, Spain

**Emilio Garcia-Tutor**
Department of Plastic and Reconstructive Surgery, Hospital de Guadalajara, Guadalajara, Spain
MD Anderson Cancer Center, Madrid, Spain

**Michael P. Chae, David J. Hunter-Smith and Warren Matthew Rozen**
Department of Surgery, School of Clinical Science at Monash Health, Faculty of Medicine, Monash University, Monash Medical Centre, Clayton, VIC, Australia

Monash University Plastic and Reconstructive Surgery Unit (Peninsula Clinical School), Peninsula Health, Frankston, VIC, Australia

**Ole Goertz, Leon von der Lohe, Adrien Daigeler, Kamran Harati, Tobias Hirsch, Marcus Lehnhardt and Jonas Kolbenschlag**
Department of Plastic Surgery, BG University Hospital Bergmannsheil, Ruhr-University, Bochum, Germany

**Ramón Martinez-Olivera**
Neurosurgical Unit, Department of Surgery, BG University Hospital Bergmannsheil, Ruhr-University, Bochum, Germany

**Thomas D. Dobbs and Iain Stuart Whitaker**
Reconstructive Surgery and Regenerative Medicine Research Group (ReconRegen), Institute of Life Science, Swansea University Medical School, Swansea, United Kingdom
The Welsh Centre for Burns and Plastic Surgery, Morriston Hospital, Swansea, United Kingdom

**Olivia Cundy and Harsh Samarendra**
Oxford University Medical School, Oxford, United Kingdom

**Khurram Khan**
Department of Plastic Surgery, Birmingham Children's Hospital, Birmingham, United Kingdom

**Ferdinand Köckerling, Marinos Damianos Botsinis and Christine Rohde**
Department of Surgery, Centre for Minimally Invasive Surgery, Vivantes Hospital Berlin, Academic Teaching Hospital of Charité Medical School, Berlin, Germany

**Wolfgang Reinpold**
Department of Surgery, Wilhelmsburger Hospital Groß Sand, Academic Teaching Hospital of University Hamburg, Hamburg, Germany

**Robert Slade**
Welsh Centre for Burns and Plastic Surgery, Morriston Hospital, Swansea, United Kingdom

**Thomas H. Jovic, Zita M. Jessop, Thomas Dobbs and Iain S. Whitaker**
Welsh Centre for Burns and Plastic Surgery, Morriston Hospital, Swansea, United Kingdom
Reconstructive Surgery and Regenerative Medicine Research Group, Institute of Life Sciences, Swansea, United Kingdom

**Nasra N. Alam, Sunil K. Narang, Ian R. Daniels and Neil J. Smart**
Exeter Surgical Health Services Research Unit (HeSRU), Royal Devon and Exeter Hospital, Exeter, Devon, UK

**Ferdinand Köckerling,**
Department of Surgery, Center for Minimally Invasive Surgery, Academic Teaching Hospital of Charité Medical School, Vivantes Hospital, Berlin, Germany

**Brian J. White**
WesternOrthopaedics,Denver,CO,USA

**Mackenzie M. Herzog**
Professional Research Institute for Sports Medicine, LLC, Chapel Hill, NC, USA

**Jungo Imanishi**
Department of Orthopaedics, St. Vincent's Hospital, Melbourne, VIC, Australia

**Lester Wai Mon Chan**
Department of Orthopaedics, St. Vincent's Hospital, Melbourne, VIC, Australia
Department of Orthopaedic Surgery, Tan Tock Seng Hospital, Singapore, Singapore

**Peter Choong**
Department of Orthopaedics, St. Vincent's Hospital, Melbourne, VIC, Australia
Department of Surgery, University of Melbourne, Melbourne, VIC, Australia

**Damien Glen Grinsell**
Department of Plastic Surgery, St Vincent's Hospital, Melbourne, VIC, Australia

**Georgios Koulaxouzidis and Filip Simunovic**
Department of Plastic and Hand Surgery, University of Freiburg Medical Center, Freiburg, Germany

**Holger Bannasch**
Department of Plastic and Hand Surgery, University of Freiburg Medical Center, Freiburg, Germany
Section for Plastic-Reconstructive Tumor Surgery, University of Freiburg Medical Center, Freiburg, Germany

**Charles M. Malata**
Postgraduate Medical Institute, Faculty of Health Sciences, Anglia Ruskin University, Cambridge and Chelmsford, UK
Cambridge Breast Unit, Plastic and Reconstructive Surgery Department, Cambridge University Hospitals NHS Foundation Trust, Cambridge, UK

**Nicholas G. Rabey**
Cambridge Breast Unit, Plastic and Reconstructive Surgery Department, Cambridge University Hospitals NHS Foundation Trust, Cambridge, UK
Department of Plastic and Reconstructive Surgery, Salisbury District Hospital, Salisbury, UK

**Ayesha Al-Sabah**
Reconstructive Surgery and Regenerative Medicine Research Group (ReconRegen), Institute of Life Science, Swansea University Medical School, Swansea, UK

**Sarah Al-Himdani, Zita M. Jessop, Emman Combellack and Iain S. Whitaker**
Reconstructive Surgery and Regenerative Medicine Research Group (ReconRegen), Institute of Life Science, Swansea University Medical School, Swansea, UK
The Welsh Centre for Burns and Plastic Surgery, Morriston Hospital, Swansea, UK

**Amel Ibrahim**
Reconstructive Surgery and Regenerative Medicine Research Group (ReconRegen), Institute of Life Science, Swansea University Medical School, Swansea, UK
The Welsh Centre for Burns and Plastic Surgery, Morriston Hospital, Swansea, UK
Institute of Child Health, University College London, London, UK

**Shareen H. Doak**
Reconstructive Surgery and Regenerative Medicine Research Group (ReconRegen), Institute of Life Science, Swansea University Medical School, Swansea, UK
In Vitro Toxicology Group, Institute of Life Science, Swansea University Medical School, Swansea, UK,

**Charles W. Archer**
Reconstructive Surgery and Regenerative Medicine Research Group (ReconRegen), Institute of Life Science, Swansea University Medical School, Swansea, UK
Cartilage Biology Research Group, Institute of Life Science, Swansea University Medical School, Swansea, UK

**Catherine A. Thornton**
Reconstructive Surgery and Regenerative Medicine Research Group (ReconRegen), Institute of Life Science, Swansea University Medical School, Swansea, UK
Human Immunology Group, Institute of Life Science, Swansea University Medical School, Swansea, UK

**Andrew M. Hart**
Canniesburn Plastic Surgery Unit, Centre for Cell Engineering, University of Glasgow, Glasgow, UK

**Zita M. Jessop, Sarah Al-Himdani and Iain Stuart Whitaker**
Reconstructive Surgery and Regenerative Medicine Research Group (ReconRegen), Institute of Life Science, Swansea University Medical School, Swansea, UK
The Welsh Centre for Burns and Plastic Surgery, Morriston Hospital, Swansea, UK

**Marc Clement**
School of Management, Swansea University, Swansea, UK
Institute of Life Science, Swansea University Medical School, Swansea, UK

**Stephanie Volpi, Francesco Doenz and Salah D. Qanadli**
Cardio-Thoracic and Vascular Unit, Department of Radiology, Centre Hospitalier Universitaire Vaudois (CHUV), Lausanne, Switzerland

**Alejandra Vilanova-Sánchez**
Pediatric Surgery, Colorectal and Pelvic Surgery Division, Hospital Universitario La Paz, Madrid, Spain
Center for Colorectal and Pelvic Reconstruction (CCPR), Nationwide Children's Hospital, Columbus, OH, United States

**Richard J. Wood, Alessandra C. Gasior, Robert E. Dyckes, Katherine McCracken, Laura Weaver, Devin R. Halleran, Karen Diefenbach, Rebecca M. Rentea, Christina B. Ching, Molly Fuchs, Daniel Dajusta, Geri D. Hewitt and Marc A. Levitt**
Center for Colorectal and Pelvic Reconstruction (CCPR), Nationwide Children's Hospital, Columbus, OH, United States

**Carlos Albert Reck**
Vienna General Hospital, Vienna, Austria

**Cristina Garcia Mauriño, Dennis Minzler and Venkata Rama Jayanthi**
Nationwide Children's Hospital, Columbus, OH, United States

**Youri P. A. Tan**
The Manchester Centre for Plastic Surgery and Burns, Manchester University NHS Foundation Trust, Manchester, United Kingdom

**Jason K. F. Wong**
The Manchester Centre for Plastic Surgery and Burns, Manchester University NHS Foundation Trust, Manchester, United Kingdom
Blond McIndoe Laboratories, Division of Cell Matrix Biology and Regenerative Medicine, University of Manchester, Manchester, United Kingdom

**Philippe Liverneaux**
Department of Hand Surgery, University Hospital of Strasbourg, FMTS, University of Strasbourg, Icube CNRS, Illkirch, France

**Ido Badash**
Keck School of Medicine of USC, University of Southern California, Los Angeles, CA, United States

**Daniel J. Gould and Ketan M. Patel**
Division of Plastic and Reconstructive Surgery, University of Southern California, Los Angeles, CA, United States

**Dustin Jon Richter**
Department of Orthopaedic Surgery, Medical College of Wisconsin, Milwaukee, WI, United States

**Roger Lyon, Scott Van Valin and Xue-Cheng Liu**
Department of Orthopaedic Surgery, Medical College of Wisconsin, Milwaukee, WI, United States
Department of Orthopaedic Surgery, Children's Hospital of Wisconsin, Milwaukee, WI, United States

**Sheeba M. Joseph**
Department of Orthopaedic Surgery, University Hospitals Cleveland Medical Center, Cleveland, OH, United States

**Michael R. Karns, Derrick M. Knapik and James E. Voos**
Department of Orthopaedic Surgery, University Hospitals Cleveland Medical Center, Cleveland, OH, United States
Sports Medicine Institute, University Hospitals Cleveland Medical Center, Cleveland, OH, United States

# Index